Entangled

How People With Serious Mental Illness Get Caught in Misdemeanor Systems

Entangled

How People With Serious Mental Illness Get Caught in Misdemeanor Systems

Edited by

Leah G. Pope, Ph.D.

Amy C. Watson, Ph.D.

Jennifer D. Wood, Ph.D.

Michael T. Compton, M.D., M.P.H.

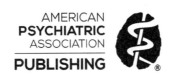

AMERICAN
PSYCHIATRIC
ASSOCIATION
PUBLISHING ®

Copyright © 2025 American Psychiatric Association Publishing
ALL RIGHTS RESERVED
First Edition

Manufactured in the United States of America on acid-free paper
28 27 26 25 24   5 4 3 2 1

American Psychiatric Association Publishing
800 Maine Avenue SW, Suite 900
Washington, DC 20024-2812
www.appi.org

Library of Congress Cataloging-in-Publication Data
Names: Pope, Leah G., editor. | Watson, Amy C., editor. | Wood, Jennifer,
    1971- editor. | Compton, Michael T., editor. | American Psychiatric
    Association Publishing, issuing body.
Title: Entangled : how people with serious mental illness get caught in
    misdemeanor systems / edited by Leah G. Pope, Amy C. Watson, Jennifer D.
    Wood, Michael T. Compton.
Other titles: Entangled (Pope)
Description: First edition. | Washington, D.C. : American Psychiatric
    Association Publishing, [2025] | Includes bibliographical references and
    index.
Identifiers: LCCN 2024025146 (print) | LCCN 2024025147 (ebook) | ISBN
    9781615375424 (paperback ; alk. paper) | ISBN 9781615375431 (ebook)
Subjects: MESH: Mentally Ill Persons--legislation & jurisprudence |
    Criminal Behavior | Crime--psychology | Incarceration--psychology |
    Public Policy | United States
Classification: LCC HV6080 (print) | LCC HV6080 (ebook) | NLM WM 33 AA1
    | DDC 364.01/9--dc23/eng/20240828
LC record available at https://lccn.loc.gov/2024025146
LC ebook record available at https://lccn.loc.gov/2024025147

British Library Cataloguing in Publication Data
A CIP record is available from the British Library.

Contents

Part 1
Understanding Misdemeanor Systems, Contexts, and Decision-Making

1 The System, the Process, and the Contexts
Misdemeanor Arrests Among People With Serious Mental Illness
> *Amy C. Watson, Ph.D.*
> *Michael T. Compton, M.D., M.P.H.*

2 Using System Maps to Understand Entanglement and Guide Change
> *Veronica Nelson, M.A.*
> *Jennifer D. Wood, Ph.D.*
> *Leah G. Pope, Ph.D.*
> *Amy C. Watson, Ph.D.*

Part 3
Toward Reform and System Improvements

Contributors

Divya K. Chhabra, M.D.
Assistant Clinical Professor, Emma Bowen Community Service Center and the New York University Grossman School of Medicine, New York, New York

Erin Comartin, Ph.D., L.M.S.W.
Professor of Social Work, School of Social Work, Wayne State University, Detroit, Michigan

Michael T. Compton, M.D., M.P.H.
Professor of Psychiatry, Columbia University Vagelos College of Physicians and Surgeons; Research Psychiatrist, New York State Psychiatric Institute, New York, New York

Brandon del Pozo, Ph.D., M.P.A., M.A.
Assistant Professor of Medicine and Health Services, Policy, and Practice (Research),The Warren Alpert Medical School of Brown University, Rhode Island Hospital, Providence, Rhode Island

Matthew L. Edwards, M.D.
Assistant Professor, Assistant Director of Residency Training, Department of Psychiatry and Behavioral Sciences, Stanford University School of Medicine, Stanford, California

Hosanna Fukuzawa, M.S.W.
Doctoral Student, Anthropology, Johns Hopkins University, Baltimore, Maryland

Jessica Gaskin, M.S.W.
Crisis Response Manager, Center for Behavioral Health and Justice, Wayne State University Center for Behavioral Health and Justice, Detroit, Michigan

Matthew L. Goldman, M.D., M.S.
Clinical Assistant Professor, Department of Psychiatry and Behavioral Sciences, University of Washington, Seattle, Washington

Megan Hicks, Ph.D.
Assistant Professor of Social Work, School of Social Work, Wayne State University, Detroit, Michigan

Elisabeth E. Jackson, M.A.
Research Assistant, Department of Psychiatry, Vagelos College of Physicians and Surgeons, Columbia University, New York, New York

Samuel W. Jackson, M.D.
Postdoctoral Clinical Fellow, Columbia University Public Psychiatry Fellowship, Columbia University, New York, New York

Athena Kheibari, Ph.D.
Assistant Professor of Social Work, School of Social Work, Wayne State University, Detroit, Michigan

Kaitlyn Kok, B.S.
Student, School of Social Work, Wayne State University Center for Behavioral Health and Justice, Detroit, Michigan

Veronica Nelson, M.A.
Doctoral Candidate, Department of Criminal Justice, Temple University, Philadelphia, Pennsylvania

Leah G. Pope, Ph.D.
Associate Professor of Clinical Behavioral Medicine, Department of Psychiatry, Columbia University Vagelos College of Physicians and Surgeons; Research Scientist, New York State Psychiatric Institute, New York, New York

Eric Rafla-Yuan, M.D.
Staff Psychiatrist, San Diego County Psychiatric Hospital, San Diego, California

Aaron Stagoff-Belfort, B.A.
Ph.D. Student, Department of Sociology, University of Chicago, Chicago, Illinois

Leonard Swanson, M.S.W.
Crisis Policy Manager, Center for Behavioral Health and Justice, School of Social Work, Wayne State University, Detroit, Michigan

Jason Tan de Bibiana, M.Sc.
Senior Research Associate, Vera Institute of Justice, Brooklyn, New York

Luis C. Torres, Ph.D.
Assistant Professor, Department of Criminal Justice, Temple University, Philadelphia, Pennsylvania

Justin E. Volpe, CPRS-A
National Association of State Mental Health Program Directors, Alexandria, Virginia

Amy C. Watson, Ph.D.
Professor, School of Social Work, Wayne State University, Detroit, Michigan

Jennifer D. Wood, Ph.D.
Professor of Criminal Justice; Vice Provost for Faculty Affairs, Temple University, Philadelphia, Pennsylvania

DISCLOSURES

The following contributors stated that they had no competing interests during the year preceding manuscript submission:

D.K. Chhabra; E. Comartin; M.T. Compton; B. del Pozo; M.L. Edwards; H. Fukuzawa; J. Gaskin; M.L. Goldman; M. Hicks; E.E. Jackson; S.W. Jackson; A. Kheibari; K. Kok; V. Nelson; L.G. Pope; E. Rafla-Yuan; A. Stagoff-Belfort; L. Swanson; J. Tan de Bibiana; L.C. Torres; J.E. Volpe; A.C. Watson; J.D. Wood

Foreword

If there were a playbook for what it looks like to become "entangled" in the criminal legal system, my early life would have followed the script perfectly. By the time I was 23 years old, I was addicted to drugs and alcohol, was diagnosed with a serious mental illness, and had cycled through a series of involuntary hospitalizations, drug rehabilitations, and eventually the county jail for a misdemeanor crime. What followed, however, was an opportunity to change my course.

While still in custody for the misdemeanor, I was approached by a member of the County Court Jail Diversion Program after being transferred to the hospital from jail. After learning about the program, I accepted admission into court-monitored treatment. I was released to a recovery house in the community and enrolled in outpatient mental health treatment. The program would monitor the treatment I received in the community and would do check-ins with me. The court's intervention was not divine. At 23 years old, I was not ready to be completely abstinent from drugs and alcohol and had many peer affiliations that supported that lifestyle. I absconded from the recovery house while on probation and stopped going to treatment.

After a brief return to using substances, I went back to treatment. I took medication that was prescribed for me by a doctor, not sold to me by someone on the corner. My outlook improved; my mood got better; I began to smile again. I completed my treatment program, and the court closed my case by a plea (which meant that the misdemeanor offense stayed on my record like a conviction). Upon leaving the courthouse to celebrate the completion of my program, I was sidetracked by an unexpected opportunity: the offer to become a county employee as a peer specialist with the jail diversion program. From this initial position, I worked to become a Certified Peer Recovery Specialist for Adults (CPRS-A). I have since become a national consultant, trained more than

3,000 Crisis Intervention Team (CIT) law enforcement officers, had articles published in major newspapers, appeared in two PBS documentaries on mental health, and been invited to the White House and the Supreme Court.

During my 14 years employed by the County Court Jail Diversion Program, I worked very hard getting thousands of people out of custody and connecting them to timely and mostly accessible resources. I also saw the unfortunate results when those resources could not be accessed. I worked with an amazing team that fought for the rights of the most vulnerable citizens living in a major city who were from all over the world. Unfortunately, as is well documented, most of the people I saw who ended up in the legal system were people of color who did not have equitable access to health care or the financial ability to fight their legal cases. Even those who ended up in the court-ordered treatment program where I worked as a peer specialist often faced barriers that led them to fail—many of which related to situations in which their basic needs were not met. For the many people who did succeed, I often reflected that they should not have had to be arrested and prosecuted to have a chance at living a meaningful life.

What happened after my life spiraled out of control was a sheer miracle. Some people believe in being in the right place at the right time, others in divine intervention, or others in just plain luck. The "miracle" that I encountered unfortunately does not happen for most people who have been diagnosed with a mental illness and who cycle in and out of the criminal legal system. Supportive and effective diversion programs like the one in which I enrolled are still few and far between compared with the number of people who could benefit from them. The problems associated with entanglement in the criminal legal system are well recognized. But tested and proven solutions are too few.

The editors of this book, Drs. Pope, Watson, Wood, and Compton—along with all the contributing chapter authors—provide a thorough overview of the problems, but they also offer solutions, in both the mental health profession and the criminal legal system. And they encourage us all to be a part of crafting more solutions.

By deciphering some of the most common misdemeanor charges that people with mental illness receive—including criminal trespass and loitering charges, shoplifting and minor retail theft, resisting arrest and officer obstruction, and misdemeanor assault—we better understand the nature of entanglement. *Entangled* articulates the ways in which contexts, behaviors, and decisions (e.g., of the client, the caller, the complainant, the police) can lead to, or move away from, arrest and processing through the misdemeanor criminal legal system. Arrest and processing result in the criminalization of those with serious mental illness. Drawing on data from a mixed method, multisite (Atlanta, Chicago, Manhattan, Philadelphia) study, the editors and authors demonstrate how people with mental illness all too often become entangled, and how underfunded social and mental health service systems result in individuals who have committed no serious crime being at the mercy of the criminal legal system. *Entangled* also illustrates efforts by those cities and others to reduce entanglement. Through case examples and first-person accounts, readers can better understand the situations in which people with mental illness find themselves—situations that initiate the cascade from a 911 call, to a police encounter, to being behind bars, where recovery is impeded if not forever halted.

The opportunity of recovery that was given to me so freely needs to be as easily accessed at every street corner in this country. I invite the readers of this book to learn more about the complex issues related to misdemeanor arrests among people with serious mental illness and to become part of the much-needed solutions today and in years to come. I have committed my life to becoming part of the solution; I encourage you to join me.

Justin Volpe, CPRS-A
Senior Peer Support Coordinator
National Association of State Mental Health Program Directors
Alexandria, Virginia

Preface

Leah G. Pope, Ph.D.
Amy C. Watson, Ph.D.
Jennifer D. Wood, Ph.D.
Michael T. Compton, M.D., M.P.H.

We are an interdisciplinary team of researchers from the fields of anthropology, social work, criminology, and psychiatry, with a unified mission. Driving our scholarly work is the goal to help individuals with mental illness, especially serious mental illness, embrace a life of recovery that includes hope, empowerment, and integration and is supported by effective and equitable mental health and social services, while minimizing criminal legal system involvement to the largest extent possible.

By criminal legal system involvement, we mean too many law enforcement encounters, including a reliance on the police for behavioral health crisis response; excessive arrests usually for minor, low-level charges; and the resulting excessive jail detention, court monitoring, fines and fees, and probation requirements. We are generally interested in misdemeanor charges as opposed to felonies or violent crimes, and we are especially focused on specific misdemeanor charges such as criminal trespass, shoplifting, obstruction, and minor assault, as well as all the variations on those general types, which might include loitering, vagrancy, petit larceny, resisting arrest, disorderly conduct, and the like (and eventually additional charges such as failure to appear to court and probation violation). These are the charges that set the stage for the criminalization of serious mental illness, and it is this criminalization that we seek to clearly define, and then collaborate with others—including, most importantly, policymakers—to find solutions for. This criminalization is what we refer to as being "entangled"—entangled in the criminal legal system, or the misdemeanor processing system more specifically, which stifles hope rather than promotes it, disempowers rather than empowers, and segregates rather than integrates.

In writing *Entangled* (and in coordinating the writing of a cadre of colleagues committed to our mission), we have provided what we hope is a nuanced account of how the misdemeanor criminal legal system intervenes in the lives of individuals with mental illness, both generally and in relation to specific types of behaviors resulting in specific misdemeanor charges. Taking quantitative and qualitative data that we collected from four major cities as a foundation, and looking across the continuum of criminal legal involvement from the point of police contact to incarceration, *Entangled* examines how decision-makers within the criminal legal continuum operate within dynamic and interrelated contexts that both facilitate and frustrate attempts to address the mental health needs of defendants while balancing considerations of public order and safety. We examine how decision-making occurs across intercepts and from a systems-level perspective, showing readers how decisions at one stage impact decisions at subsequent stages.

Although our approach is academic, to serve as an authoritative reference on the intersection of serious mental illness and misdemeanor criminal legal system involvement, we also provide first-person accounts and case examples to illustrate our points. These accounts and case examples are drawn from and informed by interviews and focus groups with people with serious mental illness and a range of criminal legal and behavioral health professionals. Some case examples are partly fictional or serve as composite descriptions of specific but all-too-common situations that lead to entanglement with misdemeanor systems. Across the United States, such systems vary in aspects of their structures and functioning, but the problem of entanglement is universally felt. Our hope is to provide a comprehensive source of information on how certain behaviors and contexts bring individuals with serious mental illness into the fold of the criminal legal system and what we can do to adequately address this complex challenge.

We have divided the book into three parts. The first part provides four chapters to describe various facets of the misdemeanor criminal legal system. The goal is to set the stage for the specific content covered in subsequent chapters. These initial chapters provide a historical perspective on how shifts in social, mental health, and criminal legal system policies have put individuals with serious mental illness at risk for criminal legal system involvement; an overview of the misdemeanor case-processing system; and a summary of recent quantitative research that led to our qualitative work (Chapter 1, "The System, the Process, and the Contexts"). We also depict, in Chapter 2 ("Using System Maps to Understand Entanglement and Guide Change"), both the common features of misdemeanor systems and differences in how systems in different places have created so-called off-ramps in efforts to reduce entanglement. We draw from a multisite systems mapping exercise from four cities (Atlanta, Chicago, New York [Manhattan], and Philadelphia) to illustrate the value of producing system maps to guide system change efforts. In Chapter 3 ("Decision-Making Contexts of Misdemeanor Charges"), we show the contexts that shape decision-making across misdemeanor systems—with a specific emphasis on the decisions of police, prosecutors, and defense counsels—and the ways in which a chain of decisions across the criminal legal continuum come together to produce case outcomes. This chapter highlights the importance of context and variability in decision-making and the ways in which altering decision-making contexts might reduce misdemeanor system entanglement. Chapter 4 ("Common Themes and Tensions") details results from in-depth interviews at the four research sites, including 17 focus groups and in-depth interviews involving 94 stakeholders in the criminal legal and mental health service systems. Here, we articulate how the focal concerns and organizational values of different agencies involved in misdemeanor case processing create points of both alignment and divergence in decisions about how to resolve cases involving people with serious mental illness, including decisions about what counts as the "best outcome."

The second part of the book provides four chapters on specific misdemeanor charges that are historically among the most common for individuals with serious mental illness entangled in the criminal legal system. Chapter 5 ("Being in the Wrong Place") covers misdemeanor charges related to the management of space and place (such as criminal trespass); Chapter 6 ("A $25 T-Shirt From the Bargain Store") details misdemeanor charges related to minor theft (shoplifting, petit larceny, retail theft); Chapter 7 ("Noncooperation With Officers and Using 'Fighting Words'") explores misdemeanor charges related to poor interactions with police officers, including resisting arrest, giving false information, other types of obstruction, and disorderly conduct; and Chapter 8 ("That's Scary Because Now They're Showing Violence") describes misdemeanor assault and battery charges, highlighting how these charges are often handled differently from misdemeanor charges that do not involve physical harm. Each of these chapters provides insight into the reasoning or logic behind the use of such charges in different situations and contexts. These chapters also reveal varying levels of ambivalence among criminal legal actors as to the long-term value of such charges in effecting public safety and improving the life trajectories of people with mental illness. Together, the chapters in this second part of the book offer ideas for reforms in both the mental health system and the criminal legal system to reduce the overuse of these charges and thus the criminalization of people with serious mental illness.

The third part of the book is even more solution focused and future oriented. The authors review reforms and policy advances in recent years in terms of alternatives to incarceration and diversion programs, attempts to imbue the criminal legal system with a rehabilitative ethos, and policies designed to reduce the footprint of the misdemeanor criminal legal system altogether (Chapter 9, "The Current Era of Multifaceted Criminal Legal System Reform"). Chapters in this third section address reforms and policy advances in recent years in terms of a reimagining of mental health crisis response systems and services, including changes at the federal level to help states and local communities improve mental health care access and reform crisis systems (Chapter 10, "Reform in an Era of Mental Health and Crisis Services Innovation"). Finally, in Chapter 11 ("Equity in Mental Health and Criminal Legal System Reform"), because of the intertwined problems of racial and health inequities in both the criminal legal and mental health systems, the authors emphasize the need for multisystem collaboration with a specific focus on advancing, and ensuring, racial equity in all reforms.

The problems we face are large, complex, and fraught with inequities. The solutions must be even larger and more complex. If our mission—helping individuals with mental illness embrace recovery while minimizing criminal legal system involvement—is to be achieved, we will need your help: help in the nature of care and treatment of your clients, education for those both within and outside of your own profession, and advocacy across sectors and levels of government for change that will advance the lives of individuals with serious mental illness in a fair and just way.

Acknowledgments

The project that inspired this book and the writing and editing of these chapters was made possible by a series of collaborations for which we are grateful. We thank Laura Roberts, M.D., M.A.; Simone Taylor, Ph.D.; Erika Parker; and Annie Birge at American Psychiatric Association Publishing for their support of this project from the beginning. We thank the National Science Foundation and the National Institute of Mental Health for their commitment to interdisciplinary scholarship. We thank all our chapter authors—many of whom are long-term collaborators—for their willingness to join us in extending the work of several of our studies into a book that clearly articulates what we see so often in our research and what we endeavor to change: the entanglement of people with mental illness in misdemeanor systems. We are grateful for members of our original study team who worked to collect data reported in this book, including Oluwatoyin Ashekun, Tehya Boswell, Samantha Ellis, Nili Gesser, Ronni Nelson, Aaron Stagoff-Belfort, Jason Tan de Bibiana, Amanda Warnock, and Adria Zern. We owe deep appreciation to our study partners in Atlanta, Chicago, Manhattan, and Philadelphia who facilitated our collaboration with dozens of police officers, public defenders, prosecutors, judges, mental health service providers, and people with lived experience of mental illness. The agencies, organizations, and individuals are numerous, and this book would not have been possible without their willingness to share with us their perspectives about how their local criminal legal systems work and how they have forged innovative pathways to reform. We remember especially Flo Messier, a former public defender and then supervisor for the mental health unit of the Philadelphia District Attorney's Office, who passed away unexpectedly during this project; she was an extraordinary advocate for people with behavioral health issues and an inspiration for further reforms. We are grateful for the collaboration with our cover artist, Joy Majors, and to the Returning Artists Guild, which facilitated our connection to Joy and which works tirelessly to support practicing artists directly impacted by incarceration. Finally, we thank the many colleagues, friends, and family members who have been patient with us during the countless hours we spent writing and editing this book and who have supported our efforts to produce scholarship that reflects our personal commitments to justice and recovery for people with mental illness.

Part 1

Understanding Misdemeanor Systems, Contexts, and Decision-Making

Understanding the Researcher
System: Context, and
Decision Making

The System, the Process, and the Contexts

Misdemeanor Arrests Among People With Serious Mental Illness

Amy C. Watson, Ph.D.
Michael T. Compton, M.D., M.P.H.

At a recent staff meeting at a certified community behavioral health clinic (CCBHC), the assertive community treatment (ACT) teams staff discussed the fact that many of their clients have been cycling in and out of the local jail, often on minor charges. A housing specialist from one of the ACT teams shared that he had finally located housing for one of their newer clients, but before she could move in, she was arrested on charges of criminal trespass and resisting arrest. By the time she was re-leased, the landlord had found another tenant, leaving her unhoused and at risk of another arrest for being in a place where others viewed her as needing to move along. Staff members shared their frustrations about how disruptive arrests are for their clients and how their arrest histories often create barriers to benefits enrollment and housing. The clinical director decided to look further into the frequency of criminal legal system involvement for the agency's clients and very quickly became convinced that the CCBHC should be seeking out ways to reduce their entanglement with the system. Through talking with other providers, the clinical director learned about the newly established local Stepping Up Initiative, a national initiative to guide counties in strategies to reduce the number of people with serious mental illness (SMI) in jails. The CCBHC soon joined the local initiative as a new partner.

The overrepresentation of people with SMI in the criminal legal system has received significant research and policy attention in recent decades, and substantial resources have been focused on addressing the problem. Despite these efforts, people with SMI continue to be overrepresented across all points of the criminal legal continuum. Although some of these individuals have committed violent or other serious crimes, the majority have become entangled in the criminal legal system following arrests for minor offenses. In this book, we examine the contexts and behaviors that lead to the arrest and processing of people with SMI through the misdemeanor criminal legal system. We explore how decision-makers, operating within dynamic and interrelated contexts, both facilitate and frustrate attempts to address the mental health needs of arrestees while balancing considerations of public safety and order. We use data from our four-site study of misdemeanor processing among people with SMI, as well as related projects, to gain an understanding of how—despite significant resources, commitment, and effort—individuals with SMI remain entangled in misdemeanor systems. We also explore developments in the criminal legal and mental health systems that hold promise for advancing solutions for what has proven to be an intractable problem.

In this chapter, we set the context for the rest of the book. First, we examine the overrepresentation of people with SMI in the criminal legal system and offer explanations for why this has happened. Second, we briefly discuss misdemeanor legal systems generally, before narrowing our focus to the processing of specific misdemeanor charges among those with SMI. Third, we summarize the methods used to generate the data discussed in some of the subsequent chapters.

Overrepresentation of People With Serious Mental Illness in the Criminal Legal System

Overrepresentation of people with SMI occurs at every level of the criminal legal system. More than 30% of those with SMI have lifetime histories of arrest (Kennedy-Hendricks et al. 2016), and analysis of population data indicates a relationship between psychiatric disorders and arrests (Swartz and Lurigio 2007). Most of these arrests are for minor offenses, and this population is overrepresented in survival-type crimes associated with poverty and homelessness.

Jails house people awaiting trial (pretrial detention) as well as those serving jail sentences of <1 year. Among the jail population, prevalence rates of having a current SMI are several times higher than those of the general population, estimated at ~15% for males and 29%–31% for females (Lynch et al. 2014; Steadman et al. 2009). In state prisons, where those convicted of more serious crimes serve sentences of 1 year or more, prevalence rates are a bit lower, 8%–14% (Prins 2014). Individuals with SMI are also overrepresented among probationers and parolees, with estimates of 11%–19% (Prins and Draper 2009; Vaughn et al. 2012). There is evidence that once arrested, people with SMIs are at higher risk of re-arrest; serve more days in pretrial detention; if convicted, serve more of their jail or prison sentences; and are more likely to have their probation or parole revoked than are offenders without SMI (Baillargeon et al. 2009; Cloyes et al. 2010; Magee et al. 2021; Prins and Draper 2009; Skeem et al. 2006). Hence, once arrested, they become *entangled*.

Causes of Overrepresentation

Many point to deinstitutionalization and the failure to create a robust community mental health system as driving the criminalization of SMI. According to early versions of this explanation, people with SMI, who in prior eras would have been institutionalized in state hospitals, now live in the community, often without adequate mental health treatment. Their symptomatic behavior brings them into contact with law enforcement and the criminal legal system because these behaviors are defined as criminal matters rather than mental health issues. Following this line of thinking, addressing the problem involves providing more or better mental health treatment to manage symptoms. There is some evidence that deinstitutionalization has contributed to prison population growth, termed *transinstitutionalization*. Although they did not find evidence of transinstitutionalization for the period 1950–1980, Raphael and Stoll (2013) estimated that 4%–7% of prison population growth for the period 1980–2000 was attributable to deinstitutionalization. They further estimated that 14%–26% of those with mental illness (or 40,000–72,000 people) incarcerated in the year 2000 would have likely been patients in psychiatric hospitals in prior periods.

Critics of the criminalization perspective argue that although deinstitutionalization has left many with SMI in the community without adequate supports, their involvement in the criminal legal system is more complex than simply being arrested for symptomatic behavior. Skeem et al. (2011) suggested that a plausible alternative to the "criminalization hypothesis" is that risk factors for criminal legal system involvement are generally the same for people with and without SMI. However, SMI may increase one's exposure to and burden of these risk factors. They pointed to criminological perspectives that emphasize a person's position within the social hierarchy and access to normative institutions, as well as social and personality psychology models that focus on more proximal individual risk factors for offending, such as antisocial cognitions and criminal associates.

Broadly defined, the criminological perspective maintains that poverty increases exposure to neighborhood conditions that are conducive to a person engaging in criminal behavior and becoming entangled in the criminal legal system (Skeem et al. 2011). These conditions include high rates of adverse childhood experiences, criminal activity, victimization, illicit drug use, homelessness, and unemployment. Further, those who are marginalized, including individuals with SMI, tend to be concentrated geographically in neighborhoods rife with these conditions. This increases opportunities for criminal behavior, association with others engaged in criminal behavior, and substance misuse. Poverty impacts the propensity for offending by interfering with access to normative systems and institutions (social, educational, occupational, civic) that exert formal and informal social control. Individuals with SMI may be at heightened risk for offending because the onset and chronicity of their illnesses can create barriers to inclusion, interfere with important life transitions (e.g., pursuing education, entering the workforce, marrying, buying a home), cause frequent disruptions in their living situation due to hospitalizations and arrests, and (given high rates of unemployment in this population) leave people with abundant unstructured time (Fisher et al. 2006b). The subsequent declining economic status forces many with SMI to live in poor, high-crime neighborhoods, contributes to homelessness, and increases risks for criminal legal system contact. This perspective might lead to interventions that address (in addition to mental health treatment needs) poverty, housing stability, social inclusion, and support of people with SMI in navigating social, educational, and occupational transitions.

Social and personality psychology models focus on individual criminogenic risk factors for offending such as antisocial cognitions (criminal thinking) and criminal associates. Bonta et al. (1998) suggested that criminal behavior is learned by early modeling and reinforcement patterns. The behaviors are maintained by a history of benefiting from criminal activity, social circumstances that encourage criminal activity, personal attitudes supportive of criminal behavior, and a personality style that finds impulsivity rewarding. Skeem et al. (2011) suggested that individuals with SMI may be at higher risk of being in adverse environments that expose them to the modeling and reinforcement of criminal behavior. Andrews et al. (2006) suggested that the association between mental illness and criminal legal system involvement is due to its association with antisocial cognition, antisocial personality patterns, and substance abuse. However, although antisocial attitudes and personality patterns can be present in individuals with SMI, they are not characteristic phenomena or defining features of SMI. Comorbid substance use disorders are common among people with SMI who are involved in the criminal legal system, and there is evidence that the relationship between SMI and system involvement is largely mediated by substance use (Abram et al. 2003; Baranyi et al. 2022; James and Glaze 2006; Swartz and Lurigio 2007).

Building on these frameworks, the risk-needs-responsivity (RNR) model is a widely accepted approach to offender assessment and treatment that includes the tailoring of the intensity of supervision and treatment to risks and needs associated with criminality (called *criminogenic risk/needs*), taking into consideration factors that may impede a person's ability to successfully participate in treatment (*responsivity*). The model identifies eight empirically established risk/needs for recidivism (Andrews and Bonta 2010). Four have the strongest association with recidivism and are considered the "big four": history of antisocial behavior, antisocial personality pattern, antisocial cognition, and antisocial associates. The remaining four, more distal, risk factors have a moderate association with continued criminal legal system involvement: substance abuse, family conflict, low educational attainment or unemployment, and lack of prosocial leisure activities. In this model, SMI is considered a responsivity factor, as it may impact participation in needs-focused interventions and is associated with other needs-related challenges. Recently, the concept of responsivity has been expanded beyond individual-level factors to include *systemic responsivity*, which includes addressing local and neighborhood characteristics that increase the risk of criminal legal system involvement (Taxman 2014).

Guided by the RNR model, strategies to reduce offending behavior have primarily targeted criminogenic needs related to the modifiable big four risk factors. Interventions based on cognitive-behavioral therapy have been developed that target antisocial attitudes, personality patterns, and criminal associates. There is emerging evidence that such interventions can reduce recidivism for individuals with SMI who are involved in the criminal legal system (Wilson et al. 2018), and some have suggested they be used in the community behavioral health system to prevent criminal legal system involvement (Bonfine et al. 2020).

Rotter and Compton (2022) pointed out the overlap of social determinants of mental health and RNR model factors, specifically adverse childhood events (family conflict, trauma), employment and educational challenges, and neighborhood disorder (lack of resources). They noted that risk factors related to antisocial attitudes, behavior, and associates have also been linked to social determinants such as adverse childhood experiences, poverty, and neighborhood disorder. The authors further pointed out that although the RNR framework is presented as race neutral, the social determinants perspective recognizes structural issues such as systemic racism that drive the social determinants of mental health and criminal legal system involvement. They argued for consideration of the impact of structural racism and social determinants when addressing the involvement of people with SMI in the criminal legal system.

In sum, the overrepresentation of individuals with SMI in the criminal legal system has been linked to myriad factors including deinstitutionalization and inadequate funding of community-based mental health services, social psychological risk factors, poverty, community-level risk factors, and a broad array of social determinants of mental health that both people with SMI and those charged with criminal offenses are more likely to experience (e.g., poverty, unemployment, housing instability) (Bronson and Berzofsky 2017; Caruso 2017; Prins 2011).

Misdemeanors

We chose to focus on misdemeanor arrests in this book because they far outnumber felony arrests for people with and without mental illness. In fact, there are four times as many misdemeanor cases as felonies filed annually in the United States, making up 80% of state court dockets (Natapoff 2018). Misdemeanor offenses are generally less serious crimes that do not result in significant harm to people or property. They can involve offenses related to public disorder such as trespass and disorderly conduct, minor theft or property damage, possession of small quantities of drugs, and assaults without a weapon and not resulting in serious injury. Although many misdemeanor charges are resolved without jail time, typically, the maximum jail sentence for misdemeanor offenses is 1 year or less.

Alexandria Natapoff (2018) argued in *Punishment Without Crime* that the misdemeanor legal system has become a fast, informal assembly line, a processing system that disproportionately targets poor and vulnerable people of color. Given that the stakes tend to be lower than in felony cases, procedural safeguards are lax, and many cases are quickly pleaded out. There is growing recognition that even when individuals receive minimal sentences, there may be long-term collateral consequences related to employment, benefits eligibility, and failure to pay fines and fees. Further, as Issa Kohler-Haussman (2018) asserted in her book *Misdemeanorland,* even when charges are dropped or defendants are found not guilty, the misdemeanor machinery exerts social control over the lives of those who become entangled by creating records of their law enforcement contacts, testing their ability to show up to court and comply with the process, and applying punitive responses for failures to comply with the court's demands. For example, a person charged with a misdemeanor assault offense may have to take time off work and find transportation to appear in court multiple times. Missing a scheduled court date may result in a warrant being issued, the person being arrested on the warrant, and spending time in jail before being released with a new court date. During that period, they may lose wages or their job altogether, and forfeit any bond that was posted after their initial arrest. Even if the case is dropped at the next court date, the harms and long-term collateral consequences resulting from being processed in the misdemeanor system are significant.

Although criminal legal system reform efforts are underway in many jurisdictions to reduce incarceration for some misdemeanor offenses, they may not prevent many of the direct and collateral harms of the misdemeanor machinery. As Natapoff (2019, p. 1056) warned,

> Even as we retract certain formal punishments—primarily incarceration—we are simultaneously expanding the system's capacity to watch, label, direct, and derail the lives of a growing population subject to arrest, conviction, and non-prison punishments.

This may be particularly true for people with SMI, who may be monitored and required to participate in mental health treatment and attend regular court dates to be released from custody pretrial and in lieu of convictions and jail sentences.

On What Charges Are People With Serious Mental Illness Being Arrested?

If we want to reduce the involvement of individuals with SMI in the misdemeanor legal system, it is helpful to understand the types of charges and situations that initiate their entanglement. The available research in this area is limited, but what does exist provides some insight into the types of charges that are common among those with SMI. For example, in an analysis of arrest records of 13,816 individuals receiving services from the Massachusetts Department of Mental Health in 1991 and 1992, 27% had been arrested in a 10-year period, almost exclusively for minor crimes such as property offenses, crimes against public order (e.g., disturbing the peace), public indecency, and motor and drug offenses (Fisher et al. 2006a). Across several studies, property offenses, including trespass, have been reported as the most common charges among individuals with SMI, followed closely by alcohol-related charges or drug possession and disorderly conduct (Baillargeon et al. 2009; Clark et al. 1999; Fisher et al. 2006a; Hiday and Ray 2010).

As an initial stage of our own work looking into misdemeanors among people with SMI, we analyzed all arrests ($N=2,224,847$) in New York State during 2010–2013 (Compton et al. 2023). Medicaid data and the state's mental health authority's records were used to create an SMI indicator for each arrest: 4.1% of arrests involved individuals with the SMI indicator (91,363 arrests), and 2,133,484 without. When rank ordering the most common charges among the two populations, two criminal trespass charges (second- and third-degree) appeared on the rank list of most common charges in arrests involving individuals with the SMI indicator but did not appear on the list of most common charges in arrests involving individuals without SMI. Simple assault was also among the most frequent charges for people with the SMI indicator, representing 14.9% of all arrests, compared with 14.0% of all arrests for people without SMI. Using the same data, we had previously shown that those with mental illness were more likely to receive a jail sentence for misdemeanor charges (Hall et al. 2019).

In a study of 240 individuals with SMI (65% with psychotic disorders and 35% with mood disorders) being discharged from inpatient psychiatric settings in southeast Georgia (mean age 35.9±11.6 years, 65% male), we found that 171 (71%) had been previously arrested, and among them, the mean number of lifetime arrests was 8.6±10.1, with a mean number of lifetime charges of 12.6±14.6 (Compton et al. 2022). The four most common lifetime charges were criminal trespass, willful obstruction of law enforcement officers, disorderly conduct, and theft by shoplifting, all misdemeanors. Evidence of entanglement is present in how the most common charges changed over time. The earliest arrests occurred at an average age of 20–21 years and commonly involved marijuana possession, driving under the influence, shoplifting, and burglary charges. Recent arrests occurred at an average age of 33–35 years and more commonly involved probation violations, obstruction of an officer, disorderly conduct, and failure to appear in court.

Taken together, available research suggests that most arrests among those with SMI are for minor charges that are often the targets of initiatives, ranging from pre-arrest to court diversion programs, that connect people to behavioral health and other social services. However, despite significant attention and investment in such programming, the entanglement of people with SMI in the criminal legal system persists.

Our Work to Understand the Charges and System Processes Driving Entanglement

Policymakers, advocates, and practitioners in the criminal legal and mental health systems all want to address the problem of criminal legal system entanglement among individuals with SMI. It is generally understood that these arrests typically involve misdemeanor charges used to address behaviors that stem from circumstances in which people with SMI find themselves (e.g., a person with limited financial resources and homelessness could be charged with criminal trespass, loitering, panhandling, or other misdemeanor charges) or that are associated with manifestations of their illness (e.g., a person with disorganized thinking and disorganized behavior stemming from schizophrenia could be charged with disorderly conduct or another public nuisance misdemeanor). However, remarkably little research has been done to describe and explain how, why, and in what contexts misdemeanor charges get applied. Without this foundational knowledge, current efforts to reduce entanglement are weakened by a limited understanding of how behavior, context, and logic for applying charges—and the nature of subsequent misdemeanor processing—are together producing the entanglement problem.

In pursuit of this understanding, the editors of this book designed a study to identify and understand the use and processing of the most frequent and overrepresented misdemeanor charges among people with SMI. The results of that study are featured across the various chapters of this book. The study objectives were to 1) identify the two to five misdemeanor charges that appear to be most overrepresented among individuals with SMI; 2) understand the use and processing of those specific misdemeanor charges in various contexts by conducting *system mapping exercises* in four cities; 3) gain a rich, in-depth understanding of the use of those charges by conducting focus groups in each of the four cities; and 4) create an explanatory understanding of the use of misdemeanor charges among people with SMI that will serve as a foundation for further definitive research, as well as policy and program development to address the problem of overrepresentation, or what we call *entanglement*.

We relied on two different quantitative approaches to identify the most common misdemeanor charges among individuals with SMI. As noted above, the first involved using a large administrative data set that included all arrests in New York State across 3 years (Compton et al. 2023). The second used data from a clinical study involving 240 patients with SMI and a history of two or more inpatient stays in Georgia (Compton et al. 2022). Findings from those analyses helped us identify the following misdemeanor charges as frequent or overrepresented among people with SMI: criminal trespass, retail theft, willful obstruction of law enforcement officers, disorderly conduct, and simple assault.

Next, we wanted to gain an in-depth understanding of how and when these misdemeanor charges are applied to people with SMI, how people are processed through the criminal legal system, and how decisions are made by actors in the criminal legal system during this process. Working in four jurisdictions—Atlanta/Fulton County, GA; Chicago/Cook County, IL; the borough of Manhattan, New York City, NY; and Philadelphia, PA—we conducted misdemeanor system mapping exercises, followed by focus groups and in-depth interviews with professionals working in misdemeanor systems and at the interface of criminal legal and behavioral health services. For the system mapping exercises, the team selected three charge types based on our prior analysis: trespassing, retail theft/shoplifting, and simple/misdemeanor assault. Each site had the opportunity to examine additional charges of interest. In Atlanta, for example, willful obstruction of a law enforcement officer and disorderly conduct charges were also discussed. Before the mapping session, we developed draft maps of misdemeanor case processing for each site based on available reports and consultation with site contacts. During the mapping sessions, which included participants representing law enforcement, prosecutors, public defenders, the judiciary, and mental health professionals working in the criminal legal space, we started at the beginning of the draft maps for each charge type and asked them, "What happens next?"

Through this process, we developed detailed maps with explanatory notes on decision-making points and case flows in relation to misdemeanor charges generally as well as our identified misdemeanor charges of interest. Inspired by the maps that were produced from each of the four systems mapping exercises, we provide in Chapter 2 ("Using System Maps to Understand Entanglement and Guide Change") a generic misdemeanor system map to depict key case processes and potential case flows depending on jurisdiction. The chapter also provides examples of efforts to reduce entanglement, in the form of so-called off-ramps created by jurisdictions to move people out of criminal legal systems and into systems of community-based care and support. In general terms, Chapter 2 is meant to illustrate the value of system maps in generating a common visual reference point and diagnostic tool for identifying entanglement-reduction opportunities.

Based on our analysis of the explanatory notes related to decision-making points, case flows, and real or hypothetical examples of cases, the study team found that despite jurisdictional variation, decision-makers across all sites experience contexts that shape how, when, and where they intervene. These contexts relate to 1) the law and policy environment; 2) the location of the behavior; 3) the expectations of stakeholders; 4) knowledge of mental illness; and 5) access to community resources (Wood et al. 2023). Chapter 3 ("Decision-Making Contexts of Misdemeanor Charges") expands on what was learned in the study by incorporating insights from the literature on criminal legal decision-making.

After the misdemeanor system mapping sessions, we conducted focus groups and in-depth interviews with system professionals to obtain a rich understanding of how our selected misdemeanor charges are used and processed in relation to people with SMI in each of the four jurisdictions. (Quotes in this book that are otherwise unattributed are from this study.) Discussed in Chapter 4 ("Common Themes and Tensions") are the data from this phase of the project (also detailed in Pope et al. 2023b) that revealed that although criminal legal system stakeholders across agencies shared a commitment to reducing system contact among people with SMI, they differed on how to make good on that commitment owing to the distinct values and goals they brought to the table.

As such, in Chapters 2–4, we elaborate on what we learned from our work in the four cities, describing overall findings from system mapping exercises and focus groups/interviews. We then look more closely at several specific charges in Chapter 5 ("Being in the Wrong Place"), Chapter 6 ("A $25 T-Shirt From the Bargain Store"), Chapter 7 ("Noncooperation With Officers and Using 'Fighting Words'"), and Chapter 8 ("'That's Scary Because Now They're Showing Violence'"). Where useful, we also draw on data from a related project examining the criminal legal system experiences of individuals with SMI specific to our charges of interest (Pope et al. 2023a). We close the book with chapters discussing current criminal legal and mental health system efforts to reduce the criminal legal system footprint generally and more specifically in the lives of people with SMI. The final chapter reflects on the intersection of race and health inequities in the criminal legal and mental health systems and argues that stakeholders must pursue racial equity at every level and across systems as we work to reduce the involvement of individuals with SMI in the criminal legal system. Taken together, the chapters in this book are meant to serve as a resource for describing, explaining, and acting on the problem of entanglement.

KEY POINTS

- Overrepresentation of people with serious mental illness (SMI) occurs at every level of the misdemeanor criminal legal system: police encounters, arrests, likelihood and duration of jail detention, and extent of probation involvement and violation.

- Beyond symptomatic behavior and substance use, causes of this entanglement include—among many other factors—psychosocial circumstances associated with the mental illness (e.g., low education, unemployment, low income or poverty, housing instability, neighborhood disorder, poor social supports).

- Misdemeanors are by far much more common than felonies among individuals with SMI, and they often stem from behaviors related to either the mental illness or the associated psychosocial circumstances.

- Some of the most common misdemeanor charges—and those that are a focus in subsequent chapters—are criminal trespass, retail theft, willful obstruction of law enforcement officers, disorderly conduct, and misdemeanor assault.

- The book's editors conducted system mapping exercises and focus groups/interviews with diverse criminal legal system professionals in four cities to create an explanatory understanding of the use of misdemeanor charges among people with SMI. Results were given in prior publications and are discussed in subsequent chapters.

References

Abram KM, Teplin LA, McClelland GM: Comorbidity of severe psychiatric disorders and substance use disorders among women in jail. Am J Psychiatry 160(5):1007–1010, 2003 12727711

Andrews DA, Bonta J: Rehabilitating criminal justice policy and practice. Psychol Public Policy Law 16(1):39–55, 2010

Andrews DA, Bonta J, Wormith JS: The recent past and near future of risk and/or need assessment. Crime Delinq 52(1):7–27, 2006

Baillargeon J, Binswanger IA, Penn JV, et al: Psychiatric disorders and repeat incarcerations: the revolving prison door. Am J Psychiatry 166(1):103–109, 2009 19047321

Baranyi G, Fazel S, Langerfeldt SD, et al: The prevalence of comorbid serious mental illnesses and substance use disorders in prison populations: a systematic review and meta-analysis. Lancet Public Health 7(6):e557–e568, 2022 35660217

Bonfine N, Wilson AB, Munetz MR: Meeting the needs of justice-involved people with serious mental illness within community behavioral health systems. Psychiatr Serv 71(4):355–363, 2020 31795858

Bonta J, Law M, Hanson K: The prediction of criminal and violent recidivism among mentally disordered offenders: a meta-analysis. Psychol Bull 123(2):123–142, 1998 9522681

Bronson J, Berzofsky M: Indicators of Mental Health Problems Reported by Prisoners and Jail Inmates, 2011–12 (Special Report NCJ 250612). Washington, DC, U.S. Department of Justice, 2017

Caruso GD: Public Health and Safety: The Social Determinants of Health and Criminal Behavior. Burnley, UK, ResearchersLinks Books, 2017

Clark RE, Ricketts SK, McHugo GJ: Legal system involvement and costs for persons in treatment for severe mental illness and substance use disorders. Psychiatr Serv 50(5):641–647, 1999 10332899

Cloyes KG, Wong B, Latimer S, et al: Time to prison return for offenders with serious mental illness released from prison: a survival analysis. Crim Justice Behav 37(2):175–187, 2010

Compton MT, Graves J, Zern A, et al: Characterizing arrests and charges among individuals with serious mental illnesses in public-sector treatment settings. Psychiatr Serv 73(10):1102–1108, 2022 35378991

Compton MT, Zern A, Pope LG, et al: Misdemeanor charges among individuals with serious mental illnesses: a statewide analysis of more than two million arrests. Psychiatr Serv 74(1):31–37, 2023 35795979

Fisher WH, Roy-Bujnowski KM, Grudzinskas AJ Jr, et al: Patterns and prevalence of arrest in a statewide cohort of mental health care consumers. Psychiatr Serv 57(11):1623–1628, 2006a 17085611

Fisher WH, Silver E, Wolff N: Beyond criminalization: toward a criminologically informed framework for mental health policy and services research. Adm Policy Ment Health 33(5):544–557, 2006b 16791518

Hall D, Lee LW, Manseau MW, et al: Major mental illness as a risk factor for incarceration. Psychiatr Serv 70(12):1088–1093, 2019 31480926

Hiday VA, Ray B: Arrests two years after exiting a well-established mental health court. Psychiatr Serv 61(5):463–468, 2010 20439366

James DJ, Glaze LE: Mental Health Problems of Prison and Jail Inmates. Washington, DC, U.S. Department of Justice, Office of Justice Programs, Bureau of Justice Statistics, 2006

Kennedy-Hendricks A, Huskamp HA, Rutkow L, et al: Improving access to care and reducing involvement in the criminal justice system for people with mental illness. Health Aff (Millwood) 35(6):1076–1083, 2016 27269025

Kohler-Haussman I: Misdemeanorland: Criminal Courts and Social Control in an Age of Broken Windows Policing. Princeton, NJ, Princeton University Press, 2018

Lynch SM, Dehart DD, Belknap JE, et al: A multisite study of the prevalence of serious mental illness, PTSD, and substance use disorders of women in jail. Psychiatr Serv 65(5):670–674, 2014 24487481

Magee LA, Fortenberry JD, Rosenman M, et al: Two-year prevalence rates of mental health and substance use disorder diagnoses among repeat arrestees. Health Justice 9(1):2, 2021 33411067

Natapoff A: Punishment Without Crime: How Our Massive Misdemeanor System Traps the Innocent and Makes America More Unequal. New York, Basic Books, 2018

Natapoff A: Misdemeanor decriminalization. Vanderbilt Law Rev 68(4):1055–1116, 2019

Pope LG, Patel A, Fu E, et al: Crisis response model preferences of mental health care clients with prior misdemeanor arrests and of their family and friends. Psychiatr Serv 74(11):1163–1170, 2023a 37070262

Pope LG, Stagoff-Belfort A, Warnock A, et al: Competing concerns in efforts to reduce criminal legal contact among people with serious mental illnesses: findings from a multi-city study on misdemeanor arrests. Adm Policy Ment Health 50(3):476–487, 2023b 36717527

Prins SJ: Does transinstitutionalization explain the overrepresentation of people with serious mental illnesses in the criminal justice system? Community Ment Health J 47(6):716–722, 2011 21655941

Prins SJ: Prevalence of mental illnesses in US state prisons: a systematic review. Psychiatr Serv 65(7):862–872, 2014 24686574

Prins S, Draper L: Improving Outcomes for People With Mental Illnesses Under Community Corrections Supervision: A Guide to Research-Informed Policy and Practice. New York, Council of State Governments Justice Center, 2009. Available at: https://csgjusticecenter.org/publications/improving-outcomes-for-people-with-mental-illnesses-under-community-corrections-supervision-a-guide-to-research-informed-policy-and-practice. Accessed October 19, 2023.

Raphael S, Stoll MA: Assessing the contribution of the deinstitutionalization of the mentally ill to growth in the U.S. incarceration rate. J Legal Stud 42(1):187–222, 2013

Rotter M, Compton M: Criminal legal involvement: a cause and consequence of social determinants of health. Psychiatr Serv 73(1):108–111, 2022 34126776

Skeem JL, Emke-Francis P, Louden JE: Probation, mental health, and mandated treatment: a national survey. Crim Justice Behav 33(2):158–184, 2006

Skeem JL, Manchak S, Peterson JK: Correctional policy for offenders with mental illness: creating a new paradigm for recidivism reduction. Law Hum Behav 35(2):110–126, 2011 20390443

Steadman HJ, Osher FC, Robbins PC, et al: Prevalence of serious mental illness among jail inmates. Psychiatr Serv 60(6):761–765, 2009 19487344

Swartz JA, Lurigio AJ: Serious mental illness and arrest: the generalized mediating effect of substance use. Crime Delinq 53(4):581–604, 2007

Taxman FS: Second generation of RNR: the importance of systemic responsivity in expanding core principles of responsivity. Fed Probat 78(2):32–40, 2014

Vaughn MG, DeLisi M, Beaver KM, et al: Toward a criminal justice epidemiology: behavioral and physical health of probationers and parolees in the United States. J Crim Justice 40(3):165–173, 2012

Wilson AB, Farkas K, Bonfine N, et al: Interventions that target criminogenic needs for justice-involved persons with serious mental illnesses: a targeted service delivery approach. Int J Offender Ther Comp Criminol 62(7):1838–1853, 2018 29237311

Wood JD, Watson AC, Pope L, et al: Contexts shaping misdemeanor system interventions among people with mental illnesses: qualitative findings from a multi-site system mapping exercise. Health Justice 11(1):20, 2023 37014478

2

Using System Maps to Understand Entanglement and Guide Change

Veronica Nelson, M.A.
Jennifer D. Wood, Ph.D.
Leah G. Pope, Ph.D.
Amy C. Watson, Ph.D.

As explained in Chapter 1 ("The System, the Process, and the Contexts"), the purpose of this book is to shed light on the problem of misdemeanor system entanglement among people with serious mental illness (SMI). Across the chapters, we set out to understand how entanglement happens, what is being done to reduce it, and what more could be done. As part of this effort, this chapter addresses the complexity of the entanglement problem by illuminating the pathways through which a person enters and gets caught up in misdemeanor systems. Systems across the country have common features but also vary in their structures, processes, and pathways. This chapter illustrates the value of *system maps* that visually depict how people enter and flow through systems. Given our interest in the trajectories of people with mental illness, maps are of value in illuminating where, along system continuums, a person's mental health needs could be identified and addressed, and where pathways could be created to move people away from the harms of system entanglement.

Research has tended to focus on police interactions as the main source of entanglement. As Chapter 3 ("Decision-Making Contexts of Misdemeanor Charges") explains, the police are indeed the primary "gatekeepers" of criminal legal systems owing to the substantial discretionary authority of officers to make misdemeanor arrests. Yet the police are simply one part of a chain of criminal legal actors who, together, make decisions that are consequential to people's lives (Lum et al. 2011). Misdemeanor systems are intricate, and entanglement is a complex problem that occurs at different points along system continuums. Entanglement with police is often harmful in various ways to people with mental illness, and deeper penetration into misdemeanor systems can produce compounding, cumulative harms to a person's health and psychosocial circumstances. For those reasons, jurisdictions across the country have been working to create alternate pathways, or *off-ramps*, designed to divert or deflect people away from criminal legal interventions at the point of contact with police and beyond. This chapter highlights examples of such efforts in different jurisdictions (Philadelphia, Chicago, Manhattan, and Atlanta) to illustrate the potential for reducing entanglement at different points along the misdemeanor system continuum.

Toward the end of this chapter, we further describe the value of system maps to help us understand entanglement and guide change. System maps are useful visual aids in making sense of a complex problem. Maps have descriptive and analytic value. They can provide a visual framework for guiding entanglement reduction projects and can inspire jurisdictions committed to change by illustrating alternate pathways away from harm and toward community-based mental health and social service resources. This chapter notes the value of maps as tools that can complement other forms of research and perspectives on entanglement that are the subjects of other chapters in this book.

The Harms of Entanglement

As noted in Chapter 1, there are direct and collateral harms associated with entanglement in misdemeanor systems. Such harms come in a va-

riety of forms. Some scholars have suggested that the notion of iatrogenic harm, typically applied in the field of medicine, is useful in
understanding the deleterious consequences of criminal legal system
interventions (Anderson and Burris 2017). In simple terms, the notion
of *iatrogenesis* captures the idea that a treatment for a problem (in this
case, an officer intervening and potentially arresting a person) can
cause more harm than good. For instance, when a police officer encounters a person with an SMI, the interaction itself can be experienced by
the individual as stigmatizing, disrespectful, or threatening. At worst,
such an encounter can result in injury or even death. Researchers have
also found that negative encounters with police can produce deleterious mental health effects. Efforts to avoid police are especially notable
among young Black men (Bowleg et al. 2020). When a person with an
SMI is arrested and ultimately charged with a crime, additional harms
can ensue. Being in jail, for example, is isolating and can interrupt mental health treatment plans and healthy routines. The further a person becomes entangled, the more likely other harms will compound mental
health harms, such as loss of employment and lack of connection to
family and informal social support networks (Slate et al. 2013).

Arguably, the most decisive approach to reducing the harms of
criminal legal system involvement is to prevent it altogether, but opportunities to reduce entanglement arise at every stage of the criminal legal
continuum. In what follows, we offer a case example of Mr. Mateo Hernandez and tell a brief story of how he became entangled following a
complaint about his behavior at a bus stop. As the chapter unfolds, we
provide variations on Mr. Hernandez's story based on the availability
of different pathways away from entanglement.

Case Example: Mr. Hernandez at the Bus Stop

Mateo Hernandez was a 20-year-old Latino man with an SMI who lived
at home with his mother and two younger siblings. He had worked a
variety of jobs but had found it difficult to manage his mental illness and
maintain full-time employment. As a result, he had been unable to hold
a steady job for more than a few months consecutively. He spent much
of his time walking around the nearby neighborhoods and often could
be found sitting at the bus stop talking to himself. One afternoon, a
neighbor whose home was in sight of the bus stop observed Mr. Hernandez talking to himself and moving erratically. She called 911, reporting that she was "concerned about the children in the community."

When police officers arrived at the scene, they found it difficult to
get Mr. Hernandez to cooperate with their requests because of his level
of agitation and preoccupation with responding to the voices he heard.
The 911 caller was on the scene demanding that the officers do something. The officers initially tried to resolve the incident by simply having

Mr. Hernandez leave the area and return home. Their goal was to move him along informally and avoid making an arrest, while still meeting the wishes of the complainant. However, Mr. Hernandez appeared disorganized and did not respond to their requests to leave the area. The officers asked his name, and after mumbling under his breath, he loudly stated, "I'm not telling you!"

The officers soon grew frustrated as their instructions continued to be ignored, and they inadvertently escalated the situation by circling around him and attempting to grab him, resulting in Mr. Hernandez knocking into one of the officers while flailing his arms and trying to pull away. Mr. Hernandez was subsequently arrested for both obstruction (because of his lack of cooperation and refusal to give his name) and assault (because of his physical contact with the officer). He found himself in the county jail ahead of his arraignment, at which time he met with his court-appointed public defender and entered a not guilty plea. Because the physical contact was directed at a police officer, the assault charge was upgraded to a felony. He now faces up to 5 years in prison.

This story of Mr. Hernandez provides one illustration of how people with mental illness can become entangled in criminal legal systems. Mr. Hernandez's story, however, is not inevitable and could have ended differently based on the alternate pathways (off-ramps) available to steer him away from entanglement and toward community-based care and support. Later in this chapter, we return to Mr. Hernandez, tracing how his journey could have unfolded differently based on illustrative examples of alternate pathways in Philadelphia, Chicago, Manhattan, and Atlanta.

In the following section, we provide a general description of the misdemeanor system process, illustrated by a composite system map that we produced, informed by the specific system mapping exercises conducted in the four cities just mentioned (see Chapter 1 for a note on our study methods). The purpose of this general map is to provide a visual tool for understanding the misdemeanor system continuum as well as main points along the continuum at which mental health needs can be identified and addressed. Following this general understanding of the system continuum, we turn to variations in Mr. Hernandez's story to illustrate the potential for reducing entanglement in cases like this and other cases involving people with SMI.

Mapping Systems

Figure 2–1 depicts a general representation of a misdemeanor system and the continuum of decision-making points, recognizing that jurisdictions vary in system structures, decision-making options, and pathways leading away from entanglement. Not all decision-making options are available in every jurisdiction, and legal terminology does vary. The general map captures decision-making processes beginning with the initial incident or behavior (captured in the circle at the top/middle portion of the figure), moving through the police decision-making process, to the charging decision made by the prosecutor's office, and ultimately, the sentencing decision at the judicial stage (assuming there is a conviction, as we discuss later). Each of the sites we examined (Philadelphia, Chicago, Manhattan, and Atlanta) has been innovative in developing alternate pathways aimed at deflecting or diverting people with mental illness away from system entanglement. Examples of such alternate pathways are discussed later in the chapter (see "Illustrative Pathways Away From Entanglement").

As depicted on the left side of Figure 2–1, the initial incident or behavior that results in a police encounter can become known to the police in several ways but primarily results from either a 911 call for service or an officer's observation of the behavior while on patrol. In the case of 911 calls, the information provided by the caller and how this information is classified and transmitted by 911 call takers and dispatchers can have significant consequences for how police then respond to the call. Gillooly (2020) illustrated this in her case study of how a call taker's process of interpreting and classifying information provided by a caller influenced the police response and subsequently resulted in the arrest of Henry Louis Gates, a Harvard University professor, for "breaking and entering" into his own home. In the case of 911 calls about behaviors that may be the result of a mental health crisis, it can be especially critical for call takers to receive training on how to identify signs of a behavioral health crisis and to convey information to responding officers so that they are prepared to use crisis intervention rather than resorting to coercion or force (Feldman 2020). Some jurisdictions have worked to improve 911 call triage and dispatching services to support an expanded set of first-response options when calls are received about an incident that may involve mental health distress. These include the Philadelphia-based 911 Triage and Crisis Intervention Response Team (CIRT) program (see subsection on page 28, "911 Triage and First Response Alternatives in Philadelphia"), as well as the Chicago-based Crisis Assistance Response and Engagement (CARE) program (see subsection on page 32, "Community-Based Triage Centers in Chicago"), which dispatches a team comprising a mental health clinician, a paramedic, and a police officer to a limited set of 911 calls that have a mental health component (Casanova and McCoppin 2022). Although CARE remains primarily a police co-response model, they have begun

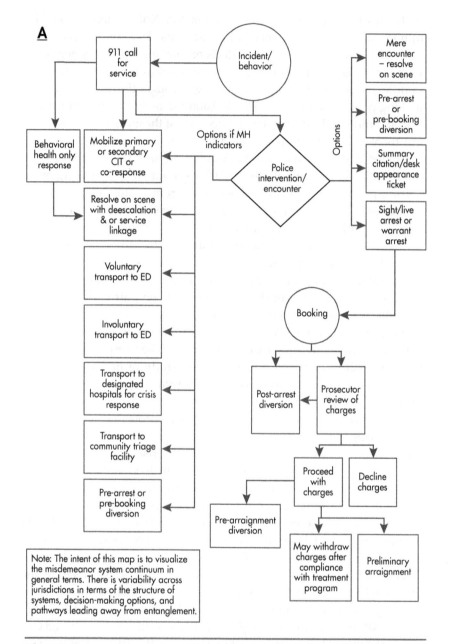

Figure 2–1. General misdemeanor system map. (A) From initial incident through preliminary arraignment.

Note. CIT=Crisis Intervention Team; ED=emergency department; MH=mental health.

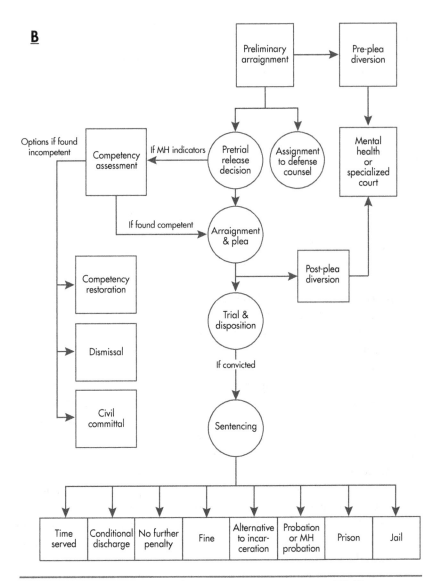

Figure 2-1. General misdemeanor system map. (B) From arraignment through sentencing.

piloting response teams made up of just a mental health clinician and a paramedic. Both programs in Philadelphia and Chicago have evolved since they were first identified during our data collection period.

As depicted in our general map, once a police officer is on the scene, they have several options available to them for resolving the situation (and to reiterate, such options vary across jurisdictions). Figure 2–1 de-

picts an expansive set of options based on our research. It is common for
an officer to first attempt to resolve an incident informally on the scene,
resulting in no further engagement with the system. This was the officers' initial approach with Mr. Hernandez when they tried to get him to
just go home. It is also possible that the police may call for emergency
medical services (EMS; what some police term *rescue*), or EMS may arrive on scene at the same time as police depending on the medical complexities that may be apparent in the call for service. In situations in
which a crime has been committed, officers may also decide to arrest
immediately or to submit an affidavit of probable cause for a future
warrant arrest. State and municipal jurisdictions have rules and procedures governing the arrest powers of police, including the circumstances under which officers can make arrests with and without
warrants. Generally, police can make arrests without warrants (also
known as *sight arrests* or *live arrests*) when the behavior occurs in the
presence of officers and in other circumstances described in state criminal procedures and police department directives.

If any indications of mental illness are observed, additional response options and diversion alternatives may become available at the
point of the police encounter and onward over the course of the criminal legal process. If the person is experiencing a mental health crisis, an
officer may choose to transport the individual to a hospital emergency
department, crisis response center, or triage facility for emergency psychiatric evaluation and crisis stabilization services. The availability of
crisis response centers (typically, in designated hospitals with psychiatric expertise) or triage facilities varies by jurisdiction. This transport
may be done on a voluntary basis if the person is agreeable or they may
take the person into protective custody and transport them on an involuntary basis if the officers believe the person needs emergency psychiatric evaluation and meets statutory criteria. Transporting the person
for psychiatric care is not always a diversion from arrest. For example,
if officers decide to make an arrest, in the case of a more serious crime,
they can first take the person to the hospital on a petition or "hold to be
evaluated" and then submit an affidavit for a warrant arrest that will
authorize them to take the person into custody once evaluated.

Other options available to police for lower-level offenses include issuing desk appearance tickets or summary citations. In New York City,
the terminology used is a *desk appearance ticket*. Citations and desk appearance tickets are used by police to order a person to appear in court
at a future date instead of being placed through the formal arrest and
booking process. In Manhattan, officers are required to issue these tickets
for class E felonies and below, which include offenses such as third-

degree criminal mischief (e.g., painting graffiti) or seventh-degree criminal possession of a controlled substance. When the suspect has an open warrant or has had a warrant in the past 2 years; when the case involves a domestic violence, sex crime, or driving while impaired/intoxicated offense; or when the suspect is experiencing medical or physical distress, officers can choose to arrest the person instead. However, officers still have the discretion to choose to issue a desk appearance ticket even if those circumstances are present.

Officers can also choose to utilize pre-arrest, pre-booking, or post-arrest diversion mechanisms depending on the decision options available in a jurisdiction. These options are captured in Figure 2–1. Pre-arrest, pre-booking, and post-arrest diversion programs are often reserved for low-level, nonviolent, or first-time offenders and are intended to divert people away from further engagement with the system and connect them with appropriate social services. In the case of pre-arrest or pre-booking diversion options, the individual also can avoid a formal arrest record that could jeopardize their housing, employment, and educational opportunities (i.e., forms of iatrogenic harm, discussed at the start of this chapter). Generally, if someone is deemed ineligible for diversion at the point of police contact or this opportunity is not available to them, their charges are then reviewed by the local prosecutor, who will choose to either decline or proceed with the charges based on the amount and quality of evidence submitted by police.

Figure 2–1 shows additional opportunities further along the misdemeanor system continuum for diverting a case with the goal of addressing a person's mental health and underlying needs. For example, charges may be dropped if the person completes a treatment program. If a case proceeds to a preliminary arraignment, in which the person is informed of the charges against them as well as their constitutional rights, they may be diverted to a specialized court before they enter a plea, such as a veterans treatment court, or after they enter a plea, such as a mental health court. A mental health court typically mandates treatment under court supervision.

Figure 2–1 also depicts a pathway to a competency assessment process if certain mental health indicators are seen between the preliminary arraignment and trial stages. If the person is deemed not competent to stand trial, several outcomes may occur, including dismissal of the case or competency restoration, in which the person receives treatment until they are able to understand the charges against them and to assist in their own defense. If the person otherwise goes through the process of arraignment, plea, or trial, there may be opportunities to address their mental health needs at the sentencing stage if they are convicted. Such options are contingent on the jurisdiction. For example, a person may be subject to mental health probation (probation overseen by a mental health unit) following disposition by a misdemeanor court, as in the state of Illinois. The state of New York offers an Alternatives to Incarceration program that, as the name suggests, seeks to avoid incarceration for people with unaddressed needs. Among these programs are those offering mental health services to people diagnosed with SMI.

In summary, the general map contained in Figure 2–1 provides a basic visualization of the misdemeanor system continuum, noting points along this continuum at which jurisdictions generally attempt to identify SMI and link people to treatment and community-based care. All four cities we examined have undertaken distinctive efforts to build alternate pathways to reduce or avoid the entanglement of people with SMI. We do not review all such efforts in the next section but rather provide examples accompanied by map figures for each novel pathway.

Illustrative Pathways Away From Entanglement

In this section, we highlight specific examples of system reforms at different points across the criminal legal continuum that are designed to reduce entanglement among people with mental illness. These reforms comprise novel pathways away from, or out of, criminal legal systems. They include the 911 call triage and CIRT program in Philadelphia, community-based crisis triage centers in Chicago, a post-arraignment pathway in Manhattan, and Misdemeanor Mental Health Court in Atlanta. We tell variations of Mr. Hernandez's story based on the availability of these pathways.

911 Triage and First Response Alternatives in Philadelphia

As previously noted, entanglement begins as early as when people call 911 to mobilize a police response to a situation (Wood and Anderson 2023). At this early stage of calling for help, there are opportunities to triage such calls in ways that identify mental health components and deploy alternative first responses. During the process of collecting the data that inform this book, the City of Philadelphia was in the early stages of developing its 911 triage and CIRT program, which began implementation in 2021. In the ensuing years, this pilot has been further refined and expanded as part of a widespread, holistic effort by the city to enhance its continuum of crisis services and mental health first-responder options, building on prior efforts, such as Community Mobile Crisis Response Teams (CMCRTs) that consist of behavioral health professionals and Crisis Intervention Team (CIT) police officers. CIRT units are a type of co-response, with each unit comprising two CIT officers and a mental health professional (see Chapter 10, "Reform in an Era of Mental Health and Crisis Services Innovation," for more information on co-response and Chapter 9, "The Current Era of Multifaceted Criminal Legal System Reform," for more on CIT programs) (Leonard 2023; Philadelphia Department of Behavioral Health and Intellectual disAbility Services 2021; Shefner et al. 2023b; Wood and Anderson 2023).

Key aims of the CIRT program are to minimize the use of arrest and the use of force, reduce injuries to police and civilians, increase time on scene to develop collaborative health-centered resolutions to the issue at hand, increase voluntary transports to psychiatric treatment, and link people to community-based care, support, and follow-up. Since November 2022, when the Philadelphia Police Department established its new Behavioral Health Unit, CIRT has been a formal program within this unit (Leonard 2023). The CIRT program is a multiagency collaborative effort involving the city's Office of Criminal Justice, the police department, and the Department of Behavioral Health and Intellectual disAbility Services, which also oversees nonpolice crisis response hotlines, a 988 suicide helpline, and community mobile crisis response units (Leonard 2023; Philadelphia Department of Behavioral Health and Intellectual disAbility Services 2021). For calls received at the suicide helpline, there is always a safety net to route the call back to 911 if police are needed.

The CIRT model was developed in tandem with a new 911 call triage process. In the emergency communications center, where 911 calls are received, call takers use a script to ascertain whether the subject of the call may be experiencing a mental health crisis. Depending on answers to scripted questions, a dispatcher can deploy a CIRT response. A CIRT unit may also be requested as a secondary response by officers who arrive on a scene and discern that there may be a person in mental health distress. CIRT units also actively monitor the mobile data terminals in their vehicles to self-deploy to available jobs if the description of the job indicates that their presence may be needed. Once a CIRT team is deployed, a follow-up team consisting of certified peer and recovery specialists helps connect people in distress to community-based services within 72 hours of their initial encounters with CIRT members.

The 911 triage and CIRT pathways were intentionally designed to complement and supplement other efforts in Philadelphia to reduce misdemeanor system entanglement, including the city's Police-Assisted

Diversion (PAD) program, which now operates under the auspices of the Behavioral Health Unit (Shefner et al. 2023a). PAD, a pre-booking diversion opportunity, was created to redirect people involved in low-level, nonviolent retail theft, drug, and prostitution offenses. Instead of being booked for a crime—a process at the point of arrest when information about a person is entered to inform the prosecution stage—individuals receive a referral from police. The referral component involves a collaboration between police and service providers to connect participants with services to address basic needs such as medical care and mental health treatment. Police officers can also proactively make social referrals to PAD for individuals they may encounter while on duty or in response to a call. In such situations, there is no potential for arrest; rather the officer recognizes a need that could be addressed through service linkage. Figure 2–2 depicts the 911 triage and CIRT program, which can be understood as a relatively new pathway away from criminal legal system entanglement and toward community-based care.

Recall that in the case of Mr. Hernandez, police were dispatched to the scene based on information provided to the call taker that he had been acting in ways that were threatening to public safety. One can imagine that the call would have been identified as a disturbance, but because the person calling 911 did not know Mr. Hernandez, they were likely not aware that Mr. Hernandez was displaying symptoms of a mental illness. As a result, a regular police unit was dispatched to the scene to address the caller's concern for public safety. However, consider this alternate version of Mr. Hernandez's story:

Case Example, continued: CIRT

On their arrival, the officers immediately recognized the signs of mental health distress. In trying to converse with Mr. Hernandez, they could tell he was hearing voices and was agitated. As such, they called dispatch to request a CIRT response. Knowing that a CIRT response was on its way, the officers chatted calmly with Mr. Hernandez, walking over to an area somewhat removed from the bus stop. Once the CIRT arrived, the mental health specialist was able to convince Mr. Hernandez to return home and committed to Mr. Hernandez that a peer specialist would visit him to follow up, connect him to mental health services, and assist with scheduling appointments. The CIRT unit gave Mr. Hernandez a ride home.

Community-Based Triage Centers in Chicago

Other jurisdictions are implementing additional strategies that make it possible for decision-makers to deflect individuals away from further en-

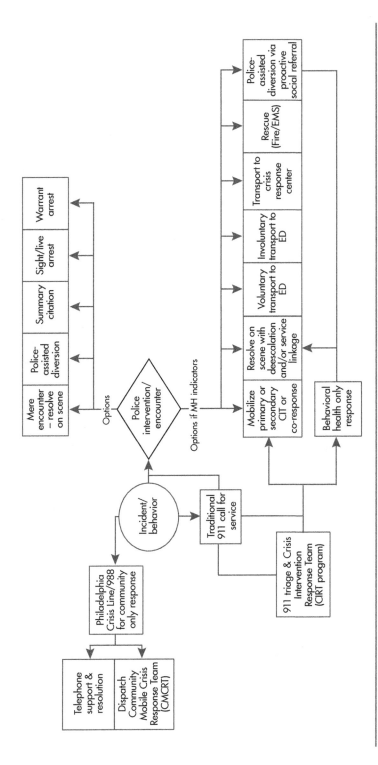

Figure 2–2. 911 triage and first response alternatives in Philadelphia.

Note. CIT=Crisis Intervention Team; ED=emergency department; EMS=emergency medical services; MH=mental health.

gagement in the system. In Chicago, one deflection option is the voluntary transport of individuals to one of several crisis triage centers instead of arrest or transport to a hospital emergency department. These triage centers provide crisis stabilization, mental health treatment, and linkage to care for those experiencing a mental health crisis. Among their goals, these centers endeavor to decrease emergency department visits and reduce the Cook County jail population. Once a person has been stabilized, the centers can provide on-site psychiatric evaluations, case management, follow-up, and referrals to other community mental health resources. Although some triage centers are hospital-based, others are community-based and may not have prescribers on-site. Figure 2–3 visually depicts this example of a pre-arrest and pre-booking diversion option.

The Westside Triage Center, one of these community-based triage centers, works closely with several police districts in Chicago, functioning as a drop-off point for Chicago police, mobile crisis teams, and other first responders. To be eligible for services at the triage center, the individual must not be under arrest and must be 18 years or older, nonviolent, and willing to go there voluntarily. An officer can transport individuals meeting these criteria directly to the triage center or contact the center for mobile crisis assistance. A Chicago police officer explained that police may also choose to "resolve the issue on the scene and to make sure that they have contact information for one of the triage centers or the NAMI [National Alliance on Mental Illness] Chicago help line," in which case that person could voluntarily walk into the triage center for assistance after resolution of the police encounter.

If we return to the story of Mr. Hernandez, had he lived in Chicago, the officers responding to the call about his behavior may have known that transport to a crisis triage center was an option. In this case, we can imagine a different scenario unfolding.

Case Example, continued: Triage Centers

After observing his behavior and struggling to calm down Mr. Hernandez enough to successfully communicate with him, the officers explained the option of transport to a triage center where Mr. Hernandez could receive some help and mental health treatment. Indicating he was not feeling well, Mr. Hernandez agreed to be taken to the triage center. Instead of being arrested, Mr. Hernandez was voluntarily transported to one of the nearby triage centers. While he was there, a crisis worker asked him how he was doing, told him about available services, and set up some appointments for him at a community mental health agency that offered psychosocial rehabilitation services. With his permission, the social worker called his mother to come in, and they discussed the plan and things that Mr. Hernandez could do next time he felt upset and

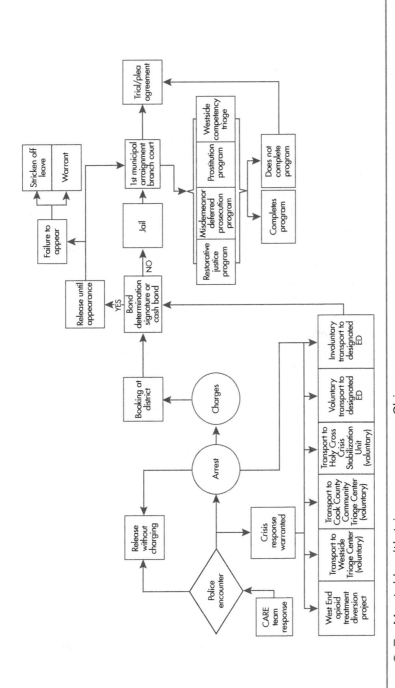

Figure 2–3. Mental health triage processes: Chicago.

Note. CARE=Crisis Assistance Response and Engagement; ED=emergency department.

agitated. The crisis counselor also provided them with a flyer from the local NAMI chapter about some of the programming and support groups they offered in the Latino community.

Pre- and Post-arraignment Pathway in Manhattan

Other opportunities exist to reduce the extended entanglement of people with SMI in the criminal legal system, even in cases where someone has already been arrested and arraigned on a misdemeanor charge. Alternative to Incarceration programs such as Manhattan Justice Opportunities provide an example, as shown in Figure 2–4. As background context, since 2015, Manhattan criminal courts have screened all individuals awaiting arraignment through the Enhanced Pre-Arraignment Screening Unit. Located in central booking, this specialized unit aims to collect timely physical and behavioral health information to provide better care to people in the arrest-to-arraignment process, improve care coordination, and widen opportunities for alternatives to traditional case processing. With a defendant's permission, the information collected can be shared with defense counsel before arraignment. Defense attorneys may then decide to use this information at arraignment or at a point further into case processing to advocate for outcomes that meet the unique needs of their clients.

Manhattan Justice Opportunities is one option that New York defense attorneys might pursue for clients who they know have an SMI and who have been arraigned on a misdemeanor charge. Launched in February 2020, this program provides an alternative to jail, fines, and sometimes convictions for people charged with misdemeanor offenses. Individuals who plead guilty or are convicted, as well as those who receive an adjournment in contemplation of dismissal (in which a judge agrees to defer the case and offers the possibility of a dismissal if the defendant complies with certain terms), can be mandated to a specific number of sessions. Program engagement begins with an individualized assessment, followed by the collaborative development of a plan for services. Mandated services can include individual counseling sessions, employment and housing support, and community service (Barrett 2022). The goal is to have a light-touch intervention that can target outstanding needs for individuals with low-level offenses (Vance 2021).

Recall that in the first version of the case example, Mr. Hernandez was arrested for obstruction (owing to his lack of cooperation) as well as assault. Let's reimagine this case example in Manhattan:

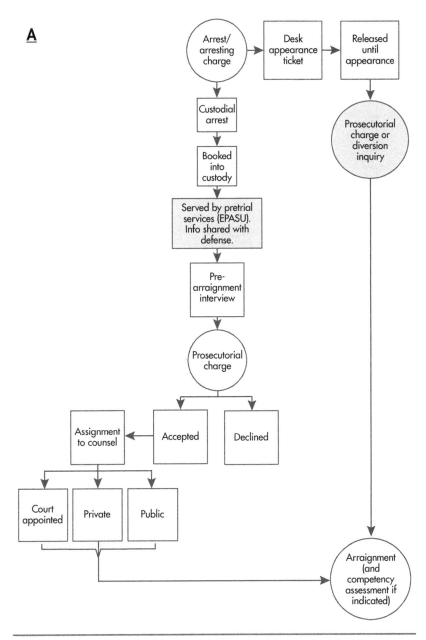

Figure 2–4.   Pre- and post-arraignment pathway in Manhattan. (A) From arrest through arraignment.

Note.   EPASU = Enhanced Pre-Arraignment Screening Unit.

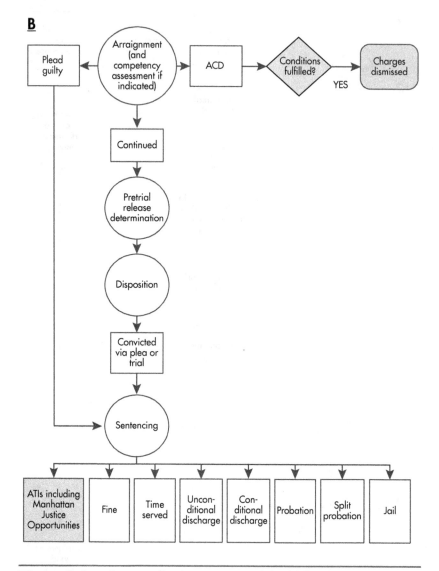

Figure 2–4.   Pre- and post-arraignment pathway in Manhattan. (B) From arraignment through sentencing

Note.   ACD=adjournment in contemplation of dismissal; ATI=Alternatives to Incarceration.

Case Example, continued: Manhattan Justice Opportunities

Mr. Hernandez had now been subjected to pre-arraignment screening, and his court-appointed public defender was aware of the Manhattan

Justice Opportunities program as an alternative to incarceration. The public defender discussed this option with the assistant district attorney, and both agreed that Mr. Hernandez was an ideal candidate for the program, which would help address Mr. Hernandez's need for community-based services and employment support. After discussing options with the public defender, Mr. Hernandez pleaded guilty and formally entered the program, beginning with an individualized assessment and a service plan designed to help him seek employment.

Misdemeanor Mental Health Court Pathway in Atlanta

Another example of a diversion opportunity that is available at the time of arraignment is the misdemeanor mental health court. All four sites in our study have mental health courts, although in Cook County (Chicago), the mental health court accepts only felony cases. In Atlanta, individuals with mental health concerns can be referred to the Fulton County Misdemeanor Mental Health Court (known alternatively as MMC) (see Figure 2–5). MMC is a voluntary, 12-month program that diverts eligible misdemeanor defendants with SMI into a supportive treatment program (Fulton County 2024). It was first established as a pilot program in July 2018 to provide support and a safer release for defendants with mental health needs detained in the Fulton County Jail. Referrals to the MMC can be made during an individual's first court appearance or at the arraignment and plea stage. Trained social workers screen for individuals in the jail who may benefit from this program. To be eligible for a referral, a prospective participant must be found to be competent, must be willing to engage in the treatment process, and must have their current misdemeanor charge connected with a diagnosed behavioral health concern (Fulton County Magistrate Court 2024). A participant can also choose at any time to opt out of the MMC program and return to the traditional prosecution process.

Once a referral has been made, the behavioral health team conducts an assessment to determine treatment and release options in lieu of the traditional trial and sentencing options. An individualized plan is developed based on each participant's needs. The behavioral health team monitors treatment goals and provides linkage to other resources to assist with housing, medical care, education, and employment. An individual's case will be dismissed once they have successfully complied with their treatment and if they do not reoffend while in the court program. Those who successfully complete the MMC program participate in a graduation that acknowledges their hard work and allows their case to be sealed to reduce the impact on future employment and hous-

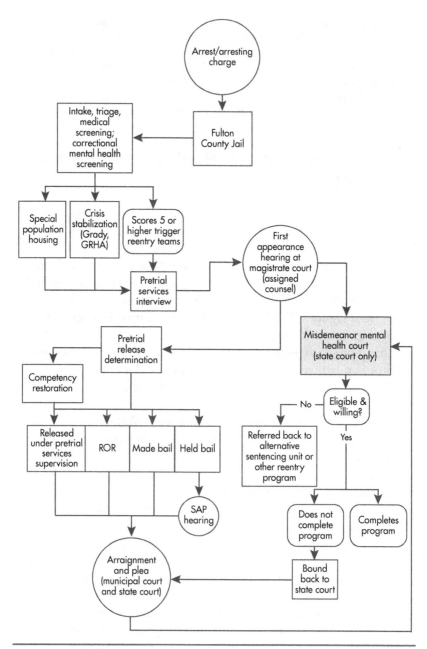

Figure 2–5. Misdemeanor mental health court pathway in Atlanta.

Note.   GRHA=Georgia Regional Hospital–Atlanta; ROR=release on own recognizance; SAP=special administrative permit.

ing. Following graduation, participants are eligible for a minimum of 3 months of ongoing support with behavioral health specialists.

Returning a final time to the story of Mr. Hernandez, had he lived in Atlanta:

Case Example, continued: Misdemeanor Mental Health Court

Mr. Hernandez was taken to the Fulton County jail following his arrest for obstruction and assault. During the intake process, he was given a brief mental health screening and received a score of 6, indicating potential mental illness and triggering a referral for mental health evaluation. Taking into consideration the indicators of mental illness and statements from the police officers involved in the arrest expressing their wishes that Mr. Hernandez not be charged with felony assault, the prosecutor decided to drop the assault charge and proceed only with the misdemeanor obstruction charge. Based on the results of the mental health screening and the behavioral health notes provided on the report from Mr. Hernandez's pretrial interview, the judge at the first appearance hearing referred him to the MMC. The assigned public defender explained the program to Mr. Hernandez, and he agreed to participate. Following his referral, he received a full mental health assessment, after which he was given an individualized treatment plan to follow and prescribed medication to take. During his ongoing meetings with his case manager, he was also linked to other community services that would help address his need for employment support. At one of his most recent meetings, Mr. Hernandez told his case manager how much he was looking forward to his graduation from the program and to inviting his mom to the ceremony.

Maps as Tools to Understand Entanglement and Guide Change

System maps are tools that can inform common understandings of complex systems as well as guide efforts to improve systems. Specifically, maps can be useful for describing and interpreting how systems function. Equally, they can inspire change by visualizing innovative system reforms. Maps can also be aspirational, providing a visual device for helping stakeholders and change agents imagine how systems might look and function differently. In what follows, we expand on the four types of value (descriptive, analytic, inspirational, and aspirational) that maps bring to the agenda of reducing misdemeanor system entanglement among people with SMI.

On a descriptive level, misdemeanor system maps provide a visual depiction of the complex pathways through which people enter and move through these systems. The general map presented in Figure 2–1 was designed to ground readers in a common understanding of *how* entanglement occurs and evolves in relation to a system's structure or architecture. Maps can also represent unique system architectures where jurisdictions have built pathways or off-ramps away from or out of systems to reduce entanglement. Figures 2–2 through 2–5 provide examples of such pathways in the jurisdictions of Philadelphia, Chicago, Manhattan, and Atlanta.

In addition to their value as descriptive tools, maps have value as tools to analyze and explain *why* entanglement happens. At each decision point along the criminal legal continuum, decision-makers have a finite set of options for how to handle a case, and each decision is consequential to how a person travels through or out of systems. Maps can therefore be used as tools to pinpoint system-limited decision options, such as the lack of options available to police in the management of mental health–related encounters. Police may have limited access to pathways out of entanglement for the people they encounter. Even before the police decision point, in which officers interact with people with SMI, there is the earlier stage of citizen mobilization of the police through 911 calls for service. System maps can help point us to such upstream processes that lead to entanglement.

As descriptive and analytic tools, maps can provide frameworks for change and help inspire reform. Figures 2–2 through 2–5 illustrate aspects of wider change efforts to reduce entanglement in the jurisdictions we studied. In this way, maps such as these have the potential to inspire change in other jurisdictions by providing examples of alternate pathways. Additionally, because jurisdictions are distinct in their system architectures, maps can be developed in customized ways to guide stakeholders at state, county, and municipal levels in change efforts. A pioneering approach to jurisdiction-specific mapping exercises and change efforts is the Sequential Intercept Mapping (SIM) framework and approach (Abreu et al. 2017; Munetz and Griffin 2006; Steadman 2007). The notion of an *intercept* refers to key points leading into and along the criminal legal continuum, where interventions could be developed to reduce entanglement and better address the needs of people with SMI. The concept of intercepts provides a clear and compelling framework for practitioners to describe their system continuums, analyze deficiencies in their systems, imagine reform efforts, and visually represent such reforms. In basic terms, the SIM framework depicts key intercepts including intercept 0 (at the community level and prior to police involvement including crisis care and response), intercept 1 (the stage of police contact), intercept 2 (the stage of courts and detention in jails), intercept 3 (jails, courts, and specialty courts), intercept 4 (reentry following incarceration), and intercept 5 (parole and probation). Chapter 9 in this book ("The Current Era of Multifaceted Criminal Legal System Reform"), which examines criminal legal system reform from a national perspective, explains the SIM framework and approach in more detail and provides a figure that depicts these key intercept points and their sequencing. Chapter 10 ("Reform in an Era of Mental Health and Crisis Services Innovation"), which examines mental health and crisis services innovation through a national perspective, also references change efforts in relation to sequential intercepts.

In essence, maps are tools to aid in strategic conversations across systems about universal entanglement problems and common change efforts. Maps can also be customized to jurisdictions to guide specific change efforts. We suggest that maps and mapping projects can be tailored to guide analyses of specific types of entanglement problems. Several chapters in this book (Chapter 5, "Being in the Wrong Place"; Chapter 6, "A $25 T-Shirt From the Bargain Store"; Chapter 7, "Noncooperation With Officers and Using 'Fighting Words'"; and Chapter 8, "'That's Scary Because Now They're Showing Violence'") examine the drivers and processes of entanglement in relation to common types of charges (i.e., criminal trespass, theft/shoplifting, noncooperation/obstruction, and assault). In theory, maps could be used as tools to analyze how such charges are processed along the misdemeanor system continuum and the unique entanglement problems that arise with each. We have argued elsewhere (Wood et al. 2023) that maps could be used to guide scenario-based exercises, centered on examples of "high-churn" cases (a term used by one of our study partners) to identify concrete barriers and facilitators affecting access to alternate pathways away from entanglement.

So far, we have suggested that maps have value in helping to describe systems, analyze systems, and inspire change by both illuminating novel pathways away from entanglement and providing a visual framework to identify opportunities or aspirations for change. That said, maps have inherent limitations. On their own, they do not "tell the story," as it were, about what happens in systems either at each decision point and intercept or about how systems function holistically. Systems consist of structures, pathways, and processes, but within those systems there are human actors making decisions, both in isolation and together at different decision-making stages and within specific decision-making contexts. Moreover, maps alone do not illuminate the ways in which racial inequities function to structure people's pathways and trajectories, limit self-determination, and produce disparate outcomes across a range of common goods (e.g., physical and mental health, education, employment).

Considering these limitations, this chapter's focus on the value of system maps should be understood in relation to the other chapters in this book. Chapter 3, "Decision-Making Contexts of Misdemeanor Charges," and Chapter 4, "Common Themes and Tensions," seek to enrich our understanding of the human decisions and contexts that make up misdemeanor system functioning and help us better understand complex drivers of entanglement. Chapter 3 aims to illuminate the contexts and factors shaping decision-making along the continuum with an emphasis on police and prosecutorial decision-making. In a complementary way, Chapter 4 highlights the plurality of values, or normative concerns, that shape the sensibilities and practical judgments of professionals making decisions about the lives of people with SMI. System maps can thus be understood as tools that can complement qualitative insights into the entanglement problem. Chapter 11 ("Equity in Mental Health and Criminal Legal System Reform") provides a thorough analysis of racism in criminal legal and mental health systems and stresses the importance of racially equitable reform across all systems concurrently. Moving forward, therefore, it is important to advance system mapping projects and efforts to create pathways away from entanglement through a racial equity lens and with the active involvement of people with lived experiences of structural racism.

KEY POINTS

- The problem of misdemeanor system entanglement must be understood as resulting from a complex set of processes and decisions along the criminal legal continuum.

- Entanglement in criminal legal systems is harmful in a variety of ways to people with serious mental illness (SMI). As such, jurisdictions across the country have created alternative pathways away from those systems. Four examples from Philadelphia, Chicago, Manhattan, and Atlanta are provided to illustrate efforts to reduce entanglement at different points along system continuums.

- System maps are useful as descriptive and analytic tools to identify how and where along system continuums entanglement occurs for people with SMI.

- Given their value as descriptive and analytic tools, maps can help guide system reform efforts by identifying potentially new pathways away from entanglement as well as showcasing the pathways created by specific jurisdictions.

- System maps and map-making activities should be understood as complements to other forms of research on why, when, and in what contexts of different misdemeanor charges entanglement occurs. Moving forward, it is important to center equity, including racial equity, in the development and interpretation of maps to guide change.

References

Abreu D, Parker TW, Noether CD, et al: Revising the paradigm for jail diversion for people with mental and substance use disorders: Intercept 0. Behav Sci Law 35(5–6):380–395, 2017 29034504

Anderson E, Burris S: Policing and public health: not quite the right analogy. Policing Soc 27(3):300–313, 2017

Barrett J: Manhattan Justice Opportunities. MJO Fact Sheet, July 2022. Available at: https://www.innovatingjustice.org/sites/default/files/media/document/2022/MJO_FactSheet_07272022.pdf. Accessed November 20, 2023.

Bowleg L, Del Río-González AM, Mbaba M, et al: Negative police encounters and police avoidance as pathways to depressive symptoms among US Black Men, 2015–2016. Am J Public Health 110(S1):S160–S166, 2020 31967888

Casanova S, McCoppin R: New 911 response alternatives find success in Chicago area but also limits. EMS1, August 3, 2022. Available at: https://www.ems1.com/mental-illness/articles/new-911-response-alternatives-find-success-in-chicago-area-but-also-limits-emzfBe0v2uhBvfeL. Accessed January 22, 2024.

Feldman N: Philly police to start flagging 911 calls that involve a behavioral health crisis. WHYY, October 9, 2020. Available at: https://whyy.org/articles/philly police-to-start-flagging-911-calls-that-involve-a-behavioral-health-crisis/. Accessed January 22, 2024.

Fulton County: Court related mental health, in Fulton County Departments: Behavioral Health and Developmental Disabilities. Atlanta, GA, Fulton County, 2024. Available at: https://www.fultoncountyga.gov/inside-fulton-county/fulton-county-departments/behavioral-health-and-developmental-disabilities/court-related-mental-health. Accessed January 22, 2024.

Fulton County Magistrate Court: Misdemeanor Mental Health Court. Atlanta, GA, Fulton County Courthouse, 2024. Available at: https://magistratefulton.org/151/Misdemeanor-Mental-Health-Court-MMC. Accessed May 16, 2023.

Gillooly JW: How 911 callers and call-takers impact police encounters with the public: the case of the Henry Louis Gates Jr. arrest. Criminol Public Policy 19(3):787–804, 2020

Leonard N: A new era of crisis response: Philly police team up with mental health experts. WHYY, July 17, 2023. Available at: https://whyy.org/articles/philadelphia-crisis-intervention-police-mental-health-emergency-response. Accessed January 10, 2024.

Lum C, Koper CS, Wu X: The influence of places on police decision pathways: from call for service to arrest. Justice Q 28(4):631–665, 2011

Munetz MR, Griffin PA: Use of the sequential intercept model as an approach to decriminalization of people with serious mental illness. Psychiatr Serv 57(4):544–549, 2006 16603751

Philadelphia Department of Behavioral Health and Intellectual disAbility Services: Behavioral Health Crisis Expansion Fact Sheet. Philadelphia, DBHIDS, September 2021. Available at: https://dbhids.org/wp-content/uploads/2021/10/BH-Crisis-Expansion-Factsheet_Sept-2021.pdf. Accessed January 10, 2024.

Shefner RT, Johnson J, Shofer FS, et al: Police officer perspectives on a pre-booking diversion program for people who use drugs in Philadelphia. J Drug Issues 54(4):576–589, 2023a

Shefner RT, Koppel R, Wood J, et al: Co-deployment is an answer, but what are the questions? Insights from officer focus groups in Philadelphia. Police Pract Res 24(6):728–734, 2023b 37981953

Slate RN, Buffington-Vollum JK, Johnson WW: The Criminalization of Mental Illness. Durham, NC, Carolina Academic Press, 2013

Steadman HJ: NIMH SBIR Adult Cross-Training Curriculum (AXT) Project: Phase II Final Report. Delmar, NY, Policy Research Associates, 2007

Vance CR Jr: Reducing the Criminal Justice Footprint in Manhattan. New York, Manhattan District Attorney's Office, 2021

Wood JD, Anderson E: Triaging mental health emergencies: lessons from Philadelphia. Law Contemp Probl 86:29–53, 2023

Wood JD, Watson AC, Pope L, et al: Contexts shaping misdemeanor system interventions among people with mental illnesses: qualitative findings from a multi-site system mapping exercise. Health Justice 11(1):20, 2023 37014478

3

Decision-Making Contexts of Misdemeanor Charges

Luis C. Torres, Ph.D.
Jennifer D. Wood, Ph.D.

This chapter features the contexts that shape decision-making across misdemeanor systems, with an emphasis on the decisions of police, prosecutors, and defense attorneys. We explain that historically, decision-making scholars have paid minimal attention to the ways in which considerations of mental illness figure into decisions about whether and when to arrest, charge, and prosecute individuals for misdemeanor offenses. As discussed in Chapter 2, "Using System Maps to Understand Entanglement and Guide Change," the problem of entanglement among people with serious mental illness (SMI) cannot simply be attributed to a single decision by one decision-maker. Rather, there is a chain of decisions across the criminal legal continuum that work together to produce case outcomes. Given this complexity of the criminal legal process, it is important to understand mental illness as one among a variety of considerations that influence how system actors—including police, prosecutors, defense attorneys, and judges—decide what to do and dictate the trajectory of a person's case. In simple terms, decision-making must be understood holistically.

We begin this chapter by discussing the importance of both context and variability in decision-making. Decision-makers, both individually and collaboratively, determine courses of action considering case-level factors as well as the constraints and pressures of the systems and sub-systems (organizational settings) within which they operate. After reviewing some key ideas from research on decision-making, we offer a case example depicting the case of an unhoused person with an SMI who is arrested for trespassing. Engaging with the themes of the example, we provide an overview of key research findings on the factors shaping the decisions of police, prosecutors, and defense attorneys. We conclude by discussing the need to advance research on place (location of behaviors), as well as on the role of SMI as one of myriad decision-making elements. We also present ideas to reduce misdemeanor system entanglement, extending on developments already occurring across the country. These ideas include changes to the law and policy environments of criminal legal systems through a *progressive prosecution* agenda, improved data collection on system outcomes for people with mental illness, and place-based, problem-oriented strategies for reducing the likelihood of police contact as well as arrests. We also stress the importance of centering the voices of people with lived experience in the research process, ensuring that people who are directly affected by decisions can help policymakers understand their needs and ways of better addressing them.

Context and Variability in Decision-Making

Decisions about whether, how, and when to enforce misdemeanor laws are not simply robotic processes governed by formal rules and check-lists. Rather, these decisions are human-made and guided by a variety of subjective considerations. Consider police officers, who are sometimes referred to as gatekeepers of the criminal legal system (Neusteter et al. 2019) because they represent the first point of contact between people and the system as a whole. Police officers wield considerable discretion in exercising the power of arrest, especially when it comes to handling minor and nonviolent offenses. Goldstein (1960, p. 543) explained that the police routinely make decisions "not to invoke the criminal process" and are selective in their enforcement actions due to competing pressures and priorities from within and outside of their agencies. The police decision to arrest is therefore consequential to the decision-making of other criminal legal actors because it determines which cases make it through the "door" of the system.

Regardless of the decision-maker, the process of making decisions is not just the product of internal cognitions but is shaped by interactive joint processes involving multiple people working across a "loosely coupled" system (Bishop et al. 2010). This decision-making process also varies across system contexts. Because of variability in both decision-makers and decision-making systems, noted in Chapter 2, differences in laws and in the application of laws and policies can be assumed (see Chapter 5, "Being in the Wrong Place"; Chapter 6, "A $25 T-Shirt From the Bargain Store"; Chapter 7, "Noncooperation With Officers and Using 'Fighting Words'"; and Chapter 8, "'That's Scary Because Now They Are Showing Violence'" that highlight variations in laws with respect to common types of misdemeanor charges). To understand decision-making, it is important to recognize that each decision-maker functions within certain social, political, legal, and cultural contexts (Ulmer 2019). For example, in the court context, *courtroom workgroups* (collectively referring to the group of individuals such as judges, prosecutors, and defense attorneys who play different roles and come together during the processing of cases) (Eisenstein and Jacob 1977) are expected to uniquely interpret and apply the law, resulting in differences in case outcomes.

Criminal legal scholars, particularly those who study decision-making and decisions within the court context, have recently pushed for researchers to treat courts as *inhabited institutions*, meaning places where court participants actively and dynamically shape decisions, and not simply places where decision-making occurs in a static, top-down manner (Lynch 2019; Ulmer 2019). From the inhabited institutions perspective, researchers have stressed the importance of understanding how organizational participants (e.g., judges, prosecutors) interpret and apply the overarching rules and structures that govern courts and the respective organizations that each represents (e.g., prosecutors represent the District Attorney's Office, public defenders speak for the Public Defender's Office).

The inhabited institutions perspective recognizes the importance of the interactive sense-making among decision-makers. From this perspective, scholars have been critical of existing research that places little emphasis on participants and courtroom workgroups—for example, by relying on large secondary administrative datasets and complex quantitative analyses to examine the effects of relevant legal (e.g., seriousness of charge) and extralegal (e.g., defendant's race and sex) factors on various decisions, including the likelihood of conviction, sentence type, and sentence length. In sentencing research, the technique is so commonly used that it is referred to as the *modal approach* (Baumer 2013). The modal approach focuses on statistical patterns, with a view to determining which factors emerge most salient in the data. This approach turns a blind eye to the important and undoubtedly insightful interactions, negotiations, and collaborative decision-making that happen within entities or subsystems of criminal legal systems, such as courts (Lynch 2019). Through the inhabited institutions lens, then, scholars place a stronger emphasis on participants and courtroom workgroups, as well as their individual and collective interpretations and applications of the law. Such scholars more heavily consider contextual factors that may guide decision-making and influence case outcomes. The perspective posits that scholars should, for example, turn to the use of more diverse data and methods (e.g., ethnographies). Lynch (2019, p. 1165) suggested that research move "away from just descriptively measuring outcomes, such as demographic disparities, and instead foreground the dynamic, contextual factors that create an operational milieu in which criminal case adjudication happens."

Although the inhabited institutions perspective has been examined predominantly in relation to courts, police organizations can also be thought of as inhabited institutions. Just as prosecutors, defense attorneys, and judges make decisions in courtroom settings, police officers engage in sense-making on the streets, interpreting each situation before them and deciding when and how to apply the rules (laws and departmental procedures) that govern their work. As scholars of police culture have observed, through experience on the job, officers develop informal rules (or forms of practical reasoning) when making decisions about how to resolve the situations before them (Ericson 1981). As is observed with other criminal legal decision-makers, variability exists in police decision-making due to the unique legal, social, political, and cultural contexts of the organizations and systems within which they function.

To illustrate the complex nature of misdemeanor system decision-making, we now turn to a case example involving the case of Mr. Kevin Thompson. Following this example, we elaborate on the contexts shaping decision-making. Table 3–1 summarizes these contexts in relation to two key decisions (e.g., arrest, charge), with a focus on the decision-making of police and prosecutors.

Case Example: Mr. Thompson at the Donut Shop

Kevin Thompson is a 54-year-old White man with schizophrenia. For the last 4 years, he has been homeless in downtown Atlanta, having last worked as a grocery store clerk in an Atlanta suburb. He lost his job owing to poor performance, coupled with customer complaints about his odd behavior, resulting from symptoms of his untreated psychiatric condition. After losing his ability to pay rent, he made his way downtown, where there was a community of other people who, like him, struggled to subsist. Over time, he gravitated to a covered sidewalk beside the storefront of a donut shop. He and his friends created a makeshift space to eat, sleep, and stay out of the elements. Mr. Thompson spent several hours a day in this spot asking for money. Much of what he collected was used to purchase beer from a store half a block away.

Over several months, Mr. Thompson's use of the space outside of the donut shop caused concern, and at times anger, on the part of patrons, surrounding business owners, the managers of the establishment, and the security guard who worked for them. Mr. Thompson sometimes sat at a table in the donut shop for hours at a time when the weather was cold or wet or when he needed to use the restroom. Employees called 911 on several occasions, enlisting city police officers to talk to Mr. Thompson and make him move along. The calls were usually precipitated by Mr. Thompson acting erratically, speaking loudly to himself, and claiming that he worked for the FBI. Mr. Thompson did not agree that there was a problem and saw the donut shop as a legitimate place for him to spend time. He did not see the need to comply with police requests to move, but usually chose to leave the premises temporarily, until public pressure waned, returning only a few hours later. He had come to dislike the police and the security guard for telling him what to do. Patrons continued to view his behavior as unusual, unpredictable, or even threatening, and the owner and managers worried about losing customers.

There were two police officers who knew Mr. Thompson best, since they regularly patrolled the area, and the district station was nearby. Knowing Mr. Thompson for many months, they knew he did not pose a real threat to public safety. He had never broken anything or hurt anyone, but their experience told them that he suffered from some kind of mental illness and needed shelter and assistance to care for himself. Their preference was not to arrest Mr. Thompson, and their usual course of action was to encourage him to move along. They had even offered multiple times to link Mr. Thompson to a nearby shelter—offering to take him there and advocate for him to get help. But after many repeat calls to 911, the business owner had had enough, wanted to press charges, and insisted that Mr. Thompson be arrested and taken to jail. The two officers acquiesced and arrested Mr. Thompson for trespassing, surmising that at least in jail he might get screened for a mental illness, avoid the temptation of alcohol, and receive three square meals a day.

After Mr. Thompson was arrested and detained in jail, he was visited by a public defender who had seen cases like his before. She had been a public defender for 10 years and was frustrated at a long institutional history of using criminal trespass charges as a catch-all charge for getting rid of people who are seen as undesirable but pose no threat to public safety. In her experience, trespassing cases such as Mr. Thompson's were common among her clients who had a mental illness. Mr. Thompson's behavior met certain criteria for the misdemeanor offense of criminal trespass in Georgia. For instance, Mr. Thompson was interfering with the use of the donut shop's property by sitting inside for long periods of time, not purchasing food, and using the customer restroom as a bathing facility without the consent of the business owner, managers, or employees. At the same time, the Georgia Code specified that such behavior must be undertaken "knowingly and maliciously," which in Mr. Thompson's case was debatable (GA Code § 16–7–21). Both the public defender and the prosecutor recognized this and were frustrated that there were few places for people such as Mr. Thompson (who was both homeless and living with an SMI) to go. They surmised that keeping him in jail for psychiatric screening and linkage to care might be in his best interests. Therefore, the prosecutor decided to pursue the misdemeanor charge, which would provide an opportunity for Mr. Thompson to be administered a mental health screening at the county jail and ideally be routed to the Misdemeanor Mental Health Court and receive community-based treatment and monitoring by the court and service providers.

In Mr. Thompson's case, the Misdemeanor Mental Health Court could have provided a tangible pathway away from traditional prosecution with the promise of both linking him to mental health and housing services and releasing him under a set of conditions designed to help him avoid future police contact and system entanglement. Yet, because Mr. Thompson did not fully understand why his behavior constituted trespassing, he declined to volunteer for the Misdemeanor Mental Health Court program. Although his defense attorney believed that the program would benefit him, she also valued his self-determination (a value discussed in Chapter 4, "Common Themes and Tensions") and supported his decision. Eventually, the judge dismissed the charge due to the absence of knowingness on Mr. Thompson's part.

In this story, there are details that help us understand how a person may became entangled with the police and the criminal legal system. In the following sections, we examine this case in relation to what is known about such contexts in the literature, beginning with the police decision point. These contexts are summarized in Table 3–1.

Police Decision-Making

In the case example, the officers decided to arrest Mr. Thompson based on their contextualized knowledge of the situation—that is, the knowledge that is specific to the situation and the events leading up to it (Thacher 2008). Consider, for example, the location of the behavior. Location is relevant because part of the police role involves managing or

Table 3–1. Factors influencing arrest and charging decisions

Actor	Key decision-making point	Case-level factors	Other factors	Factors considered in Mr. Thompson's case (+, aggravating factor; –, mitigating factor)
Police	Arrest	Incident location Offense type/seriousness Victim desires Victim characteristics Officer characteristics Suspect behavior Prior criminal history Presence of mental illness	Public pressure Policing strategies Standard operating procedures Prosecutorial policies	Incident location (+) Public pressure (+) Victim desires (+) Offense type/seriousness (–) Threat to public safety (–) Needs of those with serious mental illnesses (+) Previous unsuccessful attempts to curb similar behaviors (+)
Prosecutor	Charging	Offense type/seriousness Evidence strength Prior criminal history Defendant demographics Victim-defendant relationship Victim characteristics Presence of mental illness	Prosecutorial policies	Likelihood of conviction (–) Needs of those with serious mental illnesses (+)

brokering (del Pozo 2022) the use of public space according to the norms of the area or neighborhood (Kohler-Hausmann 2018). In this role, the police are required to serve a peacekeeping function (Bittner 1967). Mr. Thompson was spending much of his time outside of a retail business; the owner and other business owners in the area, however, had expectations that Mr. Thompson would not hang around. Both the owners and customers likely shared views about what was acceptable and normal behavior, and Mr. Thompson's behavior challenged this norm and related standards of civil behavior (Kelling 1987).

Stakeholders in this space, particularly the customers and the business owners, exerted pressure on the police to do something about Mr. Thompson's presence. In discussing a similar example of trespassing on a donut shop's property, an Atlanta-based defense attorney reflected on the pressure from stakeholders, noting "a lot of the officers say they don't really have a choice—that client is in front of that [shop] every day. And that business owner is insistent that the cops take them to jail." What frustrated the officers, however, was that Mr. Thompson was not a threat to public safety. They knew this through several prior interactions with him. They also knew that he struggled with unmet mental health needs as well as homelessness. The officers presumed he had a mental illness, but this knowledge would not have mitigated the risk of pressure by stakeholders to address the nuisance that he represented.

Another situational factor shaping the police decision in this case was Mr. Thompson's previous poor compliance with officers' directives, coupled with an assessment that the officers' previous attempts to address stakeholder complaints did not solve the problem. Such attempts only achieved "temporary solutions to chronic vulnerability" (Wood et al. 2017, p. 89). On past occasions, the officers tried to handle the matter informally, working to persuade Mr. Thompson to leave the space, but he could not accept the reasoning behind his banishment. Researchers who have studied policing in and around privately owned communal spaces, such as the donut shop in this case, have observed that banishment is a common tool for managing behavior (Kempa et al. 1999). Faced with pleas to do something once and for all, the officers chose to arrest Mr. Thompson, which would remove him from the space, at least temporarily.

Mr. Thompson's case reveals that the police weigh different factors when deciding how to handle a situation. In an Atlanta-based focus group, an officer expressed it this way:

> The reason I saw so many mentally ill people getting caught in criminal trespassing is that's their doorway. That's where they sleep. That's their

home. It's just a lot of their mental health and their addiction prevent that. I mean, the cop says move down the street to the corner. I mean, we work across the street from a donut shop that has about four people that always want to be in front of it. And it's a constant struggle between the cops, the homeless people who think they live there, and the security guard. So that's, it's still a lot of their mental illness. That's their home. That's where they're at. They don't process information.

Mr. Thompson's case illuminates the role of discretion in police decision-making. Discretion relates to the decision of whether to enforce an applicable law. When it comes to nonviolent misdemeanors, officers have the authority to enforce the law, and they also have some latitude in determining whether to do so. Officers are faced with competing demands, especially when other calls for service are waiting for their attention. Officers must decide when it is prudent to arrest and when it is just as (or more) effective to handle a matter informally. The police are, as it were, street-level decision-makers (Lipsky 2010) and criminal legal gatekeepers that, in dealing directly with the public, make discretionary decisions about whether and how to enforce the law.

The discretionary space of officers depends on the contexts of the wider systems within which they work. This includes broader policing strategies, the standard operating procedures of their police agencies, and more widely, the law and policy environments of their jurisdictions. Consider, for example, the following comments from a participant in the Manhattan systems mapping exercise that links a decline in the use of trespassing charges to a larger shift away from a strong reliance on the order maintenance agenda of former Mayor Rudy Giuliani and his Police Commissioner at the time, William Bratton (see Scrivener et al. 2020):

> If you look at the strategy papers for stop and frisk during the Giuliani administration, one of the strategies was, in fact, to make arrests in public spaces, things like the park across from Macy's, as a way of bringing in people on criminal trespass charges. Many of them were mentally ill, not necessarily SMI.... Clearly those arrests have gone down, and certainly [our agency] is seeing this extraordinary drop in criminal trespass charges, both with respect to what you're talking about, buildings, but also in public spaces. But if you go back to the enormous volume during the stop and frisk days—the beginning of the Giuliani administration—it was very much part of the [New York Police Department] strategy.

Officer discretion may also be affected by the relationships between police and the District Attorney's Office. After arrests by police, prosecutors must determine whether to formally charge individuals with crimes (decisions by prosecutors are discussed in more detail in the next section). In some instances, line prosecutors may be directed by their respective offices to stop formally charging individuals arrested for certain types of offenses, including low-level offenses (e.g., trespassing) or drug-related offenses. As a result of any shifts in prosecution practices by the District Attorney's Office, officers must then determine whether to make arrests for crimes that they know will not likely be prosecuted. This delicate interplay, as captured in Figure 3–1, is evident in jurisdictions with a commitment to reduce mass incarceration (described in the next section), whereby prosecutors have attempted to circumvent the discretion of police by refusing to formally charge certain offenses. As is discussed in the next section, this prosecutor-led practice has implications for reducing the entanglement of people such as Mr. Thompson in the system.

Prosecutorial policies, along with changes in the law, shape officer discretion by determining the legal "toolbox" available to police in managing the behaviors they are asked to manage. As Chapter 5 explains in detail, criminal trespass statutes generally emphasize the element of *knowingness* to be liable for entering or remaining on a restricted premise. There is, however, statutory variation in both the definitional criteria for trespassing and the penalty for the offense, and sometimes, there are changes to local policies and procedures down to the police department level that serve to limit the use of arrest. In Philadelphia, for example, following a high-profile case of a trespassing arrest at a Starbucks location in 2018, the Philadelphia Police Department adopted a new policy that effected a shift away from the use of arrest in favor of informal efforts to both educate people that they are trespassing and encourage them to leave. After that incident, there was a move by the City of Philadelphia to effectively decriminalize Defiant Trespass by reducing it to a Philadelphia Code violation (Wood et al. 2023). The story of Mr. Thompson would have had a different trajectory in Philadelphia because the option to arrest would likely not have been viable.

Police decision-making therefore varies by context—the context of the situation itself; the place where the behavior is occurring; and the wider organizational, legal, and policy environments within which police operate. Additionally, policing research has shown that officers' decisions can vary depending on individual-level factors, including the characteristics of the officers themselves. Such characteristics include officers' styles and preferences, years of service (known colloquially as "time on the job"), education, racial and ethnic identity, sex, and personal beliefs and attitudes, because officers' perceptions of social problems shape how they approach people in the community (Bonner 2015; Crum and Ramey 2023; del Pozo et al. 2021; Gant and Schaible 2022;

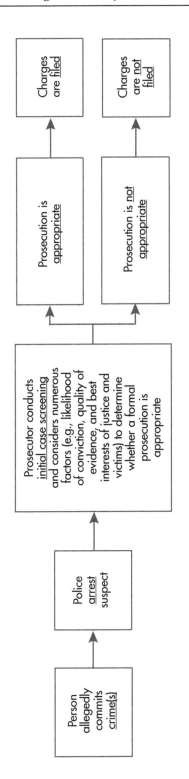

Figure 3–1. Prosecutorial case screening and charging decisions.

Grace et al. 2022; Ishoy 2015; Ishoy and Dabney 2018; Novak and Engel 2005; Slothower 2019).

Victims can influence officers' decisions. Victims may in some cases be sympathetic to an alleged offender. A victim's believability and level of cooperation with the police can play a role (Bonner 2015; Campbell 2015). The victim's sex, race (Lapsey et al. 2022), and even marital status (O'Neal and Spohn 2017) have been examined as potential factors influencing officers' decisions.

The characteristics of the alleged offender have also been the focus of police decision-making studies, as has the behavior of the alleged offender (e.g., their demeanor, expressed attitudes, perceived level of resistance to officers' directives) (Bonner 2015; Grace et al. 2022) and the presence of a weapon (O'Neal and Spohn 2017). Scholars have also studied the relevance of a person's prior arrest history and criminal legal system involvement (Campbell 2015; Franklin et al. 2022; O'Neal and Spohn 2017; Peterson 2023). Offense severity plays a clear role in officers' decisions (as it does with prosecutorial decisions). There is less discretionary authority when it comes to violent offenses, where there is an actual victim and evidence of direct, physical harm (Lamb et al. 2002).

With a few exceptions (Cotton and Coleman 2010; Novak and Engel 2005; Peterson 2023; Schulenberg 2015, 2016), the scholarly literature is limited in its analysis of the presence of a mental illness as a factor or consideration that influences decision-making, including the decision to arrest, and how that consideration interacts with other situational and contextual factors. There are mixed views on whether officers are more inclined (Teplin and Pruett 1992), or not (Engel and Silver 2001), to arrest someone presenting with a mental illness versus someone without a mental illness. What is clear is that any police encounter is a two-way interaction. An officer interprets the behavior of the individual while determining whether that individual is likely to comply with their directives. If an officer considers a person to be uncooperative, resistant, or defiant, the officer may resort to a more formal measure, such as arrest or use of force, to maintain their authority and take control of a situation.

Unsurprisingly, the ability to recognize the symptoms of mental illnesses varies by officer, in large part because of variations in officers' prior knowledge, experience, and training (Lamb et al. 2002). A lack of knowledge about mental health symptomatology can lead to an officer misinterpreting the behavior and demeanor of a person with a mental illness. It is especially challenging for an officer to interpret a person's behavior if drug or alcohol use is involved (Lamb et al. 2002). At the same time, the person interprets the behavior of the officer and considers whether the officer is treating them in a dignified manner. Researchers have observed that if a person experiences their encounter with an officer as stigmatizing or disrespectful, this can undermine their willingness to cooperate (Watson and Angell 2007, 2013). In the case of Mr. Thompson, one would need to carefully examine how he perceived his previous interactions with officers in their attempts to informally address his behavior, and whether he felt he was treated with dignity and respect.

It should be noted that the decision to arrest may be made on compassionate grounds. The officers in Mr. Thompson's case knew him to have a long-standing mental illness, coupled with homelessness. Mr. Thompson's behavior did not meet the criteria for an urgent hospital transport, nor did the officers see arrest as the best option. In the absence of other solutions to the problem, and in the face of community pressure, the only viable option, and the chosen course of action in this story, is the use of "mercy booking" (Lamb et al. 2002), so that jail-based mental health screening, evaluation, and possible treatment might address Mr. Thompson's needs. Based on research from the 1960s, police scholar Egon Bittner pointed out that officers use arrest as a last resort when there are no other apparent solutions (Bittner 1967). Decades later, Teplin and Pruett (1992) made a similar observation that officers use arrest in some instances in which hospitalization is not appropriate and there is community pressure to address disruptive behavior.

Prosecutorial Decision-Making

Once police make an arrest, cases are passed along to the court system and prosecutors. More than 80 years ago, Supreme Court Justice Robert H. Jackson stated that prosecutors have "more control over life, liberty, and reputation than any other person in America" (Jackson 1940, p. 3). Today, Jackson's statement still holds true, perhaps even more than ever before (Bibas 2001). Considered the fulcrum of the criminal justice system, prosecutors make numerous important and highly consequential, discretionary decisions that dictate the trajectory of cases through the judicial system and the subsequent punishment of defendants, including whether to accept cases for prosecution (i.e., formally file criminal charges), engage in the largely hidden and informal plea negotiation process, and provide courts with sentencing recommendations (Bibas 2001; Edkins and Redlich 2019; Ulmer 2018). Although the exact prevalence of plea negotiations is unknown owing to a lack of transparency and available data, figures show that >90% of federal and state criminal cases are resolved via guilty pleas, many of which stem from the prose-cutor-driven decision to negotiate. Altogether, this highlights the im-portant role that prosecutors and their decisions play in a criminal prosecution (Devers 2021).

Numerous studies have examined the legal and extralegal factors that influence prosecutorial decision-making throughout the different stages of a criminal prosecution, with very few considering the role of the presence of a mental illness. Generally, studies have found that prosecutorial decision-making is largely driven by legal factors such as offense type, evidence strength, and defendant culpability (see Freder-ick and Stemen 2012 for a review of the literature discussed here). How-ever, some studies have found that other factors also influence decision-making. For example, research to date is equivocal on whether the race of defendants plays a role in prosecutors' charging decisions and case dismissals (e.g., Free 2002; Kutateladze et al. 2014). The effects of race are evident in studies examining other decisions by prosecutors, includ-ing decisions to pursue the death penalty, plea negotiations (e.g., down-grading charges), and mandatory and third-strike sentences (e.g., Kutateladze et al. 2014). Other factors, such as the defendant's sex and the relationship between the victim and the defendant, have also been found to affect the decisions of prosecutors. Altogether, most studies have found that legal factors largely guide prosecutorial decision-mak-ing, and the variability of results found across studies is largely at-tributed to context, such as jurisdiction and courtroom workgroups (Johnson 2006).

Although empirical research on the effects of mental illness on pros-ecutorial decision-making is limited, some research has examined this relationship. For example, a recent study used vignette-style survey data of state and local prosecutors ($N=542$ respondents) from different regions to investigate the factors and reasons guiding their initial charging decisions and subsequent punishment recommendations (monetary penalty or term of confinement). After being presented with a fictional police report that described a minor crime, ~97% determined that filing one or more charges was appropriate, and 16% reported charging the defendant with a felony. Regarding their punishment de-cisions, ~70% of respondents did not recommend a term of confine-ment, and 60% did not recommend that monetary sanctions be imposed. The authors noted that initial charging and punishment deci-sions varied heavily across regions. When justifying their punishment decisions, >25% of respondents mentioned the defendant's mental health, 8.5% mentioned the need for counseling or treatment, and nearly 4% mentioned anger management (Wright et al. 2021). The authors also found that the presence of mental health concerns helped mitigate punishment. Specifically, they found that many of the respondents who had concerns about the defendant's mental health ultimately determined that punishment was not appropriate. Relatedly, these respondents further justified their decision to not punish defendants with mental health concerns by also highlighting the lack of physical harm caused by the crime.

In Mr. Thompson's case, it is evident how a mental illness and the seriousness of the alleged crime influenced the prosecutor's decision-making. Specifically, the prosecutor assigned to Mr. Thompson's case recognized how little danger he posed to the community, his actual needs (housing and psychiatric treatment) that should be addressed to curb similar future occurrences, and the uncertainty associated with being able to eventually secure a conviction. A public defender in an Atlanta-based focus group noted the challenge of securing criminal trespass convictions when they involve a person with a known mental illness, stating that

> criminal trespass requires that we prove an element of knowingness, that the person knew, actively knew that they were trespassing or that they were staying somewhere that they had been told to leave. And so when you talk about these mental health cases, practically, right, it is a catch-all and it's a way to quote-unquote "get rid of people that you don't want to be there," but as those cases continue, if you have someone with mental health concerns, they are gonna be very difficult cases for the state to prove should they choose to prosecute them all the way through. Because they must be able to prove some element of knowingness and that the person was aware of whatever their violation was.

Decision-Making by Courtroom Workgroup Members

As organizations, courts are governed by institutional rules and have clearly stated goals and interests, including efficient disposition of cases (Blumberg 1967). Given the competing objectives of adversaries (defense attorneys and prosecutors), these overarching goals and the rules in place ensure that the court's needs are met and play an influential role in guiding courtroom processes and decision-making. The main objectives of prosecutors and defense attorneys are to secure convictions and defend defendants from being convicted, respectively. The role of efficiency and uncertainty is evident in Mr. Thompson's case, as is the important interplay between both these actors, the judge, and other criminal legal professionals (including the police at times) who participate in the workings of courts.

In Mr. Thompson's case, both the prosecutor and the public defender expressed their frustrations about such cases involving alleged low-level offenses committed by people with SMI. Although both court actors agreed that Mr. Thompson needed adequate services and should not be formally prosecuted, this shared belief may also have been driven, at least in part, by concerns about efficiency. Specifically, given high caseloads and limited resources, prosecuting and defending defendants for such low-level offenses may hinder their own efficiency as prosecutors and defenders as well as the efficiency of their respective organizations and the court. The prosecutor's frustration in prosecuting Mr. Thompson's case may also have been guided by the high certainty of the case being dismissed by the judge and not ultimately resulting in a conviction: as discussed, legal questions surrounding Mr. Thompson's knowingness of the alleged trespassing make it difficult for the prosecutor to secure a conviction.

Given the importance of context (e.g., jurisdiction, courtroom workgroup), ample research has focused on examining how variability across these characteristics influences the court process and, ultimately, decision-making. For example, public defenders are considered *repeat players*, meaning that they, compared with private attorneys, have higher familiarity with the court's formal and informal strategies for disposing of cases and repeatedly interact with the other members of the workgroup (Blumberg 1967). These repeated interactions and the high probability of additional interactions in future cases foster cooperation and facilitate communication and negotiations (Champion 1989; Stover and Eckart 1974). Given this insider's role, Wice (1985) posited that public defenders may be better positioned than private attorneys to mitigate the punishment imposed on their clients by prosecutors.

Research has also explored how the characteristics of judges and courtroom and community characteristics influence decision-making. Some research has found that judge-specific factors, including race (Steffensmeier and Britt 2001), sex (Steffensmeier and Hebert 1999), and political affiliation (Schanzenbach 2015), influence sentencing decisions. As expected, ample research finds that characteristics on both the courtroom level (e.g., caseloads, resources) and the community level (e.g., crime rate of the county, racial composition of the community) also influence decision-making (see Johnson 2006 for a review of this literature).

Similarities across several characteristics of workgroup members, including race, sex, years of experience, where they went to college and law school, and political affiliation, influence courtroom processes and case outcomes (Haynes and Ruback 2010; Metcalfe 2016). For example, Metcalfe (2016) used administrative data to examine how similarities in the characteristics of judges, prosecutors, and public defenders influence the plea process (mode of disposition and time to disposition). Metcalfe (2016) hypothesized that cases involving workgroup members who shared similar characteristics and common pasts (Ulmer 1995) would be disposed of most efficiently owing to the elevated levels of cooperation previous research has found between similar people. The authors reported that cases in which all three primary workgroup members were of the same sex were resolved more efficiently. Specifically, cases involving all same-sex workgroup members were more likely to be disposed of via pleas of guilt and no contest (the defendant accepts penalty but does not accept or deny responsibility for the charges), as opposed to disposition via trial (Metcalfe 2016). Given that the need for trials is circumvented following pleas of guilt and no contest, both modes of disposition are viewed as most efficient. The study also found that cases involving prosecutors and public defenders of the same sex were resolved faster (fewer days to disposition).

Reducing Entanglement: What Else We Can Learn and Do

This section lays out a set of four propositions for the future of research and practice efforts aimed at preventing entanglement, streamlining decision-making, and limiting the use of coercion in misdemeanor cases involving individuals with SMI. The propositions are interconnected: 1) examine how different workgroups function in the handling of cases involving individuals with SMI; 2) center the voices of those with SMI in assessing decision-making; 3) study the effects of the progressive prosecution movement on decision-making processes and outcomes; and 4) implement place-based strategies for reducing entanglement.

Courtroom Workgroup Functioning in the Handling of Cases Involving People With Serious Mental Illness

Given that the entanglement of people with SMI cannot be solely attributed to one courtroom decision-maker, future research should consider how workgroups, rather than individual court actors, assess cases involving people with SMI. It is still essential to consider how individual actors assess and decide on such cases, particularly within the context of their respective organizations and that of the overarching court, but it is imperative to explore how courtroom workgroup characteristics and contexts may be influencing case processing and ultimately case outcomes. Through this research, a more nuanced understanding of how workgroups view people with SMI may be gathered; including, for example, how workgroups assess the dangerousness and blame-worthiness of individuals with SMI and, ultimately, how such assessments guide punishment decisions.

Workgroup functioning is important to understand across all stages of the criminal legal process. Although police officers make individual decisions, they are also part of workgroups (different from courtroom workgroups) (Kane 2023). As Kane (2023, p. 53) wrote, "the behaviors of their workgroup—who they stop, who they search, who they arrest, who they send on their way—are influenced by the types and characteristics of the people and events in their workgroup experiences in their local areas." In line with the inhabited institutions perspective, researchers should turn to more mixed-method approaches and rely more heavily on ethnographic and observational data to capture information and processes on the streets and in other decision-making settings such as courtrooms to illuminate aspects of decision-making that are not often captured in administrative datasets. These approaches should include research on the ways in which police officers interact with courtroom workgroups and potentially shape their collective decision-making. Ultimately, this more textured research on workgroup functioning may provide a more complete understanding of the role of SMI along the criminal legal continuum and how best to prevent entanglement.

Center the Voices of People With Serious Mental Illness in Assessing Decision-Making

It is crucial to elevate the voices of those who are often left out of decision-making: people with lived experience of SMI. Naturally, the experiences and perceptions of people who make decisions will be different from the experiences of those directly affected by those decisions. Ironically, the voices of people with SMI are traditionally left out of decision-making studies that directly affect them, but there is a positive shift toward research and policy efforts that move these voices from the periphery to the center. For instance, Pope et al. (2023) asked people with prior misdemeanor arrests and SMI about their experiences of arrest, their interactions with professionals within the criminal legal system, their needs during crisis situations, and their preferences for different types of first responders. Other researchers should build on this line of inquiry, because asking people who are directly affected by decisions can help policymakers understand their needs and determine ways to better address them. There may be ways in which specific decisions, or a series of decisions, result in unintended harms, such as stigma or loss of dignity, that decision-makers do not fully understand. Some important work has attempted to unlock this perspective (Watson and Angell 2013), partly because research has shown that the ways in which legal authorities treat people can affect cooperation and resistance toward them (Watson and Angell 2007). As scholars have noted in their studies of procedural justice (referring to the quality of interactions people have with authorities), the decision-making process can be just as important to people as the decisions themselves, because it affects people's perceptions of the legitimacy of the system (Tyler 1990). Much less is known about the actual experiences of individuals with SMI and whether and how they perceive the system as operating for or against their interests.

Study the Effects of Progressive Prosecution on Decision-Making

Many jurisdictions across the country are adopting the *progressive model of prosecution* that seeks, among other goals, to reduce mass criminalization, tackle the root causes of crime (such as inequalities in education, income, employment, and housing), address racial disparities, and increase diversionary opportunities (Meldrum et al. 2021). Although some research has examined the relationship between progressive prosecution and the processing and outcomes related to violent crime cases (Fogleson et al. 2022), future research should analyze the relationship between progressive prosecution and the processing and outcomes of cases involving people with SMI, including misdemeanor cases. Despite the low-level and nonserious offenses typically alleged or committed by people with SMI, such individuals are routinely entangled in a traditional punishment-first misdemeanor system that is ill equipped to adequately address their needs. Given the several important decision-making points of prosecutors that influence the trajectory of cases and the new models' prioritization of, for example, addressing the root causes of crime, the new model should improve how the needs of people with SMI are addressed and reduce entanglement. In jurisdictions where the model has been adopted, researchers should consider how the decisions of police officers, judges, defense attorneys, and courtroom workgroups are affected. For example, the decisions of police officers, particularly their decisions to arrest individuals for low-level offenses, may be conditioned by shifts in prosecutorial charging practices. Therefore, it is important to consider the role of the progressive prosecution movement in shaping how people with SMI are perceived by the entire system and how such perceptions may then shape responses.

Implement Place-Based Problem-Solving Strategies

We previously noted in the section "Police Decision-Making" that the police have the authority to invoke the criminal process by determining whether to make a misdemeanor arrest to manage a person's behavior. We noted that the location or geography of the behavior is one of the contexts shaping decision-making partly because the legal tools available to police vary by jurisdiction. Location is also a relevant feature of decision-making because stakeholders in each place exert demands on the police to resolve a behavior. Such stakeholders may mobilize the police in the hope that officers will invoke the criminal process as a problem-solving method. This conventional approach—known in the policing literature as the standard or traditional approach to policing—hinges on a reactive response to social problems.

An alternative approach to the traditional police response is to develop "problem-oriented policing" interventions to address situations such as Mr. Thompson's. The pioneer of problem-oriented policing, Herman Goldstein (1979), argued that the role of the police is best construed as problem-solver rather than law-enforcer, and that the police should harness their own local knowledge of the problems they encounter to identify root causes of issues. Furthermore, the police should work with other entities and stakeholders to identify, analyze, and respond to problems creatively rather than simply enforce the law without a high likelihood that the problem will not occur again in the future. Over time, problem-solving frameworks have been developed to guide multisector involvement in the problem-solving process. A common framework is the Scanning, Analysis, Response, Assessment (SARA) model (Center for Problem-Oriented Policing 2023), in which stakeholders identify an issue, gather data to better understand the nature and drivers of the problem, and develop a solution that does not simply rely on police authority and legal levers. For instance, Cordner (2006) recommended that as part of the analysis process, police departments and dispatchers could record data on calls to police involving mental health–related situations to help understand patterns or trends. In cases such as Mr. Thompson's, it could be that across jurisdictions, situations of this sort often result in calls for service to police. Understanding this larger trend could help stakeholders brainstorm solutions, such as providing better outreach support and homeless services to people such as Mr. Thompson or sending clinicians or peer support workers to calls for service instead of the police, especially at places—such as business establishments like the donut shop in this example—where there are high concentrations of calls or complaints. Examples of alternative first response models are discussed in Chapter 2, "Using System Maps to Understand Entanglement and Guide Change"; Chapter 9, "The Current Era of Multifaceted Criminal Legal System Reform"; and Chapter 10, "Reform in an Era of Mental Health and Crisis Services Intervention."

KEY POINTS

- Decision-making involves many criminal legal system professionals who individually and collectively interpret and apply the law in response to various contextual factors.
- The police function as early, first-contact decision-makers who have the discretion to "invoke the criminal process" in managing a behavior; however, their discretionary power is limited when dealing with more serious behavior and when pressured by the public.
- Prosecutors also have discretion with charging decisions, resulting in variability in how cases involving people with serious mental illness (SMI) are handled.
- Decision-making is not influenced by a single factor in isolation but rather must be understood holistically as shaped by different contexts and considerations at different levels of the case, workgroup, organization, misdemeanor system, and the wider environment (i.e., laws and policies, community-based resources).
- Future efforts to improve decision-making in ways that reduce entanglement could be based on the following four propositions: 1) examine how different workgroups function in the handling of cases involving people with SMI; 2) center the voices of people with SMI in assessing decision-making; 3) study the effects of the progressive prosecution movement on decision-making processes and outcomes; and 4) implement place-based strategies for reducing entanglement.

References

Baumer EP: Reassessing and redirecting research on race and sentencing. Justice Q 30(2):231–261, 2013

Bibas S: Judicial fact-finding and sentence enhancements in a world of guilty pleas. Yale Law J 110(7):1097–1185, 2001

Bishop DM, Leiber M, Johnson J: Contexts of decision making in the juvenile justice system: an organizational approach to understanding minority overrepresentation. Youth Violence Juv Justice 8(3):213–233, 2010

Bittner E: The police on skid row: a study of peace keeping. Am Sociol Rev 32(5):699–715, 1967

Blumberg AS: The practice of law as confidence game: organizational cooptation of a profession. Law Soc Rev 1(2):15–39, 1967

Bonner HS: Police officer decision-making in dispute encounters: digging deeper into the "black box." Am J Crim Justice 40(3):493–522, 2015

Campbell BA: Predictors of Police Decision Making in Sexual Assault Investigations. Doctoral dissertation, Sam Houston State University, 2015. Available at: https://www.proquest.com/docview/1696945275/abstract/220978ECB7DB4964PQ/1. Accessed May 20, 2024.

Center for Problem-Oriented Policing: The SARA Model. Phoenix, AZ, Arizona State University, 2023. Available at: https://popcenter.asu.edu/content/sara-model-0. Accessed May 20, 2024.

Champion DJ: Private counsels and public defenders: a look at weak cases, prior records, and leniency in plea bargaining. J Crim Justice 17(4):253–263, 1989

Cordner G: People With Mental Illness. Washington, DC, U.S. Department of Justice, Office of Community Oriented Policing Services, 2006. Available at: https://www.ojp.gov/ncjrs/virtual-library/abstracts/people-mental-illness. Accessed November 5, 2023.

Cotton D, Coleman TG: Canadian police agencies and their interactions with persons with a mental illness: a systems approach. Police Pract Res 11(4):301–314, 2010

Crum JD, Ramey DM: Impact of extralegal and community factors on police officers' decision to book arrests for minor offenses. Am J Crim Justice 48(3):572–601, 2023

del Pozo B: The Police and the State: Security, Social Cooperation, and the Public Good. Cambridge, UK, Cambridge University Press, 2022

del Pozo B, Sightes E, Goulka J, et al: Police discretion in encounters with people who use drugs: operationalizing the Theory of Planned Behavior. Harm Reduct J 18(1):132, 2021 34915910

Devers L: Plea and Charge Bargaining: Research Summary. Washington, DC, U.S. Department of Justice, Bureau of Justice Assistance, 2021. Available at: https://bja.ojp.gov/sites/g/files/xyckuh186/files/media/document/PleaBargainingResearchSummary.pdf. Accessed November 5, 2023.

Edkins VA, Redlich AD: A System of Pleas: Social Sciences Contributions to the Real Legal System. New York, Oxford University Press, 2019

Eisenstein J, Jacob H: Felony Justice: An Organizational Analysis of Criminal Courts. Boston, Little Brown, 1977

Engel R, Silver E: Policing mentally disordered suspects: a re-examination of the criminalization hypothesis. Criminology 39:225–252, 2001

Ericson R: Rules for police deviance, in Organizational Police Deviance, 83–110. Toronto, ON, Butterworths, 1981

Fogleson T, Levi R, Rosenfeld R, et al: Violent Crime and Public Prosecution: A Review of Recent Data on Homicide, Robbery, and Progressive Prosecution in the United States. Toronto, ON, Global Justice Lab, Munk School of Global Affairs and Public Policy, University of Toronto, 2022. Available at: https://munkschool.utoronto.ca/research/violent-crime-and-public-prosecution. Accessed May 20, 2024.

Franklin CA, Bouffard LA, Garza AD, et al: Focal concerns and intimate partner violence case processing: predicting arrest using a stratified random sample of police case file data. Crime Delinq 68(8):1402–1426, 2022

Frederick B, Stemen D: The Anatomy of Discretion: An Analysis of Prosecutorial Decision. New York, Vera Institute of Justice, 2012. Available at: https://www.ojp.gov/library/publications/anatomy-discretion-analysis-prosecutorial-decision-making-summary-report. Accessed May 20, 2024.

Free MD: Race and presentencing decisions in the United States: a summary and critique of the research. Crim Justice Rev 27(2):203–232, 2002

Gant L, Schaible L: The impact of policing styles on officers' willingness to make referrals into pre-arrest diversion initiatives. Police Pract Res 23(1):20–33, 2022

Goldstein H: Improving policing: a problem-oriented approach. Crime Delinq 25(April):236–258, 1979

Goldstein J: Police discretion not to invoke the criminal process: low-visibility decisions in the administration of justice. Yale Law J 69(4):543–594, 1960

Grace S, Lloyd C, Page G: "What discretion do you need?": factors influencing police decision-making in possession of cannabis offences. Criminol Crim Justice 0(0), 2022

Haynes SH, Ruback B: Courtroom workgroups and sentencing: the effects of similarity, proximity, and stability. Crime Delinq 56(1):126–161, 2010

Ishoy GA: Applying Focal Concerns and the Theory of Planned Behavior to the Decision-Making Process in Policing. Doctoral dissertation, Georgia State University, 2015. Available at: https://www.proquest.com/docview/1759059212/abstract/8716A7977B344E57PQ/1. Accessed May 20, 2024.

Ishoy GA, Dabney DA: Policing and the focal concerns framework: exploring how its core components apply to the discretionary enforcement decisions of police officers. Deviant Behav 39(7):878–895, 2018

Jackson H: The federal prosecutor. Journal of the American Institute of Criminal Law and Criminology 31(1):3–6, 1940

Johnson BD: The multilevel context of criminal sentencing: integrating judge- and county-level influences. Criminology 44(2):259–298, 2006

Kane R: Policing Beyond Coercion: A New Idea for a Twenty-First Century Mandate. Frederick, MD, Aspen, 2023

Kelling GL: Acquiring a taste for order: the community and police. Crime Delinq 33(1):90–102, 1987

Kempa M, Carrier R, Wood J, et al: Reflections on the evolving concept of "private" policing. European Journal on Criminal Policy and Research 7(2):197–223, 1999

Kohler-Hausmann I: Misdemeanorland: Criminal Courts and Social Control in an Age of Broken Windows Policing. Princeton, NJ, Princeton University Press, 2018

Kutateladze BL, Andiloro NR, Johnson BD, et al: Cumulative disadvantage: examining racial and ethnic disparity in prosecution and sentencing. Criminology 52(3):514–551, 2014

Lamb HR, Weinberger LE, DeCuir WJ Jr: The police and mental health. Psychiatr Serv 53(10):1266–1271, 2002 12364674

Lapsey DS Jr, Campbell BA, Plumlee BT: Focal concerns and police decision making in sexual assault cases: a systematic review and meta-analysis. Trauma Violence Abuse 23(4):1220–1234, 2022

Lipsky M: Street-Level Bureaucracy: Dilemmas of the Individual in Public Services. New York, Russell Sage Foundation, 2010

Lynch M: Focally concerned about focal concerns: a conceptual and methodological critique of sentencing disparities research. Justice Q 36(7):1148–1175, 2019

Meldrum RC, Stemen D, Kutateladze BL: Progressive and traditional orientations to prosecution: an empirical assessment in four prosecutorial offices. Crim Justice Behav 48(3):354–372, 2021

Metcalfe C: The role of courtroom workgroups in felony case dispositions: an analysis of workgroup familiarity and similarity. Law Soc Rev 50(3):637–672, 2016

Neusteter R, Subramanian R, Trone J, et al: Gatekeepers: The Role of Police in Ending Mass Incarceration. Washington, DC, Vera Institute of Justice, 2019. Available at: https://www.vera.org/downloads/publications/gatekeepers-police-and-mass-incarceration.pdf. Accessed May 20, 2024.

Novak KJ, Engel RS: Disentangling the influence of suspects' demeanor and mental disorder on arrest. Policing 28(3):493–512, 2005

O'Neal EN, Spohn C: When the perpetrator is a partner: arrest and charging decisions in intimate partner sexual assault cases—a focal concerns analysis. Violence Against Women 23(6):707–729, 2017

Peterson JR: "We handle it, I guess you'd say, the East Texas way": place-based effects on the police decision-making process and non-arrest outcomes. Police Pract Res 24(1):53–71, 2023

Pope LG, Patel A, Fu E, et al: Crisis response model preferences of mental health care clients with prior misdemeanor arrests and of their family and friends. Psychiatr Serv 74(11):1163–1170, 2023 37070262

Schanzenbach MM: Racial disparities, judge characteristics, and standards of review in sentencing. Journal of Institutional and Theoretical Economics 171(1):27–47, 2015

Schulenberg JL: Moving beyond arrest and reconceptualizing police discretion: an investigation into the factors affecting conversation, assistance, and criminal charges. Police Q 18(3):244–271, 2015

Schulenberg JL: Police decision-making in the gray zone: the dynamics of police–citizen encounters with mentally ill persons. Crim Justice Behav 43(4):459–482, 2016

Scrivener L, Meizlish A, Bond E, Chauhan P: Tracking Enforcement Trends in New York City: 2003–2008. New York, John Jay College of Criminal Justice, 2020

Slothower MP: When "Tough" Cops Divert and "Soft" Cops Charge: Trait Attitudes vs. State Situational Narratives in a Focal Concerns Process of Police Decision-Making. Doctoral dissertation, University of Maryland, College Park, 2019. Available at: https://www.proquest.com/docview/2376256618/abstract/38FCF69BEE1241FCPQ/1. Accessed May 20, 2024.

Steffensmeier D, Britt C: Judges' race and judicial decision making: do Black judges sentence differently? Soc Sci Q 82(4):749–764, 2001

Steffensmeier D, Hebert C: Women and men policymakers: does the judge's gender affect the sentencing of criminal defendants? Soc Forces 77(3):1163–1196, 1999

Stover RV, Eckart DR: A systematic comparison of public defenders and private attorneys. Am J Crim Law 3(3):265–300, 1974

Teplin LA, Pruett NS: Police as streetcorner psychiatrist: managing the mentally ill. Int J Law Psychiatry 15(2):139–156, 1992 1587650

Thacher D: Research for the front lines. Policing and Society 18(1):46–59, 2008

Tyler TR: Why People Obey the Law. New Haven, CT, Yale University Press, 1990

Ulmer JT: The organization and consequences of social pasts in criminal courts. Sociol Q 36(3):587–605, 1995

Ulmer JT: Prosecutorial discretion. Justice Q 35(7):1131–1132, 2018

Ulmer JT: Criminal courts as inhabited institutions: making sense of difference and similarity in sentencing. Crime Justice 48(1):483–522, 2019

Watson AC, Angell B: Applying procedural justice theory to law enforcement's response to persons with mental illness. Psychiatr Serv 58(6):787–793, 2007 17535938

Watson AC, Angell B: The role of stigma and uncertainty in moderating the effect of procedural justice on cooperation and resistance in police encounters with persons with mental illnesses. Psychol Public Policy Law 19(1):30–39, 2013 24920876

Wice PB: Chaos in the Courthouse: The Inner Workings of the Urban Criminal Courts. New York, Praeger, 1985

Wood JD, Watson AC, Fulambarker AJ: The "gray zone" of police work during mental health encounters: findings from an observational study in Chicago. Police Q 20(1):81–105, 2017 28286406

Wood JD, Watson AC, Pope L, et al: Contexts shaping misdemeanor system interventions among people with mental illnesses: qualitative findings from a multi-site system mapping exercise. Health Justice 11(1):20, 2023 37014478

Wright MS, Baughman SB, Robertson C: Inside the black box of prosecutor discretion. UC Davis Law Review 55(4):2133–2208, 2021

	4

Common Themes and Tensions

Misdemeanor System Perspectives on Managing Behaviors of People With Serious Mental Illness

Leah G. Pope, Ph.D.
Luis C. Torres, Ph.D.

This chapter sheds light on the plurality of values that guide action among criminal legal professionals when they encounter the case of a person with a serious mental illness (SMI) arrested for a misdemeanor offense. Building on Chapter 3 ("Decision-Making Contexts of Misdemeanor Charges"), which explores the many contexts shaping decision-making in the misdemeanor criminal legal system, here we engage questions about how system actors can at once seem both aligned and at odds about how to manage the frequent entanglement of people with

SMI in the misdemeanor system. We begin the chapter by providing a theoretical framework for understanding the interorganizational relationships across the criminal legal system and elucidating how unique orientations among the system's constituent agencies create points of alignment and divergence in case processing. We then provide a case example that illustrates a prototypical misdemeanor case and the various decision-makers who handle the case and engage with a defendant as they pass through the assembly line of case processing. The example provides an opportunity to unpack the concerns and values of police, prosecutors, and public defenders in four cities (Atlanta, Chicago, New York City [Manhattan], and Philadelphia) and, in turn, to consider possibilities for value alignment in strategies to reduce system involvement among people with SMI.

Case Processing in a "Loosely Coupled" System

Building on Chapter 3, which sets out the decision-making contexts that animate decisions across the criminal legal system, this chapter delves further into the values or—drawing from Thacher—the "value pluralism" (Thacher 2001) that shapes those decision-making contexts. Two strands of literature inform this discussion: 1) the concept of "loose coupling" and 2) the focal-concerns framework. Many scholars have called attention to the degree to which the criminal legal system and its various subsystems is a "loosely coupled system" (Bernard et al. 2005; Hagan 1989; Hagan et al. 1979; Reiss 1971). Loosely coupled systems comprise multiple, autonomous bureaucracies with low levels of interdependency. Loose coupling is "meant to evoke the image of entities (e.g., court subsystems) that are responsive to one another, while still maintaining independent identities and some evidence of physical or logical separateness" (Hagan 1989, p. 119). Thinking about police, prosecutors, and defenders as distinct entities operating within a given location's criminal legal *system* helps set the stage for understanding how the processing of cases across the various points of the system can appear random or chaotic. On the one hand, different entities across the system may share similar goals. As Bernard et al. (2005, p. 206) argued, "for each case, the goal of criminal justice processing is to change offenders into non-offenders while simultaneously satisfying both the victims and the public." As we explore later in this chapter (see the section "The Shared Goal of 'Getting People Out'"), in processing misdemeanor cases involving people with SMI, the commitment to getting this population out of the criminal legal system is shared. On the other hand, "there may be multiple, overlapping, and contradictory ideas about how to achieve the 'completed product' of non-offenders" (Bernard et al. 2005, p. 206). Thus, even if different decision-makers want to reduce the disproportionate contact that people with SMI have with the criminal legal system, they may be influenced by different rules or mandates—or interpret the same institutional rules differently—and may also have other goals that influence their decision-making. The result is that these agencies often seem uncoordinated and incompatible.

The *focal-concerns framework* is also helpful in elucidating the values and normative orientations that different decision-makers hold across stages of the criminal legal system. Originally developed by Steffensmeier et al. (1998) to explain judicial sentencing decisions, the focal-concerns perspective has become a dominant framework to explain race-, gender-, and age-related disparities in the criminal legal system—with scholars extending the framework to apply to police (Ishoy and Dabney 2018), prosecutors (Spohn et al. 2001), and the juvenile justice system (Bishop et al. 2010; Ericson and Eckberg 2016). The focal-concerns perspective posits that when making discretionary punishment decisions, decision-makers consider three focal concerns: 1) the offender's blameworthiness or culpability (e.g., related to the degree of harm caused to the victim, the severity and seriousness of the charges, the offender's criminal history); 2) protection of the community (related to the prevention of future offending); and 3) practical constraints and consequences (related to organizational concerns such as case flow or jail overcrowding as well as individual concerns, such as the potential negative consequences for the offender [e.g., their health or family ties]). More recently, Ulmer et al. (2022, p. 816) proposed a fourth focal concern: 4) *rehabilitation potential* or *redeemability*—"a concern not just with preventing future crime, but with helping defendants improve their lives as an end in itself." They argued that although some have suggested that rehabilitation potential fits within the focal concerns of community protection or practical considerations, recent changes toward a more reform-oriented stance in the criminal legal system suggest that judges increasingly focus on rehabilitation, and that it should be considered a distinct sentencing concern.

Furthermore, the focal-concerns framework posits that judges operate within an environment constrained by numerous organizational factors (e.g., large caseloads, limited resources) and, therefore, have little time and available information to make fully informed decisions. Because of these limitations and the heightened uncertainty associated with determinations of dangerousness and future offending, judges develop and use "perceptual shorthands" to guide their decision-making (Albonetti 1991; Hawkins 1981). *Perceptual shorthands* refers to an attribution process whereby decision-makers consider and rely on, for example, the visible demographic characteristics (e.g., race) of defendants and the associated stereotypes to streamline blameworthiness and dangerousness determinations. Some stereotypes related to race include perceptions that people from minority groups (Black and Latinx) are more aggressive, dangerous, lazy, and overall, more criminogenic than White people (Bridges and Steen 1998; Johnson and Dipietro 2012; Tittle and Curran 1988). Given these negative stereotypes, decision-makers may unconsciously treat minority group members more punitively than similarly situated White people. Research demonstrates that perceptual shorthands are linked not only to race but also to gender and age (Bishop et al. 2010; Galvin and Ulmer 2022; Steffensmeier and Demuth 2000; Steffensmeier et al. 1998).

Given the focal-concerns framework and its emphasis on stereotypes, it is important to consider how SMIs and related stereotypes and stigmas may be influencing the decisions of system actors. Although potentially not as visible as the characteristics (e.g., race, gender) previously discussed, people with SMI may similarly signal to decision-makers their illness through, for example, the display of symptoms and appearance. Alternatively, their case may be flagged for mental health concerns early in processing because of documentation from arresting police officers or previous cases. Similar to the way race and gender stereotypes influence criminal legal decisions, the negative stereotypes associated with people with SMI—including heightened dangerousness and criminality—may be influencing the decisions of system actors, resulting in discriminatory behavior (Corrigan 2000; Parcesepe and Cabassa 2013; Penn and Martin 1998).

Although no literature has explicitly examined the role of mental illness in shaping the focal concerns of various criminal legal stakeholders, there is some evidence of sentencing disparities related to mental illness. For example, a study by White (2016) demonstrated that compared to youth without mental health problems, youth with mental health problems are more likely to be sentenced to correctional confinement. Also consistent with the idea that stereotypes associated with mental illnesses may be influencing punishment decisions, another study found that adults with SMI arrested on misdemeanor charges are more likely to receive a jail sentence, even after controlling for other relevant case characteristics (Hall et al. 2019). Conversely, Kaiser and Spohn (2018) presented evidence from federal sentencing data that judges pay attention to a defendant's mental health when determining an appropriate sentence and that mental health is more likely to be cited as a reason for a downward departure from sentencing guidelines (i.e., below the guideline range for a sentence).

Following the thinking of Bishop et al. (2010), this chapter integrates the loose coupling perspective and the focal-concerns framework as a stage for examining the plurality of values guiding interventions among people with SMI in the criminal legal system. Such integration allows for attention to both the interorganizational dynamics and the decision-making that occurs across stages of the criminal legal system, as well as to the goals and values that inform that decision-making. We present a case example that draws on myriad examples that surfaced in our focus groups with system stakeholders in Atlanta, Chicago, Manhattan, and Philadelphia. We then examine the example from the perspectives of police, prosecutors, and public defenders, highlighting three central questions: 1) Who are the decision-makers at each processing stage? 2) What orientations do they bring to the table? 3) What is the role of the criminal legal system in connecting people to mental health treatment?

Case Example: Mr. Carter at the Bodega

Mr. Carter is a 43-year-old Black man with an SMI who was arrested at a local bodega in Manhattan for petit larceny (i.e., shoplifting) when the store owner caught him leaving with Skittles, crackers, batteries, and a thermometer under his sweatshirt. The store owner called the police, and when two officers arrived on the scene, Mr. Carter appeared disheveled and disorganized. The police offered to remove Mr. Carter from the store and take him to the hospital for evaluation and potential treatment, citing Mr. Carter's appearance and the somewhat bizarre combination of items he tried to steal. However, the owner was adamant that the officers arrest Mr. Carter, telling them, "I pay taxes. I want this person arrested. I want to press charges." Mr. Carter was known to both the store owner and the police. He usually spent his nights at a shelter a few blocks away. He spent his days moving around a several-block area near the store, and he had four previous arrests—two for criminal trespassing and two for petit larceny. The store owner explained that although he had been able to mediate situations with Mr. Carter in the past—often without making an arrest—he had lost patience and wanted to move forward with pressing charges. The officers arrested Mr. Carter. Although his charge was eligible for a desk appearance ticket (i.e., a written order requiring him to appear for arraignment in criminal court at a future date), the police officers made a custodial arrest because they knew Mr. Carter had a prior history of failing to appear in court and because they considered that appearing before the court could help address Mr. Carter's mental health needs.

When Mr. Carter appeared at arraignment, he met briefly with his court-appointed public defender and pleaded not guilty. His case was

adjourned for a future court date. At his next court date, the assistant
district attorney (ADA) offered Mr. Carter an Adjournment in Contemplation of Dismissal (ACD) with conditions. (An ACD is a process by
which the court defers the disposition of a defendant with a view to ultimately dismiss the charge after 6 months if the defendant stays out of
trouble.) In Mr. Carter's case, the ACD was offered with the condition
that he would also attend three sessions with Manhattan Justice Opportunities—an alternatives-to-incarceration program that offers individualized assessments and service plans including counseling, case
management, and connection to mental health services. This route offered Mr. Carter a way to receive a noncriminal disposition under the
condition that he successfully completed programming and stayed out
of trouble for 6 months. The public defender asked for time served instead. Beyond valuing the efficiency of a guilty plea with time served,
the public defender reasoned that it was more advantageous for Mr.
Carter to plead guilty and have the case disposed of immediately with
time served (which accounted for the time he spent in jail waiting for his
court dates) rather than making him attend programming. Mr. Carter
had stated that he did not want to keep coming back to court, and his
defender was worried that he would have trouble attending the three
required program sessions, which could extend his criminal legal involvement and result in more serious consequences.

The ADA reminded the judge that Mr. Carter had four previous arrests and a history of mental illness; therefore, he argued, Mr. Carter
could benefit from the programming offered by Manhattan Justice Opportunities. The judge looked at the ADA incredulously, and asked,
"Why are you making this person do Manhattan Justice Opportunities
on a simple petit larceny case?" Rather than accept the ACD offer, Mr.
Carter pleaded guilty, and the judge sentenced him to time served. Mr.
Carter left court with a new criminal conviction on his record but no
mandated programming or service connections.

The Shared Goal of "Getting People Out"

Mr. Carter's case provides an entry point for considering the complex
mix of values and orientations that come into play during the processing of misdemeanor charges. Before further exploring how and why
these values conflict, understanding points of underlying alignment in
the actions of police, prosecutors, defenders, and judges in this prototypical petit larceny case is worthwhile. Well-established initiatives
across the United States address the overrepresentation of people with
SMI in the criminal legal system (Bonfine et al. 2020). (See Chapter 9,
"The Current Era of Multifaceted Criminal Legal System Reform" for
an overview of interventions developed to divert individuals with SMI
out of the criminal legal system.) The cities in our study are no exception. In Atlanta, Chicago, Manhattan, and Philadelphia, there are multiple "off-ramps" to divert people with SMI—particularly those who

are charged with low-level misdemeanors—out of the criminal legal system. Chapter 2 ("Using System Maps to Understand Entanglement and Guide Change") provides examples with visual depictions of off-ramps, ranging from nonpolice triaging of mental health situations in the community to post-arraignment diversion. As the case example shows, the actions of each criminal legal actor at play here can be understood as an attempt to get Mr. Carter out of the system. Police offered to take Mr. Carter to the hospital, prosecutors offered the possibility of dismissing the charges if he completed treatment, and the public defender argued for disposing the case with time served. The judge concurred with the latter. Thus, insofar as criminal legal system agencies are united around a common goal of turning offenders into nonoffenders (Bernard et al. 2005), they are likewise aligned in trying to disrupt the disproportionate contact that people with mental illnesses have with the system. And yet, as we see in the example and explore further (see the section "Alternate Approaches to 'Getting People Out'"), agreement is minimal on how to achieve these common goals. As Bernard et al. (2005, p. 206) wrote,

> Even when considering the most obvious group of people that the system processes—offenders—there may be multiple, overlapping, and contradictory ideas about how to achieve the "completed product" of nonoffenders. Thus, even if this is the common goal of system processing, it appears that different parts of the system frequently do not work together to achieve it.

In the following section, we explore these contradictory ideas and the agency values from which they stem by looking at the perspectives of different system actors in turn: police, prosecutors, and public defenders.

Alternative Approaches to "Getting People Out"

The Police: Providers of Temporary Remedies

Police in all four cities in our study shared variations on the story of Mr. Carter as examples of how they serve, in the words of one Chicago police sergeant, as "front-line triage" in responding to people with SMI. This police function is well established in the literature (Bittner 1990; Thacher 2022; Wood et al. 2017), and limiting this function is a central part of the current agenda for progressive police reform (Okeowo 2020; Quattlebaum and Tyler 2020; Vitale 2017). As Thacher (2022, p. 63) has written, "Police are a residual institution, invested with the authority to manage the crises that other institutions cannot handle on their own.... Because police officers are systematically exposed to the limitations of other organizations' routines…they become experts in institutional breakdown." But if the police were such a residual institution in the case of Mr. Carter, their options for managing that crisis remained limited. Police in our four study sites articulated having four primary options in handling incidences such as Mr. Carter's: 1) resolving the incident at the scene; 2) issuing a ticket or citation at the scene; 3) transporting the person to the hospital; or 4) arresting the person and taking them to jail for further processing.

Police described that as the initial point of contact in a longer decision-making chain, they try to avoid making arrests for low-level misdemeanors and resolve situations at the scene. Often, this involves "moving people along" or issuing a warning or ticket to satisfy complainants. Police justify this in a variety of ways. First, because these misdemeanor offenses rarely involve harm to a person or property, police may be less concerned with assessing the blameworthiness of the offender or protecting the community than they are with devising short-term solutions to disturbances. As an officer in Chicago noted when reflecting on criminal trespassing, "[complainants] generally just want the person away from their property…so optimally if we remove them from the situation, the complainant is happy." This short-term prevention focus of policing makes sense: police officers are often concerned with the influence they can have over the course of their shift since they are not the final arbiters of how a case ultimately will be processed if they make an arrest (Ishoy and Dabney 2018). Although they may yearn for long-term solutions to calls such as the one involving Mr. Carter, they also know that such long-term solutions are largely beyond their control. Second, as the quoted officer's remark suggests, police at a scene must consider the concerns or issues presented by the offender as well as the concerns of the complainant. In many situations, removing offenders from the scene or issuing a warning or ticket may be enough to satisfy complainants. As seen in the story of Mr. Thompson in Chapter 3 ("Decision-Making Contexts of Misdemeanor Charges"), the police officers in our study spoke about the pressure they face to satisfy complainants and the public when minor crimes take place, especially when they happen repeatedly. Thus, even if an officer doesn't believe that a ticket will be particularly useful in changing behavior in the future, "it's useful," one Chicago sergeant reflected, "in the sense that we've taken action. We won't be accused of not having taken action."

When resolution at the scene is not possible, officers may be faced with deciding whether to make an arrest and take the person to jail or transport the person to the hospital. These options involve different sets of criteria even if officers consider them subjectively and use their discretion accordingly. The decision for an arrest is whether a crime was committed; the judgment for a hospital transport is whether the person meets statutorily defined criteria for a psychiatric assessment. Despite the differences, both options may be perceived as inefficient and ineffective. On the one hand, many officers in our study articulated that their best option in a case such as Mr. Carter's was to take the person to the hospital. "I don't want them to go to jail. I just want them to go to the hospital," remarked a Chicago sergeant. Another Chicago police officer commented that even when "store owners are adamant about locking somebody up for a bag of chips," officers will spend time with business owners "trying to convince [them] that this is not going to help this person." On the other hand, officers lamented the enormous barriers to getting people care within the hospital systems in these cities. The same Chicago police sergeant reflected, "It's a revolving door between police interacting with them because citizens are calling, going to an emergency room, not getting adequate treatment, and then [they] come right back to the street where they run into police again." This was echoed by a police supervisor in Atlanta who admitted that they take people to the hospital knowing that it is only a short-term fix. "We take 'em to [the local emergency department] and within an hour, she's right back out.... it's like a cycle that will never stop. No matter what you do." Bittner (1967, p. 281) similarly documented that taking someone to the hospital is "a tedious, cumbersome, and uncertain process." It is not surprising then that some officers described opting to pursue an arrest rather than a hospital transport. "It takes a lot less time to arrest the people and say, get it over with, than to actually take them through the mental health route," one Atlanta police officer told us. "It's a lot more difficult to actually try to get them help and get them resources. And it ties us up a lot longer than if we would just take them to jail." Even then, however, officers in Philadelphia noted that an arrest may fail to provide even a medium-term solution. "We can arrest them but from that point on...we don't know what happens to them because they're out pretty much as we're coming out." This was echoed by a Chicago officer: "You know, it's a misdemeanor, and they're always right back on the street."

Seen through the lens of focal concerns, police decision-making in responding to misdemeanor offenses involving people with SMI seems focused less on the blameworthiness or dangerousness of the offender and more on the practical constraints they face in a system with limited resources. In Mr. Carter's case, although we might expect some responding officers to take signs of Mr. Carter's mental illness as a shorthand for potential criminality, the information they had about Mr. Carter from previous encounters allowed them to enter the encounter and make an informed, pragmatic decision in response to the bodega owner. Other studies have likewise demonstrated the influence of practical constraints and extralegal factors on police decisions, including officers' needs, departments' priorities, and availability of cooperating witnesses (Ishoy and Dabney 2018; Lapsey et al. 2022). Although police officers may be inclined to consider a "strict liability perception of offender blameworthiness whereby evidence of wrongful behavior means it is fair game to affix blame and consequences to the responsible party" (Ishoy and Dabney 2018, p. 890), few police officers in our study thought arresting people with SMI for these low-level crimes would "stick" down the line. Rather, their focus was primarily on short-term solutions, centered on satisfying the public through their responsiveness, even if they were unsure what effect their actions would have in the medium to long term.

Returning to the case of Mr. Carter, and as noted in Chapter 3, we saw that the officers navigated through various layers of context as they exercised their discretion in the field. On the one hand, they were trying to avoid arrest given the low-level nature of the offense and the fact that they believed Mr. Carter met the criteria for hospital transport and psychiatric assessment. On the other hand, on top of the pressure from the store owner, the officers recognized that the linkage to the hospital may be ineffective or, at best, a temporary solution because Mr. Carter lacked stable housing or a social support network. Faced with these competing concerns, the officers arrested Mr. Carter and passed his case down the line to the next decision-makers: prosecutors.

The Prosecutors: Leveraging the System to Activate Treatment

Prosecutors, too, are influenced by several focal concerns when dealing with a case such as Mr. Carter's. It is notable that the prosecutors in our study came from large cities with relatively progressive prosecutors' offices. As the ADA demonstrated in his offer to give Mr. Carter an ACD rather than continue the case or ask for jail time, prosecutors in the four cities we studied were generally not inclined to pursue "punitive" approaches such as jail time on such low-level misdemeanors (even if some, including Mr. Carter's public defender, may consider an ACD and the potential consequences of violating its terms as more punitive than a guilty plea, conviction, and time served). This can be explained by at least two factors. First, taking the idea of blameworthiness from the focal-concerns literature and a prosecutor's desire to impose a sentence that is "just" in relation to the severity of the crime, there is little support for retribution when the seriousness of the offense is low (Steffensmeier et al. 1998). This was explained at length by a prosecutor in Atlanta:

> A retribution model looks to the past and says, well, based on the harm that this person caused in the past, we're going to visit some harm upon them. So it's backward-looking instead of forward-looking. We can't really get our judges to think about things that way. And why would they? I mean, if it's a minor crime, you really can't; it's hard to argue societal vengeance or retribution to get anybody to do anything. So you have to look forward.

Second, and in line with this idea that punishment should be forward-looking in low-level cases (i.e., focused on deterrence of future offenses), prosecutors recognized that a "traditional" punitive approach to misdemeanor offenses with jail time was likely ineffective in stopping cycles of criminal behavior. "Unfortunately, the traditional way of dealing with something like that—which is, you know, arrest, charge, conviction, sentence—doesn't do anything to help the situation of the seriously mentally ill person," remarked an ADA in Philadelphia. "It's not going to improve life for anybody."

Given the lack of support for retributive justice and a focus on deterring people from committing future crimes, it is not surprising that prosecutors described making use of diversion options in their cities when processing misdemeanor cases involving people with SMI. As illustrated in Chapter 2, communities across the United States are adopting diversion programs, or off-ramps, for people with and without mental illnesses as alternative approaches to addressing community safety and keeping people out of further entrenchment in the criminal legal system (Johnson and Ali-Smith 2022). Diversion programs occur at different stages of the criminal legal system. For example, they may be pretrial and involve the deferment of traditional case processing pending successful completion of a program. Alternatively, they may be located at the court phase—generally through "problem-solving courts" or "accountability courts" (see Chapter 9 for examples of interventions such as law enforcement–assisted diversion and mental health courts). If programs operate at the court phase, they may employ a pre-plea model (in which charges are dropped on successful program completion) or post-plea model (in which participation requires an admission of guilt and often a conviction). Regardless of the specific model, such diversion programs involve managed supervision and reporting as well as defined criteria for determining program success or failure (Center for Health and Justice at TASC 2013). Figure 4–1 shows a simplified schematic of case processing after the point of arrest in Manhattan. Opportunities for diversion are shaded in gray.

Prosecutors in our study articulated how they rely on diversion opportunities as a means of connecting people with the treatment they need and catalyzing a recovery process that will hopefully prevent future recidivism. Some of this may reflect an attempt to shift responsibility back to the mental health system. As a Philadelphia ADA reflected, "Our whole purpose is to treat the underlying mental illness," noting how important it is in the mental health court context for services in the city to be provided "that these defendants need and might not be in our system if these were readily available." This was echoed by a prosecutor in Manhattan who described diversion as a means to "make people get the health care they neglected to get before." Prosecutors were also generally optimistic about the possibilities for people who entered and completed diversion programs. "I've seen firsthand that we can bring people back from the edge," said one ADA in Manhattan, "and a lot of us … are advocating for these solutions whenever we see them so that we can bring people to a place of health and safety."

On the other hand, some prosecutors also saw diversion programs as—in the words of an Atlanta prosecutor—a "corrective measure" to "hold individuals accountable for their behavior." In this view, the value of the court system is that it can help to foster compliance with treatment as an alternative to more traditional forms of punishment such as jail that most people want to avoid. An ADA in Philadelphia described this approach:

> One of the benefits of the treatment court is we won't have to actually prosecute them in trial and have them found guilty. We can keep them in the court system, and that's I think one of the big benefits in cases like that, in situations like that. It's not just they, you know, dismissed the charges or let's go to trial. We're kind of that middle ground and say, listen, I want to keep this here for a while, have them engage in treatment, come back to you and you know, at the end of the day, we all get what we want where hopefully this person will be in a better place and will continue to take their medication and at the same time not have a criminal record as a result.

The idea that this "middle ground" of mandated treatment is necessary to ensure connection with needed services was further supported by a prosecutor in Atlanta who reflected that people with SMI entangled in the criminal legal system generally cannot correct their behavior

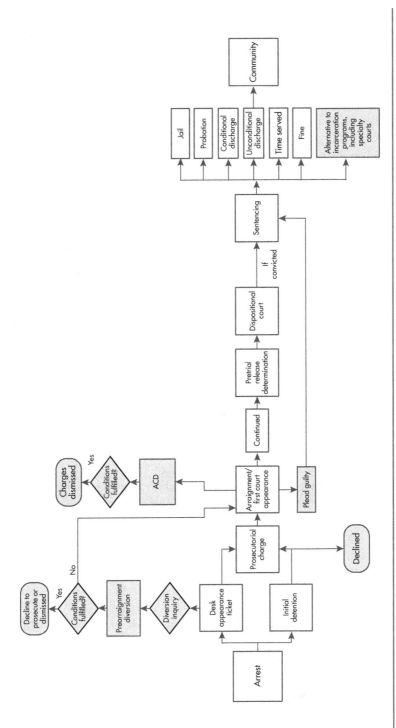

Figure 4–1. An example of post-arrest case processing and diversion opportunities for misdemeanor charges.

Note. ACD=adjournment in contemplation of dismissal.

without enforced compliance. As he said, "In my experience, those ones who've suffered from mental health don't generally self-correct, you know? There's not something that happens, and then all of a sudden they have an epiphany and then they self-correct."

Prosecutors admitted that there are challenges to using diversion and programming as a primary approach in cases such as Mr. Carter's. First, as discussed in Chapter 3 and in line with the pressures we described previously for police, prosecutors are faced with balancing the concerns of multiple stakeholders, including victims and complainants who may want a harsher response to misdemeanor offenses, particularly those committed by repeat offenders. Even if prosecutors believe that getting a defendant into a mental health program is going to get the person the services they need to stop offending, they may have a hard time convincing a victim of this approach. One assistant state's attorney in Chicago noted that "victims oftentimes just focus on jail time or conviction or whatever it might be.... So it's hard to have those conversations with people who want the outcome of a case to be a certain way that isn't necessarily the most productive from a public safety standpoint." In Mr. Carter's case, the fact that the store owner was so adamant about an arrest suggests that it is likely he thought there would be some sort of consequence for Mr. Carter's repeated offenses that would deter future behavior—not just a guilty plea with time served and the ability to walk out the courtroom door.

Second, there may be individuals who do not want to engage in treatment, who refuse to take an offer of diversion, or who repeatedly get arrested. Prosecutors in our study acknowledged that they have less leverage to offer diversion with mandated treatment when someone is not facing significant jail time. Indeed, they lacked such leverage in Mr. Carter's case—a point that we return to in the next section when reviewing the perspective of defense attorneys on these types of cases. Nonetheless, prosecutors in all cities described a preference for seeking diversion, when possible, because of their belief that it could connect someone with services, reduce recidivism, and decrease the inevitable backlog of cases. "I think it kind of benefits the system in the long run," noted a prosecutor in Manhattan. "Because then we have less cases to deal with because hopefully, they're not getting rearrested and it's less work for us too."

The perspectives offered by prosecutors in Atlanta, Chicago, Manhattan, and Philadelphia directly engage the focal-concerns framework. Prosecutors explicitly take up the focal concern of community protection when they frame treatment mandates as a mechanism for breaking cycles of recidivism. Although the offense severity is low in these cases—and thus attributions of blameworthiness likely muted—prosecutors must grapple with the best way to deter would-be offenders. In cases where a misdemeanor offense is committed by someone with an SMI, prosecutors in our study often framed untreated (or inadequately treated) mental illness as the direct cause of offending behavior and appropriate treatment as capable of reducing problematic behavior. The notion of rehabilitation or redeemability as a focal concern is also relevant here. Changes in court policies and practices point to an increased focus on rehabilitation, and recent research supports the idea that redeemability should be treated as a distinct focal concern (Galvin and Ulmer 2022; Kaiser and Spohn 2018; Ulmer et al. 2022). Thus, it is not surprising that prosecutors reflected a concern "with helping defendants improve their lives as an end in itself" (Ulmer et al. 2022, p. 816).

On the other hand, one could also interpret this welfarist approach articulated by prosecutors as reinforcing the very "managerial model" of criminal law administration that Kohler-Hausmann (2018, p. 4) has written about—one "concerned with managing people through engagement with the criminal justice system over time." Kohler-Hausmann's study of one of New York City's criminal courts describes how the technique of "performance" is a primary mechanism for social control in place of conviction and carceral sentences—in which "defendants must prove some capacity for self-governance by performing certain actions laid out by the court" (e.g., arrive to court on time, attend a program, complete community service) and "earn either leniency or sanctions depending on how they perform" (Kohler-Hausmann 2018, p. 255). As she writes, misdemeanor criminal courts can be understood as "'people-changing' organizations. They actively engage their subjects in an effort to modify or produce new sensibilities through various transformative techniques" (Kohler-Hausmann 2018, p. 223). One of these techniques is to mandate a "program" such as the mental health treatment programs that prosecutors advocated for in our study. Indeed, in Mr. Carter's case, he is presented with the option to "earn" a noncriminal disposition if he can successfully complete the required programming and prove his capacity for rule-following over the next six months. Whether such programs are tools to break the cycle of offending or widen a net of social control is one of the reasons that prosecutors and defenders can become so adversarial. The next section looks at the perspective of defenders.

The Defenders: Balancing Efficiency and Self-Determination

In contrast to the approach articulated by prosecutors in the previous section—in which diversion programming is pursued to enforce com-

pliance with treatment in ways that are seen as beneficial for the offender with an SMI and potentially for the system if treatment can
reduce future criminal legal involvement—the public defender in Mr.
Carter's case sought time served with a criminal conviction. What can
explain this willingness to plead guilty and receive a criminal conviction over the option of attending mandated programming and staying
out of trouble for the next six months?

Defenders in all cities articulated how the requirement to do what is
best for their client often means rejecting an offer of diversionary programming for low-level misdemeanors. "If it's a choice between jail or
programming," one public defender in Manhattan reflected, "we're always gonna go for the programming." But people in some places across
the United States no longer face the threat of significant jail time for an
arrest or conviction on a minor misdemeanor. In cases in which the
threat of a jail sentence is no longer a motivator for misdemeanants,
mandated programming can seem particularly onerous. One of the
most common perspectives that public defenders held in our study was
that mandated programming "set clients up for failure." An Atlanta
public defender asked the following:

> Realistically, somebody who has a serious mental illness, who's been in
> and out of the system as much as they have, are they going to succeed
> in the program? And if they don't, then it's a revocation of their proba-
> tion, right? And their mental illness is not taken into account. So now
> they're going to prison, right?

The repercussions for failing to complete noncustodial sanctions
therefore lead many clients and their attorneys to take a plea to a new
criminal conviction. A Chicago defender reflected the following:

> I don't want [programming] because they want to attach supervision to
> it, usually a conditional discharge for, like, six months to ensure that the
> person follows through with these resources given to them. And usually
> the person would be like, "No, that's a lot hanging over me. I just want
> to TCS [time considered served]."

An Atlanta defender shared a similar calculus: "Do you want time
served, or do you want to get a year's probation on the condition that
you don't ever get high again?" The perspectives of these defenders
suggest that there may be some stereotypes at play here with respect to
how public defenders consider clients with mental illnesses and their
ability to successfully complete court-mandated programming. At the
same time, such statements begin to shed light on how public defenders
must weigh competing concerns in a system where representation is a

scarce resource (Van Cleve 2016). As Van Cleve (2016) has described in writing about how the "worthiness" of clients is shaped by racialized understandings of defendants, public defenders assess the "value" of a case in determining how much advocacy they want to do. Public defenders must decide whether to pursue a short- or long-term strategy with respect to aiding their clients. This may end up being related to how much advocacy a public defender is willing to do on behalf of their client but can also be determined by the simple calculus of what it takes to avoid time in jail. One Manhattan public defender explained this as follows: "I mean, we'd like to help very much. But [you do] whatever is ultimately going to be best for the client in the moment and having less court interaction—if it's a matter of that versus time served—it's always going to be time served that wins the day."

This is not to say that public defenders in our study didn't worry about clients racking up a high number of misdemeanor cases in a short period of time. Depending on the way state statutes are written, repeated misdemeanor offenses can lead to being charged with felonies. Rather, defenders seemed to doubt the efficacy of state intervention in helping their clients. One public defender in Chicago explained this position:

> I don't like bringing a mental illness to either the prosecutor or the judge because it depends on what you believe about state intervention. But they usually make a lot more requirements of people...if there were more resources to help them, maybe they could think of a better way to help them. But usually, it's no better than when they walked in that door. And usually worse.

Meanwhile, defenders expressed that their case strategy is guided by what their clients want. "It's their case. It's 100% what they want," reflected a Philadelphia public defender. Another defender from Manhattan shared the following: "At the end of the day, whether it was programming or not, it really has to come down to the client's choice.... It's not for me to try to convince, persuade, or cajole or do whatever it is, thinking that I'm doing the best for the client. That's not my role, that's not my function."

The way public defenders frame the issue of mandated treatment for misdemeanor cases involving people with SMI reinforces the point previously mentioned in this chapter about the technique of "performance" for maintaining social control (Kohler-Hausmann 2018). This inevitably raises the question of net widening that Kohler-Hausmann (2018) describes and that was also raised by our study participants. As one example, in Manhattan, study participants described how one of the unanticipated consequences of bail reform in New York State is that more misdemeanor defendants are being placed on Supervised Release at arraignment rather than being released on their own recognizance (Center for Court Innovation 2022). While Supervised Release is intended primarily to ensure that a defendant returns to court and secondarily to connect the defendant with voluntary services, it can create burdens with respect to compliance that complicate a defendant's case even before their case proceeds. And, as described previously, as cases proceed and defendants are placed on various forms of noncustodial supervision, there are heightened consequences for failure to comply with the terms of that supervision.

The perspectives of public defenders also reengage the focal-concerns literature and demonstrate how these concerns are weighed quite differently in an adversarial system in at least two ways. First, defenders rejected prosecutors' notion that mandated programming can break cycles of recidivism and thereby serve as a means of community protection. As data in this section and previously cited suggest, defenders lacked confidence in the efficiency and the efficacy of court-mandated programming and preferred that their clients engage with treatment on their own terms and outside of the court system. Part of this strategy was related to the fact that defenders did not believe quality treatment was available through the court system or that mental health treatment alone was enough to reduce the involvement of their clients in the criminal legal system. In the absence of solutions that target broader social determinants of health, such as housing, jobs, access to resources, and community support, defenders weren't inclined to connect their clients with treatment through the criminal legal system.

Second, as advocates for their clients, defenders understandably weighed the practical constraints that their clients would face resulting from their case disposition. One defender in Manhattan framed weighing of these concerns as follows:

> I often like to pose that question explicitly, "Can you come back to court? Is this a reasonable possibility for you, or should we just try to get the best thing today, and is that better for you?" And I mean especially people who are charged with [petit larceny] a lot, they know, they know what's best for them and they're able to accurately say what works for them and what doesn't.

Returning to the case of Mr. Carter and the choice to reject an offer of an ACD with mandated programming, one can understand how Mr. Carter's defender was weighing not only what the case was worth (confident that the case could be resolved via a dismissal or time served)

(Van Cleve 2016), but also what Mr. Carter could realistically manage back in the community as someone who was homeless and had an SMI.

The notion of "rehabilitation" and "redeemability" as a fourth focal concern is also relevant here. Defenders, too, believe in rehabilitation as an end in itself. As one Manhattan defender said, "You would hope that they get that intervention that obviously breaks the cycle. So whether it's drug treatment or whether it's counseling for mental health issues, or something as basic as trying to get the person into the shelter system or a means of legitimate financial support. I think that's the strategy for the most part." The difference for defenders, however, is they remain focused on the "best disposition" as the one that entails the least continued court involvement. As a Manhattan public defender said, "To the extent possible, you know, we want to help our clients break that cycle. But we also want to have whatever the best disposition is going to be." As the case of Mr. Carter and the multiple perspectives offered by public defenders above suggest, burdensome programs are often not considered the best disposition in a misdemeanor case.

Weighing Focal Concerns: Consequences for Research and Practice

The disparate perspectives of police, prosecutors, and defenders in deciding how to proceed in misdemeanor cases among people with mental illnesses such as Mr. Carter vividly demonstrate how actors within the criminal legal system may be oriented toward different values and goals. On the one hand, system actors in different cities and across decision-making points articulated a shared commitment to reducing the entanglement of people with SMI in the criminal legal system. This objective sits neatly within the larger goal of the criminal legal system to "close cases that stay closed" (Bernard et al. 2005, p. 206). On the other hand, police, prosecutors, and defenders have different strategies for achieving this goal. This is in part because they answer to different sets of stakeholders and in part because their positions in the criminal legal system not only give them different understandings of mental illnesses and their relationship to underlying offenses but also because they provide them with different perspectives on the utility of any single approach over another. The concept of loose coupling informs us that contextual, extralegal characteristics are more likely to affect decision-making in loosely coupled stages of the criminal legal system where there are diverse organizational players with different goals and values (Bishop et al. 2010; Ericson and Eckberg 2016). Seeing mental illness as one of many contextual variables that influence decision-making may help explain why decision-making across police, prosecutors, and public defenders can seem to lack internal consistency; diverse organizational players are trying to make decisions based on goals and values that may compete with each other.

Three additional points are worth further reflection as they relate to understanding the value pluralism that guides decision-making in the life of a case. First, returning to our earlier point about how stereotypes about people with mental illnesses may influence decision-making in case processing, it is apparent that stereotypes may lead to different—even contradictory—assessments of blameworthiness and redeemability. On the one hand, the knowledge that police, prosecutors, and defenders had about Mr. Carter's mental illness led them to consider a variety of alternatives to traditional case processing, including taking Mr. Carter to the hospital and diverting him to mental health treatment. These considerations were driven by some sense that Mr. Carter's mental illness might be responsible for his behavior, that Mr. Carter himself was less culpable, and that he could be rehabilitated through appropriate treatment. On the other hand, negative attributions about people with mental illness also circulate and influence action. The public defenders wanted to avoid mandated treatment, but they did so, in part, because of their assumptions about Mr. Carter as a person with mental illness who was homeless: that he would be unable to successfully complete a treatment program. And prosecutors may have pursued diversion because of the assumption that a "corrective approach" was needed—that Mr. Carter would not "self-correct" his behavior without court-mandated intervention. The "perceptual shorthands" that criminal legal stakeholders develop about people with mental illnesses require further investigation, particularly as they relate to how negative stereotypes about people with mental illnesses (e.g., that they are dangerous or unpredictable) may further compound stereotypes about race and gender in the criminal legal system. Evidence on sentencing disparities, for example, has demonstrated that Black defendants are significantly less likely to receive downward departures from sentencing guidelines that include alternatives to incarceration (Painter-Davis and Ulmer 2020). Additional research is needed on the extent to which rehabilitative ideals are pursued for people with mental illnesses across different races and genders, as well as across different disorders (e.g., those with depression versus those with schizophrenia).

Second, the discussion of blameworthiness and stereotypes associated with mental illnesses raises important questions about how criminal legal system actors understand the relationship between mental illnesses and criminal behavior. To the extent that these actors see mental illness as the direct cause of offending behavior—and mental health treatment as the solution to stopping it—they are likely to advocate for diversion to treatment as the appropriate course of action for people with SMI. Epperson et al. (2011, 2014) have described how this framing led to a generation of system interventions premised on the belief that mental health treatment alone would curb cycles of offending. More recent research, however, suggests that the relationship between mental illness and crime is confounded by myriad factors including poverty, homelessness, and substance use, and that people with SMI encounter the criminal legal system for many of the same reasons as those without SMI (Draine et al. 2002; Epperson et al. 2014; Fisher et al. 2006). A narrow view of treatment solutions that are disconnected from larger systems of social support is likely to fall short of meeting the needs of people with mental illnesses entangled in the criminal legal system. More work is needed at the practice level to articulate the specific elements that make diversion programs successful and to then support jurisdictions in integrating such elements into existing programming. Referring to Chapter 2, it is clear that there are many innovative examples of off-ramps from the criminal legal system and also that we need to know more about what makes them viable and effective off-ramps leading to better outcomes for people with SMI.

Third, it is worth reflecting on the apparent shift by prosecutors when dealing with low-level cases involving people with SMI. Our data suggest that prosecutors have shifted from the traditional, backward-looking approach that emphasizes punishment to a more rehabilitative, forward-looking approach that better recognizes and addresses the complexity of the relationship between SMI and criminal behavior. In this shift, prosecutors set aside their short-term concerns surrounding their individual pursuit of efficiency and success (e.g., rapid case resolution, high conviction rates, reduced uncertainty) and are more open to alternative methods (e.g., ACD) in hopes of successfully curbing future offending. In Mr. Carter's case, for example, rather than seek a traditional criminal disposition, the ADA recommended programming that not only attempted to address the underlying causes of the behaviors but also guaranteed Mr. Carter a noncriminal disposition (if completed successfully). The ACD alternative recommended in Mr. Carter's case seems inconsistent with the traditional interests of prosecutors and their respective offices—it slows down final case resolution (the case remains open or pending until program completion or failure), does not ensure a conviction (the defendant may successfully complete the program), and may ultimately fail in preventing future offending (the defendant may commit another offense after successful program completion). Despite this, prosecutors in our study consistently expressed a willingness to provide people with SMI accused of low-level offenses with an opportunity to redeem themselves and avoid criminal punishment. Future research should seek to more fully assess the driving force behind the progressive prosecution agenda, the extent to which it has influenced prosecutors' perceptions of mental illnesses and how to deal with offenses involving people with SMI, and the effectiveness of shifting to a more "rehabilitative" approach to low-level misdemeanors.

On a practical level, the competing concerns and goals articulated by different criminal legal system stakeholders suggest that prospects for continued reform in the system depend critically on bringing together criminal legal decision-makers from different parts of the system to engage in cross-system learning and exchange. As we have discussed elsewhere (Pope et al. 2023; Wood et al. 2023), one possibility is to invite stakeholders across the stages of misdemeanor case processing to participate in scenario-based exercises in which they walk through the processing of "typical" misdemeanor cases involving people with mental illnesses to better understand the decision-making contexts and focal concerns at play. As Thacher (2001, p. 398) has written in describing how police confront a broad range and mix of ambiguous values in their work, "Working amidst value pluralism means that problem setting—figuring out which values are important in a situation and deciding how to evaluate different courses of action—is at least as important as problem-solving." Providing space for decision-makers to articulate the orientations of their agencies and allowing multiple values to bear on a particular situation could create opportunities for new points of intervention. Indeed, as Thacher (2001, p. 395) wrote, it is through such "situated decision-making," that "it is sometimes possible to arrive at solutions that strike most people as legitimate, even when the same people cannot agree on the relative worth of each value in the abstract." At a time when people with mental illnesses continue to have disproportionate contact with the criminal legal system and experience worse outcomes, it is worth reconsidering how such a project could move toward reducing system entanglement and advancing equity and justice.

KEY POINTS

- The focal-concerns framework has become a dominant framework to explain race-, gender-, and age-related disparities in the criminal legal system. It suggests that decision-makers consider three focal concerns when making decisions: blameworthiness, protection of the community, and practical constraints. Scholars have recently proposed a fourth focal concern: rehabilitation potential.

- Police officers are the initial point of contact in a longer chain of decision-makers within the criminal legal system. They face practical constraints in making decisions about how to resolve situations involving misdemeanor offenses by people with serious mental illnesses: the presence of complainants who want action taken, the availability of resources (or lack thereof), and the fact that most solutions are short-term.

- Progressive prosecutors have embraced a shift toward a more rehabilitative and forward-looking approach to addressing the intersection of mental illness and criminal behavior. The increasing reliance on alternatives-to-incarceration programs suggests a belief that the criminal legal system can be leveraged for treatment purposes, even if it means sacrificing goals of efficiency with respect to rapid case resolution. It also leads to net widening.

- Alternatives to incarceration may be perceived as more punitive by public defenders and defendants if they involve treatment mandates that extend criminal legal entanglement beyond the time that their client would be involved in the system with a guilty plea.

- More research is needed about the extent to which mental illness amplifies or diminishes concerns about blameworthiness when motivating decision-makers across the criminal legal system. Such research must also investigate the intersectionality of mental illness with marginalized racial, ethnic, and gender identities.

References

Albonetti CA: An integration of theories to explain judicial discretion. Soc Probl 38(2):247–266, 1991

Bernard TJ, Paoline EA, Pare P-P: General systems theory and criminal justice. J Crim Justice 33(3):203–211, 2005

Bishop D, Leiber M, Johnson J: Contexts of decision making in the juvenile justice system: an organizational approach to understanding minority overrepresentation. Youth Violence Juv Justice 8(3):213–233, 2010

Bittner E: Police discretion in emergency apprehension of mentally ill persons. Soc Probl 14(3):278–292, 1967

Bittner E: Aspects of Police Work. Boston, MA, Northeastern University Press, 1990

Bonfine N, Wilson AB, Munetz MR: Meeting the needs of justice-involved people with serious mental illness within community behavioral health systems. Psychiatr Serv 71(4):355–363, 2020 31795858

Bridges GS, Steen S: Racial disparities in official assessments of juvenile offenders: attributional stereotypes as mediating mechanisms. Am Sociol Rev 63(4):554–570, 1998

Center for Court Innovation: Expanding Supervised Release in New York City: An Evaluation of June 2019 Changes. New York, Center for Court Innovation, June 2022. Available at: https://www.innovatingjustice.org/sites/default/files/media/document/2022/NYC%20ISLG%20Report_FINAL_June22.pdf. Accessed April 18, 2023.

Center for Health and Justice at TASC: No Entry: A National Survey of Criminal Justice Diversion Programs and Initiatives. Chicago, IL, Center for Health and Justice at TASC, December, 2013. Available at: https://www.centerforhealthandjustice.org/tascblog/Images/documents/Publications/CHJ%20Diversion%20Report_web.pdf. Accessed February 28, 2023.

Corrigan PW: Mental health stigma as social attribution: implications for research methods and attitude change. Clin Psychol 7(1):48–67, 2000

Draine J, Salzer MS, Culhane DP, et al: Role of social disadvantage in crime, joblessness, and homelessness among persons with serious mental illness. Psychiatr Serv 53(5):565–573, 2002 11986504

Epperson M, Wolff N, Morgan R, et al: The Next Generation of Behavioral Health and Criminal Justice Interventions: Improving Outcomes by Improving Interventions. New Brunswick, NJ, Rutgers University Center for Behavioral Health Services and Criminal Justice Research, 2011

Epperson MW, Wolff N, Morgan RD, et al: Envisioning the next generation of behavioral health and criminal justice interventions. Int J Law Psychiatry 37(5):427–438, 2014 24666731

Ericson RD, Eckberg DA: Racial disparity in juvenile diversion: the impact of focal concerns and organizational coupling. Race Justice 6(1):35–56, 2016

Fisher WH, Roy-Bujnowski KM, Grudzinskas AJ Jr, et al: Patterns and prevalence of arrest in a statewide cohort of mental health care consumers. Psychiatr Serv 57(11):1623–1628, 2006 17085611

Galvin MA, Ulmer JT: Expanding our understanding of focal concerns: alternative sentences, race, and "salvageability." Justice Q 39(6):1332–1353, 2022

Hagan J: Why is there so little criminal justice theory? Neglected macro- and micro-level links between organization and power. J Res Crime Delinq 26(2):116–135, 1989

Hagan J, Hewitt JD, Alwin DF: Ceremonial justice: crime and punishment in a loosely coupled system. Soc Forces 58(2):506–527, 1979

Hall D, Lee L-W, Manseau MW, et al: Major mental illness as a risk factor for incarceration. Psychiatr Serv 70(12):1088–1093, 2019 31480926

Hawkins DF: Causal attribution and punishment for crime. Deviant Behav 2(3):207–230, 1981

Ishoy GA, Dabney DA: Policing and the focal concerns framework: explore how its components apply to discretionary enforcement decisions of police officers. Deviant Behav 39(7):878–895, 2018

Johnson A, Ali-Smith M: Diversion Programs, Explained. Washington, DC, Vera Institute of Justice, 2022. Available from: https://www.vera.org/inline-downloads/diversion-programs-explained.pdf. Accessed February 28, 2023.

Johnson BD, Dipietro SM: The power of diversion: intermediate sanctions and sentencing disparity under presumptive guidelines. Criminology 50(3):811–850, 2012

Kaiser K, Spohn C: Why do judges depart? A review of reasons for judicial departures in federal sentencing. Criminology, Criminal Justice, Law and Society 19(2):44–62, 2018

Kohler-Hausmann I: Misdemeanorland: Criminal Courts and Social Control in an Age of Broken Windows Policing. Princeton, NJ, Princeton University Press, 2018

Lapsey DS Jr, Campbell BA, Plumlee BT: Focal concerns and police decision making in sexual assault cases: a systematic review and meta-analysis. Trauma Violence Abuse 23(4):1220–1234, 2022 33583357

Okeowo A: How to defund the police. The New Yorker. June 26, 2020. Available from: https://www.newyorker.com/news/news-desk/how-the-police-could-be-defunded. Accessed February 28, 2023.

Painter-Davis N, Ulmer JT: Discretion and disparity under sentencing guidelines revisited: the interrelationship between structured sentencing alternatives and guideline decision-making. J Res Crime Delinq 57(3):263–293, 2020

Parcesepe AM, Cabassa LJ: Public stigma of mental illness in the United States: a systematic literature review. Adm Policy Ment Health 40(5):384–399, 2013 22833051

Penn DL, Martin J: The stigma of severe mental illness: some potential solutions for a recalcitrant problem. Psychiatr Q 69(3):235–247, 1998 9682287

Pope LG, Stagoff-Belfort A, Warnock A, et al: Competing concerns in efforts to reduce criminal legal contact among people with serious mental illnesses: findings from a multi-city study on misdemeanor arrests. Adm Policy Ment Health 50(3):476–487, 2023 36717527

Quattlebaum M, Tyler T: Beyond the law: an agenda for policing reform. Boston Univ Law Rev 100(3):1017–1045, 2020

Reiss AJ: The Police and the Public. New Haven, Yale University Press, 1971

Spohn C, Beichner D, Davis-Frenzel E: Prosecutorial justifications for sexual assault case rejection: guarding the "gateway to justice." Soc Probl 48(2):206–235, 2001

Steffensmeier D, Demuth S: Ethnicity and sentencing outcomes in U.S. federal courts: who is punished more harshly? Am Sociol Rev 65:705–729, 2000

Steffensmeier D, Ulmer J, Kramer J: The interaction of race, gender, and age in criminal sentencing: the punishment cost of being young, black, and male. Criminology 36(4):763–798, 1998

Thacher D: Policing is not a treatment: alternatives to the medical model of police research. J Res Crime Delinq 38(4):387–415, 2001

Thacher D: Shrinking the police footprint. Crim Justice Ethics 41(1):62–85, 2022

Tittle CR, Curran DA: Contingencies for dispositional disparities in juvenile justice. Soc Forces 67(1):23–58, 1988

Ulmer JT, Silver E, Hanrath LS: Back to basics: a critical examination of the focal
    concerns framework from the perspective of judges. Justice Q 40(6):813–
    836, 2022
Van Cleve NG: Crook County. Palo Alto, CA, Stanford University Press, 2016
Vitale AS: The End of Policing. New York, Verso, 2017
White C: Incarcerating youth with mental health problems: a focus on the inter-
    section of race, ethnicity, and mental illness. Youth Violence Juv Justice
    14(4):426–447, 2016
Wood JD, Watson AC, Fulambarker AJ: The "gray zone" of police work during
    mental health encounters: findings from an observational study in Chi-
    cago. Police Q 20(1):81–105, 2017 28286406
Wood JD, Watson AC, Pope L, et al: Contexts shaping misdemeanor system in-
    terventions among people with mental illnesses: qualitative findings from
    a multi-site system mapping exercise. Health Justice 11(1):20, 2023
    37014478

Part 2

Common Types of Misdemeanor Charges for People With Serious Mental Illness

PART 2

5

Being in the Wrong Place

Criminal Trespass and Criminal Legal System Entanglement

Aaron Stagoff-Belfort, B.A.

Jason Tan de Bibiana, M.Sc.

Criminal trespass is a misdemeanor offense that occurs when someone knowingly enters property without permission or remains in a location without authorization from the owner or occupant. It establishes a legal right for private and public property owners to exclude or banish people for violating rules of entry (Kempa et al. 1999). Criminal trespass is a legal tool for managing people's behaviors in spaces, and it is a charge that grew in popularity after the downfall of so-called status crimes such as vagrancy and loitering in the second half of the twentieth century (Beckett and Herbert 2010; Goluboff 2016). Similar to those

offenses, which were used to criminalize certain types of people rather
than defined behaviors, the use of criminal trespass in some jurisdictions has declined in recent years because of legal challenges against
vague statutes and broad, discriminatory policing practices (Legal Defense Fund 2010; Morgan and Thompson 2021). However, the charge of
criminal trespass remains in many jurisdictions as a critical tool that legal systems use to meet the demands of everyday people and business
entities that desire to remove people from spaces for a variety of concerns stemming from standards of civility, business interests in attract-
ing customers, and perceived threats to public safety (Beckett and
Herbert 2010; Natapoff 2018).

This chapter explores the scenarios in which people with serious
mental illness (SMI) encounter the criminal legal system because of
criminal trespass charges. We begin by exploring specific criminal trespass statutes in Georgia, Illinois, New York, and Pennsylvania, the
states where the previously described study (see Chapter 1, "The System, the Process, and the Contexts") was carried out. We briefly summarize historical perspectives and recent notable public controversies
involving the enforcement of criminal trespass laws and describe what
we currently know about people with SMI and criminal trespass
offenses. We then proceed to discuss how police officers use criminal
trespass as a charge vis-à-vis the demands that other interested stakeholders place on them to solve problems. We also discuss how racial
and other social inequalities are implicated in its use. Throughout, we
draw on case studies and interview and focus group data from our
study to illuminate how both criminal legal system stakeholders and
people with SMI who have been arrested for criminal trespass make
sense of the charge in resolving various social problems and trouble-
some encounters that arise from the competing interests of individuals.
We close with a discussion of criminal legal and mental health system
reforms, as well as prevention-based approaches that exist outside of
these systems and have the potential to reduce the entanglement of people with SMI and criminal trespass charges within the legal system.

Criminal Laws Relating to Criminal Trespass

Across the states of Georgia, Illinois, New York, and Pennsylvania,
the statutes for criminal trespass require that someone has *knowingly* entered or remained on the premises of a forbidden location (see Table 5–
1 for state criminal trespass statutes). The statutes across the four states
also include terms about whether there is a posted notice forbidding en-

Table 5–1. Criminal trespass statutes in the states included in the study

State and statute	Offense	Definition for misdemeanor offense, and escalating penalties
Georgia, Ga. Code § 16–7–21 (2021)	Criminal trespass	Trespassing is a misdemeanor offense when someone knowingly enters or remains on the premises of another person or into any part of any vehicle, railroad car, aircraft, or watercraft of another person after receiving notice from the owner, occupant, or authorized representative of the owner or occupant that entering or remaining is forbidden. Or without notice, knowingly entering or remaining on the premises or vehicle for an unlawful purpose.
Illinois, 720 ILCS 5 / 19–4; 21–2; 21–3 (2022)	Criminal trespass section 19–4; criminal trespass to a residence; section 21–2: vehicle; section 21–3: real property	Sec. 19–4. Criminal trespass to a residence. Criminal trespass to a residence is a misdemeanor offense when someone knowingly and without authority enters or remains within any residence. The offense escalates to a felony when someone enters or remains within any residence while knowing that someone else is present in the residence. Sec. 21–2. Criminal trespass to vehicles. Knowingly and without authority entering or operating any vehicle, aircraft, or watercraft is a misdemeanor offense. Sec. 21–3. Criminal trespass to real property. Knowingly and without authority entering or remaining within a building is a misdemeanor offense. Knowingly and without authority entering or remaining upon land or agricultural fields that have a conspicuously posted printed or written notice forbidding such entry or after receiving notice from the owner or occupant that the entry is forbidden is a misdemeanor offense.

Table 5–1. Criminal trespass statutes in the states included in the study *(continued)*

State and statute	Offense	Definition for misdemeanor offense, and escalating penalties
New York, NY Penal Law § 140 (2022)	Criminal trespass	Trespassing is a violation (140.05–Trespass) when someone knowingly enters or remains unlawfully in or upon premises. The violation escalates to a class B misdemeanor offense (140.10–Criminal Trespass in the Third Degree) if the premises is fenced/otherwise enclosed; elementary or secondary school; railroad or rapid transit yard; or public housing project building with conspicuously posted rules or regulations governing entry or communication to leave the premises by a housing police officer. This offense escalates to a class A misdemeanor offense (140.15–Criminal Trespass in the Second Degree) when it pertains to someone who is required to maintain a level one or level two sexual offender registration. The offense escalates to a felony (140.17–Criminal Trespass in the First Degree) when someone enters or remains in a building and possesses, or knows that another participant in the crime possesses, an explosive or a deadly weapon.
Pennsylvania, 18 Pa. C.S. § 3503 (2022)	Criminal trespass; see Defiant trespasser and Agricultural trespasser for misdemeanor offenses	Trespassing is a summary offense (simple trespass) is when someone enters or remains on a property for the purpose of threatening the owner or occupant of the premises or starting a fire or defacing or damaging the premises—without any of the verbal or posted communication to leave, as in defiant trespass. Trespassing is a misdemeanor offense (labeled as defiant trespass, or agricultural trespass when the property is agricultural land) when someone enters or remains on a property after being told they should not in one of the following ways: posted signs; being verbally notified by anyone on the property; fencing or any other enclosure; or being told to leave, in any manner, by school officials, government facility officials, or law enforcement officers. Trespassing is a felony offense when someone enters a building or occupied structure by breaking into locks or gaining entry by subterfuge.

try or if the notice has been communicated verbally by the owner, occupant, or others. For example, in Georgia, trespassing is a misdemeanor offense when someone enters or remains on a property after receiving notice that this is forbidden by the owner, occupant, or authorized representative of the owner or occupant (Criminal Trespass, Ga. Code § 16–7–21). Pennsylvania's statute specifies that trespassing is a misdemeanor offense when someone enters or remains on a property after receiving a verbal notice or if the property has posted signs forbidding entry, fencing, or other enclosures (Criminal Trespass, 18 Pa. C.S. § 3503).

Criminal trespass charges can also escalate from a violation or summary offense into more serious misdemeanor and felony offenses if certain conditions are present. For example, in Illinois, criminal trespass in a residence escalates to a felony when someone enters or remains within any residence while knowing that someone else is present in the residence (720 ILCS 5/19–4). In Pennsylvania, trespassing is a felony offense when someone enters a building or occupied structure by breaking into locks or gaining entry by subterfuge (18 Pa. C.S. § 3503). In New York, trespassing escalates to a felony when someone who is trespassing either possesses an explosive or a deadly weapon or is knowingly trespassing with another person possessing an explosive or a deadly weapon (NY Penal Law § 140.17). And, as discussed further in Chapter 6 ("A $25 T-Shirt From the Bargain Store"), a person can be charged with Burglary in the Third Degree in New York when they knowingly enter or remain unlawfully in a building with intent to commit a crime (NY Penal Law § 140.20).

Some state statutes also include conditions related to specific types of locations. For example, in New York, trespassing can escalate from a violation to a misdemeanor offense if it occurs at an elementary or secondary school, railroad or rapid transit yard, or a public housing project building with conspicuously posted rules or regulations governing entry or communication to leave the premises by a housing police officer.

The present-day application of criminal trespass laws is preceded by a sordid history, in which their passage and enforcement has been inextricably linked to efforts to criminalize the everyday life of Black Americans and other marginalized groups. In the colonial era (pre-1783), trespassing was not a criminal offense in the United States, but rather a tort that allowed property owners to sue for damages. Individual states adopted common law definitions of criminal trespass after the Revolutionary War (Lewis 1982). Until 1865, criminal trespass was rarely charged as a crime. One nationwide review found only two lawsuits that could be broadly classified as meeting the modern definition of criminal trespass, both involving a landowner suing hunters who would not leave his land in South Carolina in 1818 and 1820 (Sawers 2022).

After the Civil War and the end of chattel slavery (1865), states across the South codified the Black Codes, which were a series of laws, rules, and regulations that governed the lives of newly freed Black people (Du Bois 2017; Foner 2014). This allowed the Southern states to preserve systems of spatial segregation, social control, and labor discipline that the institution of slavery provided even after it had formally ended. Criminal law was an essential tool to achieve this end (Cohen 1976; Du Bois 2017).

As Brian Sawers (2018) showed, criminal trespass statutes were common among the laws that proliferated to criminalize the everyday life of Black Americans. States including Georgia, South Carolina, and Louisiana passed new penalties. Alabama's law sanctioned 3 months of hard labor, and Florida permitted 39 lashes as punishment. In the South, where most people of color lived and worked on land that was owned by White people, trespass laws were a tool for labor discipline. They facilitated employer and landlord control of the freedom of movement and social relations of Black people (Sawers 2022). In the absence of the formal system of chattel slavery, restricting access to private land and outlawing public hunting and fishing made communities of color reliant on the planter class. These laws eventually traveled north, becoming more common in the early twentieth century and often serving similar purposes. For example, one Pennsylvania law was enacted expressly to create new restrictions on the ability of recent immigrants to hunt in the state.

In the Civil Rights Era (1954–1968), criminal trespass laws played a prominent role in the lunch counter sit-in cases and faced sustained legal scrutiny for the first time. Important Supreme Court decisions at the time included those in which civil rights activists challenged segregation policies at lunch counters, amusement parks, and other private accommodations. In these cases, private individuals and businesses perpetuated racial segregation by harnessing the power of local police and courts to enforce state trespassing laws. In cases such as *Bouie v. City of Columbia* (1964), *Bell v. Maryland* (1964), and *Griffin v. Maryland* (1964), the Supreme Court reversed criminal convictions for trespassing, but sometimes declined to rule on broader 14th Amendment and equal protection issues (Johnston 1965). In *Bouie*, two college students were arrested at a lunch counter in Columbia, South Carolina, and were charged with violating the same 1866 criminal trespass statute the state passed after the Civil War (Sawers 2022).

Goluboff (2016) noted that criminal trespass was one of a suite of statutes similar to vagrancy that were essential to the policing of the culture wars of the 1960s and 1970s. Law enforcement used the substantial discretion these laws provided to enforce broader codes of morality against not only Black people but also sex workers; lesbian, gay, bisexual, transgender, or queer people; beatniks (a counterculture movement that began in the 1950s) and hippies; Vietnam War protestors; and communists. These statutes served to criminalize groups of people rather than individual conduct itself and targeted groups including those who were considered "idle," people who lived in poverty, or people who "wander[ed] about with no purpose" (Goluboff 2016; Wood 2016). Many of these statutes were ruled unconstitutional by the Warren Court (1953–1969, when Justice Earl Warren was the chief justice of the U.S. Supreme Court) because of their sweeping and vague language and the virtually unfettered authority they granted police to stop and search people (Goluboff and Sorensen 2018). Broader changes in American cultural norms buttressed the efforts of civil liberties advocates who argued that these laws did not serve any genuine public safety purpose but functioned instead to maintain social order and hierarchy in a society otherwise striving to become more tolerant of difference.

Although loitering and vagrancy laws were largely consigned to the dustbin of history, more narrowly tailored statutes, including many criminal trespass laws, survived into the present and demonstrate the blurry line between the policing of personal identity and morality and the policing of behaviors that threaten public order and safety. The increased popularity in the 1990s of controversial policing tactics such as the broken windows theory of policing, as well as civility codes that many municipalities passed, demonstrate the contemporary relevance of these tensions (Beckett and Herbert 2010; Gibson 2003; Vitale 2008).

In recent years, criminal trespass laws and arrests have continued to spark public controversy. For instance, in 2018, in a high-profile incident in Philadelphia, two Black men were arrested for defiant trespass while sitting at a Starbucks coffee shop and waiting for a third person to arrive for a business meeting. They spent 8 hours in jail. Philadelphia Police Commissioner Richard Ross apologized to the two men, who subsequently reached a settlement with Starbucks and the city, and the Philadelphia Police Department issued a revised policy for officers responding to trespass calls (Sanchez 2018). The new policy requires officers to engage in additional steps before making an arrest: explaining to the person that they are on private property, engaging in mediation and de-escalation between both parties, and finally calling a supervisor to the scene to make a final arrest determination if the complainant wants to press charges (Irizarry-Aponte 2018; Winberg 2018).

Other police departments have garnered criticism for trespass enforcement strategies or agreements with local businesses that have served to perpetuate racial disparities in arrests. In Grand Rapids, Michigan, the police department recruited business owners in "high-crime" areas to sign generalized "No Trespass Letters" that would allow police to make trespass arrests on commercial property without first talking to business owners or employees about whether a person belonged on the property (Williamson 2015). In some cases, these policies inspired backlash. In 2010 in New York, a group of residents and visitors to New York City Housing Authority (NYCHA) buildings filed a class action lawsuit protesting an unconstitutional pattern of stops and arrests for criminal trespass (Legal Defense Fund 2010). The case *Davis v. City of New York* (2011) challenged the New York City Police Department's practice of conducting "vertical sweeps," which concentrated enforcement in the common areas of NYCHA buildings where residents were disproportionately people of color and involved police officers making stops without reasonable suspicion. A settlement reached in 2015 played an important role in the sizeable decline in criminal trespass arrests in New York City in recent years, although racial disparities in criminal trespass arrests persist (Scrivener et al. 2020).

Understanding the Use of Criminal Trespass Charges Among People With Mental Illness

In a recent study, Compton et al. (2023) examined a dataset that included all arrests for a misdemeanor or felony in New York State between 2010 and 2013—more than 2 million total arrests. Two criminal trespass charges (second and third degree) were on the list of the 15 most common misdemeanor charges for people with an SMI (representing 2.5% of all arrests when the charges were combined), but they did not appear on the list of the 15 most common charges in arrests for individuals without an SMI (1.7% of all arrests when the charges were combined). Compton et al. (2023) called for further research to disentangle how social factors, such as mental illness and housing instability, interact and make people with SMI more likely to be arrested for criminal trespass. We draw on the results of subsequent qualitative research—case studies, interviews, and focus groups—further in this chapter to demonstrate the link between SMI and criminal trespass and how and why the charge is used and processed in the legal system.

Case Example: Mr. Harper Arrested for Sleeping in a Vacant Store

Dennis Harper is a 37-year-old Black man with an SMI, who was arrested by Chicago police officers for sleeping in a vacant store. One of the arresting officers, who had patrolled the neighborhood for the past few years, explained that they knew Mr. Harper well and "dealt with [him] quite frequently." The officer elaborated that Mr. Harper was "mentally ill and his family kicked him out of the house maybe 5 years ago." Since then, Mr. Harper spent time in homeless shelters and short-term respite housing but got into a few fights with other clients and staff at one shelter. He also had his belongings stolen at a shelter, and so did not go to shelters anymore. Instead, he slept in parks and other places outdoors around the neighborhood. During the cold winters in Chicago, he found a few different vacant homes and storefronts to sleep in, like the one he was arrested in. In the past, police officers took Mr. Harper to the hospital instead of arresting him, and that helped Mr. Harper reconnect with an outpatient mental health treatment program. However, the program was not successful in helping him secure stable housing, and the treatment program often lost contact with him.

The police officers explained that they preferred not to arrest Mr. Harper because they knew he was just seeking shelter from the cold and that arresting him was not going to change his situation. However, the property owner of this store called the police and was adamant that they needed to arrest Mr. Harper because he repeatedly entered and slept in the store, even after the property owner kicked him out and boarded up the store again. The officers explained that they talked to their sergeant, who instructed them, "Well, this guy has been breaking into this place on and off. At this point, we have to lock him up."

Space and Criminal Trespass

As emphasized in Chapter 3, "Decision-Making Contexts of Misdemeanor Charges," and Chapter 4, "Common Themes and Tensions," police officers are on the frontlines of criminal law enforcement and often have discretion in deciding whether to handle matters formally with an arrest or informally through discussion, negotiation, or persuasion with community members. The lens of location and the management of space illuminates how police officers use this discretion and why they make criminal trespass arrests that often ensnare people with SMI. Similar spaces were mentioned throughout our focus groups and interviews with a variety of criminal legal system stakeholders in all four cities: public transportation sites, apartment buildings and complexes (both occupied and vacant), and private businesses.

Our research documented that train stations and bus terminals are common sites where police make criminal trespass arrests due to a combination of heightened police presence, the concentration of homeless encampments, and pressure from elected officials and the public to "maintain order" (Diamond et al. 2021; Wood et al. 2023). However, police also exercise substantial discretion in these public spaces, frequently declining to make arrests for a host of violations including trespassing until they feel a person's behavior has transgressed a particular social norm. A prosecutor in Atlanta suggested that "how [a person] criminally trespassed," rather than the mere act of trespassing, is the critical factor. For example, "if this person becomes, for lack of a better word, a nuisance.... [If] they are consistently and continuously coming back," there is increased pressure from the public to make an arrest, and this pressure affects police decision-making.

A police supervisor in Atlanta explained that when police encounter someone in a public transit station who they suspect has an SMI, they typically try to assess the person's mental status and whether the person understands they are trespassing. Often, they consider taking the person to the local hospital rather than making an arrest. However, the police supervisor also said that officers may be more likely to make an arrest if they believe the person understands they are trespassing (in which case the element of the criminal law for "knowingly" trespassing can be applied) or if the person "acts out"—for example, bothers commuters: "they're like either yelling on the trains or they're throwing items … they're constantly just approaching people who are on their daily commute."

Whether an officer decides to make an arrest at or around a private business is shaped by pressures and demands from people in the area, such as the owners and patrons. A familiar cycle ensues: police repeatedly move along the same person who continues to return to a business, owners eventually get frustrated and ask for more coercive police action, and officers feel like they have no choice but to arrest. This dynamic is illustrated by a quote from a police officer in Atlanta:

> We get calls about people disrupting businesses—certain people with [SMI]—and they find a particular business or location that they like to go to, and they go there multiple times. So sometimes, they'll disrupt that business and then interact with people or cause some sort of commotion, whether it be dancing in the road, intimidating their customers, or yelling profanities, and the business wants them criminally trespassed. So that's when we issue that criminal trespass warning so that if they do come back, it makes it easier to deal with them because they have no reason to be there since they've been warned not to.

A criminal trespass arrest is often also used if an individual is suspected or known to have committed another misdemeanor offense such as retail theft (as described further in Chapter 6, "A $25 T-Shirt From the Bargain Store") or has a prior criminal history. For example, a Chicago public defense supervisor said that people will often be arrested for criminal trespass at stores like Target, Walgreens, or Subway where they have committed a prior retail theft and come back.

Police make arrests in private buildings when people are asked to leave the residence but refuse. Often, individuals encounter law enforcement because of the desperation of poverty: they enter a building they may or may not know they aren't allowed to be in because they need shelter to survive (Diamond et al. 2021; PBS News Hour 2020). Legal system professionals in several cities reported that homelessness and a preference for avoiding the shelter system contribute to these encounters. Police often make an arrest if someone is not compliant and refuses to leave, although the scenarios that police and other criminal legal system stakeholders encounter that lead to arrests in private residences differ across jurisdictions. For instance, an assistant district attorney (ADA) in Philadelphia described a man who lived in an apartment for years after the previous owner, his grandmother, died, and he refused to leave after he stopped paying taxes and was evicted. He wasn't aware that he didn't own the property ("his mental illness ... doesn't allow him to accept that the property is no longer his," said the ADA). Eventually, the new owner asked police to remove him.

Legal system professionals in a few cities also noted that police are called to remove people, usually adult children or spouses, from private spaces in the context of domestic disputes. If a person is violating a no-contact order (i.e., restraining orders or protective orders), police will generally make an arrest for the violation of the no-contact order rather than a criminal trespass charge. In certain cases, such arrests are mandatory, thereby constraining the options available to police. These scenarios are difficult when they involve a person with an SMI. An assistant state's attorney in Chicago remarked that "we're the court of last resort" for families who have tried to get a loved one with an SMI into treatment but have had that person cycle through hospitals and psychiatric facilities and continue to return and cause disturbances. Legal system professionals desire to address an underlying mental health issue that may be the reason the person violated a no-contact order, but police must contend with complainants who are "fed up" and want the person removed.

Managing Expectations About the Use of Space

As discussed earlier, criminal trespass laws serve as a formal tool for police to remove people who transgress the behavioral norms of a space. Some spaces are public property, whereas others are privately owned communal spaces such as retail stores (Kempa et al. 1999). As noted by a service provider in Chicago, the decision of police officers to pursue an arrest in lieu of a more informal approach is contingent on features of the place combined with concerns about the seriousness of the behavior and perceptions of the individual's mental state. Officers balance this calculus in relation to other people's sense of order and safety and the threshold of "disorderly" behavior they will tolerate. But officers may also lack awareness about the symptoms of mental illness. The same service provider described how this can present challenges for officers in the field:

> I would think ... probably part of it might depend on the business or place that they are at, whether or not that's kind of a high-profile spot, but then also perhaps the individual's response.... It can get more complicated if the person is combative in some way or really psychotic or under the influence of drugs or alcohol that may make it more complex. And I think just in the work that we've been doing with officers, some officers are not informed about mental illnesses. And so, if somebody is having psychotic symptoms, an officer could assume that they're on some sort of a substance as opposed to them being ill.

Police officers and other criminal legal system stakeholders cited two core purposes of criminal trespass law for their work: 1) it operates as a tool to move people along and remove them from public spaces where they are not wanted, and 2) it allows officers to resolve incidents with people who repeatedly don't cooperate with police orders and instructions. As the scenarios above reveal, these two rationales are critical elements of the officers' decision to use their discretion to arrest in each circumstance.

"Moving people along" (using the threat of a charge and potential arrest) and removing people (when they are arrested) are especially prevalent in the accounts legal system professionals provided, in which business owners or concerned community members pressured police officers to remove someone from a space. For example, sports arenas were mentioned as an example of a privately owned space where property owners can leverage their influence to get police to crack down more harshly and clear out people who are homeless and sleeping outside. Police and other legal system professionals had few choices in the face of the demands of businesses to get someone out of a space immediately. Responding to the desire to maintain the public image and status of these businesses often meant pursuing the path of least resistance and removing someone from a space immediately, which is what makes criminal trespass law an effective tool to resolve these complaints even if it does not address a person's underlying mental health or substance use issue. Police officers in several cities recounted a familiar rhythm produced by using criminal trespass to perform short-term space management—they continually encountered the same people in the same spaces again and again. In essence, both moving people along through the threat of a criminal trespass arrest and arresting people under certain circumstances accomplished the short-term goal of maintaining order and reasserting temporary control over a space. Moving people along and making arrests are not necessarily intended to solve the problems that necessitated criminal legal system contact, and nearly identical repeat encounters are likely.

The use of criminal trespass law also functions to temporarily incapacitate both those who do not cooperate with police orders and repeat offenders who may carry out another crime. Other community members eventually tire of seeing the same individuals repeatedly, and they call the police to ask them to arrest the individual rather than "move the person along" more informally. Prosecutors in Atlanta and police in Chicago both spoke about the problem of repeat encounters. The example of a gas station was given as a site that generates this recurring cycle: a station owner or employee asks someone to leave, they return the next week, the police are called, the police issue a warning and an order to disperse, and, finally, a criminal trespass arrest is made when complainants become exasperated by the ineffectiveness of softer approaches to enforcing rules and public order. While an individual may not have yet caused a major disturbance, the use of criminal trespass law allows officers to address the individual's history of rule breaking or their lack of cooperation with less coercive measures. The perceptions of community stakeholders can be critical, because they provide officers with knowledge of an individual's prior behavior and criminal history at that location.

Criminal trespassing statutes have some conceptual overlap with other legal tools that can be used to manage people's use of space, including disorderly conduct laws, public sleeping bans, or violations of no-contact orders. For example, a police supervisor in Atlanta spoke about their approach to reducing the large number of people sleeping at bus stops. They received a directive to move people along more aggressively, and made criminal trespass arrests, but also used an urban camping statute in cases that didn't meet the threshold of criminal trespass.

Officer Ambivalence Toward Criminal Trespass Enforcement

Police and other legal system professionals in our study expressed a broad sense of ambivalence toward the efficacy of using criminal trespass, even as they found it to be a useful short-term tool at times. Much of their ambivalence and frustration was based on the repetitive cycles of police being called to remove the same people from the same spaces and the lack of useful options to resolve the underlying issues of people who are homeless or dealing with an SMI. Whether officers convince a person to voluntarily leave the scene, or they take them to the hospital for an evaluation, the outcome is generally the same: that person returns to spaces where local stakeholders exert pressures for removal or banishment.

In Chicago, police officers described the gaps in systems of behavioral health care:

> There's absolutely zero resources that I'm aware of other than a hospital emergency room where these people can get any sort of treatment. So basically, it's a revolving door between the police interacting with them because citizens are calling, going to an emergency room, not getting adequate treatment, and then com[ing] right back to the street where they run into police again.

Officers in Chicago also explained that because criminal trespass is a misdemeanor offense, they usually do not expect that arresting someone for this misdemeanor will address any issue besides temporarily removing them from the scene. An assistant state's attorney in Chicago elaborated on how the process of encountering the same people repeatedly can wear down and desensitize officers, making them lose faith in the ability of the legal system to make a difference:

> A lot of times the officers are ... familiar with the person's issues or mental health issues just based upon repeated contacts. Depending on the officer, they're either going to just accept it, as, you know, just a pain and move on, or they're going to actually start pushing us to try and get some kind of resolution or solution to the problem.

These legal system stakeholders, both police and individuals working in criminal courts, were generally aligned in believing that the charge is a short-term solution that does not address the underlying issues or meet the material needs of system-involved people.

Risk of Racial Inequity and Other Social Inequities in the Enforcement of Criminal Trespass

As discussed in this chapter, people are arrested for criminal trespass because a confluence of circumstances—time, space, and other contextual factors including local standards of behavior and order—has occurred. In addition to symptoms of SMI, important dimensions of racial and social inequities may contribute to someone's vulnerability to arrest for being in the wrong place at the wrong time. Criminal legal system professionals in all four sites, as well as people with SMI who have been arrested for criminal trespass and other misdemeanor offenses, shared concerns about the role that bias and inequity plays in decisions about why particular public and private spaces are subject to scrutiny as opposed to others and how aggressively they are policed by law enforcement. For example, stakeholders from the Manhattan District Attorney's office explained that before the 2015 settlement of *Davis v. City of New York*, police conducted vertical sweeps of NYCHA residences and arrested individuals for criminal trespass as a strategy to dissuade drug selling and buying. One ADA highlighted how the policing of the specific type of building (public housing) as well as the specific type of drug (crack cocaine) contributed to the disproportionate criminalization of Black and Brown New Yorkers for criminal trespass and related drug possession offenses:

> They're also extremely racialized, crack and NYCHA housing. Both of those are, just because of the way society is and racism in the system, we're going to see more Black and Brown defendants coming in with a crack pipe case or a NYCHA-related case. Like, the people being policed are being overpoliced compared to non-NYCHA buildings, obviously, and a crack pipe is a much easier way to charge someone than a bag of already snorted powdered cocaine or used heroin—we're not charging residue for baggies, we're only charging it for crack pipes.

As a second example, the wife of a Black man arrested for criminal trespass in Atlanta explained that their landlord racially profiled her husband because of his dreadlocks and physical appearance. The landlord called the police on the husband when they were sitting and eating with their neighbors on their own property, and the police arrested him for criminal trespass without giving the couple an opportunity to explain that they lived on the property. This encounter illustrates that criminal trespass's fraught history is still relevant because the application of criminal trespass laws is still so dependent on the interests of business owners, property owners, and other private civilians, as well as the discretionary judgment of law enforcement. These actors have the power to decide whose and what conduct is acceptable in public and privately owned communal spaces. In many scenarios when police consider making an arrest for criminal trespass, the line between the policing of specific conduct and the policing of identity—racial and otherwise—can be easily transgressed.

Homelessness and a lack of stable and safe housing is the underlying issue for many cases in which someone is arrested for criminal trespass, and these issues are intertwined with racial and other systemic inequities (Homeless Hub 2023d; National Alliance to End Homelessness 2023e). Black, Indigenous, and other racialized populations are more likely to experience homelessness and extreme poverty compared with White people (Homeless Hub 2023e; National Alliance to End Homelessness 2020; National Alliance to End Homelessness 2023a; Olivet et al. 2021). In many cases, the lack of acceptable housing options—even when shelters are available—can create circumstances ripe for criminal trespass charges. This was described by a service provider in Manhattan:

> You'll find an overwhelming rate of homelessness for some folks charged with trespass. And a lot of them, that I can speak anecdotally about, don't want to go to the shelter system and will find other ways of maintaining a place to stay. And sometimes that's not in a place that's lawful or, you know, where someone else wants them to be.... An overwhelming rate of homelessness, of folks that just don't want to go into other shelter systems they don't feel safe in, there's other people around, and they'll find their other means of survival, where to stay, we'll see that a lot.

As the quote illustrates, many people experiencing homelessness do not feel safe or welcomed within the shelter system and may prefer to sleep outside on the streets. Queer and transgender youth and adults experiencing homelessness, for example, may feel safer sleeping outside on the streets than in shelters where they fear violence and discrimination (Fraser et al. 2019; Homeless Hub 2023b). A 2020 survey of 383 people experiencing homelessness in the city of Portland, Oregon, found racial disparities in the experiences of those surveyed; respondents who were Black, Indigenous, and people of color were less likely to access shelters and more likely to sleep on the streets without a tent, than White respondents (Zapata 2020).

For criminal legal system stakeholders and others who seek to address the harms of our existing systems, it is critical to be attuned to the potential risks of racial and other social inequities that may contribute to someone's vulnerability to being arrested for being in the wrong place at the wrong time. Policy and practice reforms must be designed, implemented, and evaluated with a focus on reducing these disparities and inequities.

Criminal Justice Reforms to Reduce the Use of Criminal Trespass Charges Among People With Serious Mental Illness

Individual Law Enforcement Officer Reforms

As the case study of the lawsuit *Davis v. City of New York* illustrates, jurisdictions can substantially reduce their use of criminal trespass arrests as a part of policing strategies like stop-and-frisk without major public safety concerns. Cities that are highly reliant on criminal trespass as a method to maintain public order—and particularly those cities whose data suggest that there are racial disparities in how criminal trespass is applied—should consider reevaluating their reliance on this tool to police public space. Jurisdictions might consider putting formal limits on the discretionary judgment of police officers to make arrests for criminal trespass, as the Philadelphia Police Department did through its policy change after the Starbucks incident. New training and procedures could emphasize de-escalation as well as mediation between the parties involved in a trespassing case.

Pre-arrest diversion programs, such as Atlanta's Policing Alternatives and Diversion Initiative, can serve as a substitution for arrest and criminal legal system sanctions for low-level offenses including criminal trespass. For example, 37% of the referrals that officers in Atlanta made to the city's Policing Alternatives and Diversion Initiative in 2022 were related to allegations of criminal trespass, the most frequent offense type (Harrell and Nam-Sonenstein 2023).

Larger Criminal Legal System Reforms

In addition to limiting the discretion of individual police officers and expanding pre-arrest diversion programs, jurisdictions might consider broader criminal legal system reforms. Several chapters in this book discuss the role that pretrial diversion programs, specialty treatment courts, and policies that can reduce failure-to-appear rates might play in reducing the harms of criminal legal system entanglement, as well as the trade-offs and potential challenges of these approaches. Chapter 10,"Reform in an Era of Mental Health and Crisis Services Innovation," also covers 911-dispatched, civilian crisis response programs that can respond to people experiencing homelessness and mental health issues as an alternative to police entirely. These programs aim to support people and make relevant referrals and connections to services. They often respond to calls for service that are low risk but account for a disproportionate number of 911 calls. For example, two of the most common 911 call types in many cities are calls involving a "suspicious person" and calls that are coded as a "business check," meaning they typically involve businesses calling 911 to respond to conduct near their business (Vera Institute of Justice 2022).

It is also worth monitoring legal changes initiated by the progressive prosecution movement, referenced in Chapter 3, which might shrink the scope of case processing for criminal trespass. In recent years, district attorney offices in cities such as New York, Baltimore, Philadelphia, and Los Angeles have issued policies that they will decline to prosecute cases for a host of low-level offenses (known as declination policies), including criminal trespass (ABC7.com 2020; ACLU Massachusetts 2019; Davis 2021; Mannarino and Cook 2022). When district attorney offices are less inclined to seek charges for certain offenses, it can have an upstream effect on police arrest practices. One recent study found that for the marginal defendant, nonprosecution of certain nonviolent misdemeanor offenses led to a 53% reduction in the likelihood that a defendant would receive a new criminal complaint and a 60% reduction in the number of new criminal complaints for a defendant over the next 2 years (Agan et al. 2023). This finding demonstrates that prosecutors' offices may improve public safety by simply declining to prosecute low-level misdemeanor cases and shrinking the scope of criminal legal system entanglement for those so charged in the process.

Mental Health Reforms to Reduce the Use of Criminal Trespass Charges Among People With Serious Mental Illness

Looking upstream of law enforcement and criminal legal system reforms, the housing and mental health sectors can focus on better meeting the underlying needs of people experiencing homelessness and living with an SMI through outreach and engagement efforts and increasing access to permanent, stable housing and mental health and other services. Doing so will reduce the reliance on criminal legal system tools, such as criminal trespass, to remove people from public spaces.

Outreach and Engagement Services

As part of a continuum of strategies to prevent and end homelessness and support people living with SMI, communities typically invest in some form of outreach and engagement services. Outreach services are important for engaging people experiencing homelessness who are disconnected from other services (for example, those who prefer not to access shelters) and should be "designed to help establish supportive relationships, give people advice and support, and hopefully enhance the possibility that they will access necessary services and supports that will help them move off the streets" (Homeless Hub 2023c). For outreach and engagement services to be successful at an individual and system level, they must be responsive to the individual needs of each person, grounded in an understanding of the barriers that have prevented people from accessing existing services, and focused on connecting people to the resources and services that will support them in accessing and maintaining permanent, stable housing (Homeless Hub 2023a; National Alliance to End Homelessness 2023b).

Outreach and engagement services can also target specific locations, including public spaces where homelessness may be more likely to be criminalized. For example, communities have considered investing in outreach workers and services for transit systems instead of deploying more law enforcement officers (McCann and Stagoff-Belfort 2022). An evaluation of policy options for Los Angeles County suggested that outreach services operated by a homelessness service provider could be more cost-effective than hiring police to handle the issue (Dembo 2020).

Philadelphia has also been developing a drop-in center model to reach community members experiencing homelessness and poverty, located in the concourse of one of the city's busiest commuter rail stations. The drop-in center, called the Hub of Hope, began as a temporary service during the coldest months of the year in 2011, expanded to a year-round program in 2018, and is operated by Philadelphia's Project HOME, a nonprofit service provider, in partnership with the city of Philadelphia and SEPTA, the Philadelphia region's transit agency. According to 2023 reporting by VICE, the Hub of Hope is "the only homeless drop-in center with food, medical, and hygiene facilities on transit property in the country" (Gordon 2023). A representative from Project HOME explained, "[t]he purpose of programs like the Hub of Hope is to provide a pathway into housing, but also to try to meet people's immediate needs for food, clothing, and shelter.... It's to have a place to be where they're not going to get kicked out" (Gordon 2023). In addition to meeting the needs of people experiencing homelessness, outreach and engagement services like the Hub of Hope offer a meaningful alternative to the tools of law enforcement and potential use of criminal trespass to remove people from public spaces who have nowhere else to go.

Improved Access to Supportive Housing

The overarching goal of reforms, strategies, and interventions to reduce criminal legal system entanglement for criminal trespass should be to increase access to permanent, stable housing and a range of mental health and other services. Key strategies, which can be linked to outreach and engagement services, include rapid rehousing and Housing First interventions that pair shorter-term and/or longer-term housing supports (for example, housing case managers or navigators, and rental assistance) with other health and supportive services (Homeless Hub 2023a; National Alliance to End Homelessness 2023c; National Alliance to End Homelessness 2023d). Importantly, these types of housing supports are provided without any preconditions (such as sobriety), and services are voluntary (Homeless Hub 2023a; National Alliance to End Homelessness 2023c; National Alliance to End Homelessness 2023d).

KEY POINTS

- Criminal trespass statutes were rarely applied before the Civil War, but they became popular during Jim Crow to enforce racial segregation and restrict the freedom of movement of Black people. As demonstrated by recent controversies, such as the cases of the Philadelphia Starbucks and the NYCHA lawsuits, and comments from some of our focus group respondents, concerns remain around the use of trespassing statutes that allow for racial profiling and exacerbate disparities.

- Criminal trespass is a common charge in the United States for people with and without serious mental illness. There is substantial police discretion to make an arrest for criminal trespass or to resolve issues informally. Mention of similar spaces recurred throughout our study as likely sites where trespass arrests are made, particularly public transportation, apartment buildings and complexes (both occupied and vacant), and private businesses.

- Police officers and other criminal legal system stake-holders offer two core purposes of criminal trespass law for their work: it operates as a tool to move people along or to remove them from public spaces where they are not wanted by making an arrest, and it allows officers to resolve incidents with people who repeatedly do not co-operate with police orders and instructions.

- The interests of private civilians—particularly business and other property owners—and their demands to po-lice asking that unwanted people be removed from the privately owned communal spaces, are a critical factor in whether police are compelled to make arrests.

- The repetitive cycle of criminal trespass law enforce-ment—the same people in the same places—may be one reason that police and other legal system professionals expressed a broad sense of ambivalence toward the ef-ficacy of arresting people for criminal trespass, even as they found it to be a useful short-term tool at times. Po-lice described how the process of encountering the same people repeatedly can wear down and desensitize officers, making them lose faith in the ability of the legal system to make a difference.

- A variety of reforms to criminal legal tools (limiting offi-cer discretion, new training procedures, pre-arrest di-version, and nonpolice crisis response), mental health systems (outreach and engagement services), and so-cial services (supportive housing) may limit the scenar-ios that often lead to criminal trespass arrests as well as disparities in application of the charge.

References

ABC7.com: New DA Gascon to decline prosecution on range of low-level crimes. ABC7 Los Angeles, December 10, 2020. Available at: https://abc7.com/george-gascon-los-angeles-district-attorney-lada-misdemeanor-crimes/8674095/. Accessed November 5, 2023.

ACLU Massachusetts: Facts over fear: benefits of declining to prosecute misde-meanor, low-level felonies. ACLU Massachusetts, March 19, 2019. Available at: https://www.aclum.org/en/press-releases/facts-over-fear-benefits-declin-ing-prosecute-misdemeanor-low-level-felonies. Accessed May 20, 2024.

Agan A, Doleac JL, Harvey A: Misdemeanor prosecution. Q J Econ 138:1453–1505, 2023

Beckett K, Herbert S: Penal boundaries: banishment and the expansion of punishment. Law Soc Inq 35:1–38, 2010

Bell v. Maryland, 378 U.S. 226, 84 S. Ct. 1814 (1964)

Bouie v. City of Columbia, 378 U.S. 347 (1964)

Cohen W: Negro involuntary servitude in the South, 1865–1940: a preliminary analysis. J South Hist 42:31–60, 1976

Compton MT, Zern A, Pope LG, et al: Misdemeanor charges among individuals with serious mental illnesses: a statewide analysis of more than two million arrests. Psychiatr Serv 74(1):31–37, 2023 35795979

Davis P: State's Attorney Mosby defends decision to not prosecute some classes of crimes, says city preparing 911 call diversion system. Baltimore Sun, April 14, 2021. Available at: https://www.baltimoresun.com/news/crime/bs-md-ci-cr-mosby-prosecution-committee-hearing-20210414-trg6iil3rvhv5mh3jgedg2n4gu-story.html. Accessed November 5, 2023.

Davis v. City of New York, 10 Civ. 0699 (SAS) (S.D.N.Y. May 5, 2011)

Dembo M: Off the Rails: Alternatives to Policing on Transit. Los Angeles, UCLA Institute of Transportation Studies, 2020

Diamond B, Burns R, Bowen K: Criminalizing homelessness: circumstances surrounding criminal trespassing and people experiencing homelessness. Crim Justice Policy Rev 33:563–583, 2021

Du Bois WEB: Black Reconstruction in America: Toward a History of the Part Which Black Folk Played in the Attempt to Reconstruct Democracy in America, 1860–1880. Abingdon, U.K., Routledge, 2017

Foner E: Reconstruction Updated Edition: America's Unfinished Revolution, 1863–1877. New York, HarperCollins, 2014

Fraser B, Pierse N, Chisholm E, et al: LGBTIQ+ homelessness: a review of the literature. Int J Environ Res Public Health 16(15):2677, 2019 31357432

Gibson TA: Securing the Spectacular City: The Politics of Revitalization and Homelessness in Downtown Seattle. Lanham, MD, Lexington Books, 2003

Goluboff RL: Vagrant Nation: Police Power, Constitutional Change, and the Making of the 1960s. New York, Oxford University Press, 2016

Goluboff RL, Sorensen A: United States vagrancy laws, in The Oxford Encyclopedia of American Urban History. New York, Oxford University Press, 2018

Gordon A: "They just need a safe place to be:" how public transit became the last safety net in America. Vice, May 4, 2023. Available at: https://www.vice.com/en/article/y3wvq5/they-just-need-a-safe-place-to-be-how-public-transit-became-the-last-safety-net-in-america. Accessed November 5, 2023.

Griffin v. Maryland, 378 U.S. 130, 84 S. Ct. 1770 (1964)

Harrell L, Nam-Sonenstein B: Unhoused and under arrest: how Atlanta polices poverty. Prison Policy Initiative, June 8, 2023. Available at: https://www.prisonpolicy.org/blog/2023/06/08/atlanta-poverty. Accessed November 5, 2023.

Homeless Hub: Housing first, in Homeless Hub: Solutions. Toronto, ON, Canadian Observatory on Homelessness, 2023a. Available at: https://www.homelesshub.ca/solutions/housing-accommodation-and-supports/housing-first. Accessed November 5, 2023.

Homeless Hub: Lesbian, gay, bisexual, transgender, transsexual, queer, questioning and two-spirit (LGBTQ2S), in Homeless Hub: About Homelessness. Toronto, ON, Canadian Observatory on Homelessness, 2023b. Available at: https://www.homelesshub.ca/about-homelessness/population-specific/lesbian-gay-bisexual-transgender-transsexual-queer. Accessed November 5, 2023.

Homeless Hub: Outreach, in Homeless Hub: Solutions. Toronto, ON, Canadian Observatory on Homelessness, 2023c. Available at: https://www.homelesshub.ca/solutions/emergency-response/outreach. Accessed November 5, 2023.

Homeless Hub: Population specific, in Homeless Hub: About Homelessness. Toronto, ON, Canadian Observatory on Homelessness, 2023d. Available at: https://www.homelesshub.ca/about-homelessness/topics/population-specific. Accessed November 5, 2023.

Homeless Hub: Racialized Communities, in Homeless Hub: About Homelessness. Toronto, ON, Canadian Observatory on Homelessness, 2023e. Available at: https://www.homelesshub.ca/about-homelessness/population-specific/racialized-communities. Accessed November 5, 2023.

Irizarry-Aponte C: Philly cops issue new trespassing policy in response to criticism over Starbucks arrests. The Philadelphia Inquirer, June 8, 2018. Available at: https://www.inquirer.com/philly/news/philadelphia-police-starbucks-trespass-policy-20180608.html. Accessed November 5, 2023.

Johnston H: The use of trespass laws to enforce private policies of discrimination. UC Law Journal 16:445, 1965

Kempa M, Carrier R, Wood J, et al: Reflections on the evolving concept of "private policing."European Journal on Criminal Policy and Research 7:197–223, 1999

Legal Defense Fund: Davis v. City of New York. Washington, DC, Legal Defense Fund, 2010. Available at: https://www.naacpldf.org/case-issue/davis-v-city-new-york. Accessed November 5, 2023.

Lewis A: Legal history backs British on trespass. The New York Times, July 22, 1982. Available at: https://www.nytimes.com/1982/07/22/world/legal-history-backs-british-on-trespass.html. Accessed November 5, 2023.

Mannarino D, Cook L: "Status quo is not working": Manhattan DA defends new policy on not prosecuting some crimes. Pix 11, January 9, 2022. Available at: https://pix11.com/news/politics/pixonpolitics/status-quo-is-not-working-manhattan-da-defends-policy-on-not-prosecuting-some-crimes. Accessed November 5, 2023.

McCann S, Stagoff-Belfort A: More police won't make public transit safer. Housing and social services will. Vera Institute of Justice, June 17, 2022. Available at: https://www.vera.org/news/more-police-wont-make-public-transit-safer-housing-and-social-services-will. Accessed November 5, 2023.

Morgan R, Thompson A: Criminal Victimization, 2020. Washington, DC, Bureau of Justice Statistics, 2021. Available at: https://bjs.ojp.gov/sites/g/files/xyckuh236/files/media/document/cv20.pdf

Natapoff A: Punishment Without Crime: How Our Massive Misdemeanor System Traps the Innocent and Makes America More Unequal. New York, Basic Books, 2018

National Alliance to End Homelessness: Racial Inequalities in Homelessness, by the Numbers. Washington, DC, National Alliance to End Homelessness, 2020. Available at: https://endhomelessness.org/resource/racial-inequalities-homelessness-numbers/. Accessed November 5, 2023.

National Alliance to End Homelessness: Homelessness and Racial Disparities. Washington, DC, National Alliance to End Homelessness, 2023a. Available at: https://endhomelessness.org/homelessness-in-america/what-causes-homelessness/inequality/. Accessed November 5, 2023.

National Alliance to End Homelessness: Solutions—Crisis Response. Washington, DC, National Alliance to End Homelessness, 2023b. Available at: https://endhomelessness.org/ending-homelessness/solutions/crisis-response/. Accessed November 5, 2023.

National Alliance to End Homelessness: Solutions—Permanent Supportive Housing. Washington, DC, National Alliance to End Homelessness, 2023c. Available at: https://endhomelessness.org/ending-homelessness/solutions/permanent-supportive-housing/. Accessed November 5, 2023.

National Alliance to End Homelessness: Solutions—Rapid Re-Housing. Washington, DC, National Alliance to End Homelessness, 2023d. Available at: https://endhomelessness.org/ending-homelessness/solutions/rapid-re-housing/. Accessed November 5, 2023.

National Alliance to End Homelessness: What Causes Homelessness? 2023e. Available at: https://endhomelessness.org/homelessness-in-america/what-causes-homelessness/. Accessed November 5, 2023.

Olivet J, Wilkey C, Richard M, et al: Racial inequity and homelessness: findings from the SPARC study. Ann Am Acad Pol Soc Sci 693:82–100, 2021

PBS News Hour: Cities try to arrest their way out of homeless problems. PBS News Hour, June 29, 2020. Available at: https://www.pbs.org/newshour/nation/cities-try-to-arrest-their-way-out-of-homeless-problems. Accessed November 5, 2023.

Sanchez R: Philly police issue new trespassing policy after Starbucks arrests. CNN, June 8, 2018. Available at: https://www.cnn.com/2018/06/08/us/philadelphia-police-starbucks-trespassing/index.html. Accessed November 5, 2023.

Sawers B: Race and property after the civil war: creating the right to exclude. Miss Law J 87(5), 2018

Sawers B: What lies behind that "No Trespass" sign. The Atlantic, July 2, 2022. Available at: https://www.theatlantic.com/ideas/archive/2022/07/the-true-meaning-of-no-trespass/661471/. Accessed November 5, 2023.

Scrivener L, Meizlish A, Bond E, et al: Tracking enforcement trends in New York City: 2003–2018. New York, Data Collaborative for Justice, 2020. Available at: https://datacollaborativeforjustice.org/wp-content/uploads/2020/09/2020_08_31_Enforcement.pdf. Accessed November 5, 2023.

Vera Institute of Justice: 911 Analysis: call data shows we can rely less on police. Vera Institute of Justice, April 2022. Available at: https://www.vera.org/downloads/publications/911-analysis-we-can-rely less-on-police.pdf. Accessed November 5, 2023.

Vitale AS: City of Disorder: How the Quality of Life Campaign Transformed New York Politics. New York, NYU Press, 2008

Williamson J: The Orwellian police tactic that targets Black Americans for simply existing. Salon, April 15, 2015. Available at: https://www.salon.com/2015/04/15/the_orwellian_police_tactic_that_targets_black_americans_for_simply_existing/. Accessed November 5, 2023.

Winberg M: Philly police get new rules for "defiant trespass" after Starbucks arrests. Billy Penn at WHYY. June 8, 2018. Available at: https://billypenn.com/2018/06/08/philly police-get-new-rules-for-defiant-trespass-after-starbucks-arrests. Accessed November 5, 2023.

Wood JD, Watson AC, Pope L, et al: Contexts shaping misdemeanor system interventions among people with mental illnesses: qualitative findings from a multi-site system mapping exercise. Health Justice 11(1):20, 2023 37014478

Wood M: Goluboff's "Vagrant Nation" Uncovers Rapid Revolution in Nation's Laws, Police Power. Charlottesville, VA, University of Virginia School of Law, 2016. Available at: https://www.law.virginia.edu/news/201601/goluboffs-vagrant-nation-uncovers-rapid-revolution-nations-laws-police-power. Accessed November 5, 2023.

Zapata M: Survey on Needs of People Living Unsheltered. Portland, OR, Portland State University, 2020. Available at: https://www.pdx.edu/homelessness/survey-needs-people-living-unsheltered. Accessed November 5, 2023.

6

A $25 T-Shirt From the Bargain Store

Shoplifting and Criminal Legal System Entanglement

Leah G. Pope, Ph.D.

Shoplifting—also known as retail theft and petit larceny—is a category of theft or larceny that occurs when a person knowingly takes goods from a retail establishment without paying the purchase price. It is considered perhaps the most common offense committed in the United States: the National Association of Shoplifting Prevention estimates that 1 in 11 Americans has shoplifted during his or her lifetime (National Association for Shoplifting Prevention 2021). Bob Nardelli, the former CEO of Home Depot, recently warned that shoplifting "is an epidemic … spreading faster than COVID," and several states are stiffening penalties for individuals caught stealing from stores (Lewis 2023). This chapter explores shoplifting as a type of misdemeanor offense that frequently results in system entanglement for people with serious mental illness (SMI). I begin by exploring the scope of the problem and the specifics of shoplifting charges in Georgia, Illinois, New York, and Pennsylvania, where our study was carried out. I then review historical perspectives on retail theft and describe what is currently known about who engages in shoplifting and who is arrested for shoplifting, including those with SMI. The remainder of the chapter draws on qualitative data from focus groups to illuminate the reasoning of criminal legal system stakeholders when it comes to using shoplifting charges, as well as the perspectives of professionals who work to defend people charged with retail theft. The focus group data are also used to illuminate the perspectives and experience of people with SMI who are arrested on such charges. By drawing on several case examples from study data, we can more easily understand how a seemingly trivial charge like shoplifting often leads to unexpected cycles of criminal legal system entanglement.

Scope of the Problem: Shoplifting in the United States

Shoplifting has been the focus of increasing media coverage over the past several years, with headlines across the country warning about "shoplifting hitting record highs" (McCarthy et al. 2023) and increased coverage of "smash-and-grab" incidents and "organized retail crime" (Center for Just Journalism 2023). Nonetheless, a clear picture of the extent of retail theft nationally is hindered by several problems. First, many shoplifting incidents go unreported. Second, many police departments across the country do not submit their data to the Federal Bureau of Investigation (FBI). For example, only 67% of law enforcement agencies submitted their crime data to the FBI as of January 1, 2023 (Criminal Justice Statistics Interagency Working Group of the National Science and Technology Council 2023). Third, retail theft is not an independent category in most crime data published by police departments but rather is included in broader crime categories such as larceny or burglary (Center for Just Journalism 2023; Dabney et al. 2004). Fourth, much of the cited data on retail theft comes from retail industry groups whose data are not necessarily reliable given the group's reliance on self-report surveys from only a few dozen retailers (Center for Just Journalism 2023).

These limitations notwithstanding, available crime data can be used to get a sense of broad trends in shoplifting. The FBI's Uniform Crime Reporting Program estimates that in 2019 there were 904,975 shoplifting offenses in the United States, accounting for 22% of all larceny thefts (excluding motor vehicle thefts). Larceny theft offenses declined over the decade between 2009 and 2019 but still account for the largest proportion of offenses; shoplifting remained steady at ~20% of all larceny theft offenses during the same period (Federal Bureau of Investigation 2020). A more recent study comparing shoplifting trends in the first half of 2023 to before the coronavirus pandemic in 24 cities showed a mixed picture, with reported shoplifting incidents increasing in 7 of the cities and decreasing in the remaining 17. Further, that study suggested that increases in shoplifting were driven by the large number of incidents in New York City during that period. When New York City is included in the analysis, total shoplifting incidents were 16% higher during the first half of 2023 compared with the first half of 2019. When New York City is removed from the analysis, however, there were about 7% fewer shoplifting incidents in the remaining 23 cities in the first half of 2023 compared with the first half of 2019 (Lopez et al. 2023).

Shoplifting results in substantial economic losses for retail companies. Estimates culled from recent data from the National Retail Federation (2022) indicate that "retail shrink" led to $94.5 billion in losses in 2021. Individual shoplifters do not account for this entire loss. Other sources of loss are attributable to organized retail theft, employee/internal theft, and process/control failures; individual shoplifting incidents result in comparatively low-level dollar losses. For example, survey data from 2018 revealed that 36.6% of shoplifting incidents resulted in dollar losses of less than $150, and 70.8% of incidents resulted in dollar losses of less than $300 (National Retail Federation 2019). Nonetheless, the total value of losses helps explain increasing concern over retail theft in many places across the country (see news coverage, for example, in Lewis 2023 and McCarthy et al. 2023).

Criminal Charges Related to Shoplifting

Misdemeanor shoplifting is a somewhat complicated charge to understand across locations because each state sets statutory definitions about the dollar value that distinguishes misdemeanor and felony charges, which has consequences for the imposed penalties. States also have different statutes for upgrading charges based on a person's prior history of retail theft. Table 6–1 provides the relevant statutes for "theft by shoplifting," "retail theft," and "petit larceny" in Georgia, Illinois, New York, and Pennsylvania.

Two observations are worth further explanation because they set the stage for a better understanding of how people get entangled in cycles

Table 6–1. State retail theft statutes

Statute	Offense	Threshold for misdemeanor	Escalating penalties	Additional information
Georgia, Ga. Code § 16–8–14 (2022)	Theft by shoplifting	≤$500	On conviction of fourth or subsequent offense, defendants shall be guilty of a felony.	Additional provisions for felony charges occur when aggregate value of theft exceeds $500 in 180 days.
Illinois, 720 ILCS 5/ § 16–25 (2022)	Retail theft	<$300	Felony offense occurs when person was previously convicted of any type of theft, robbery, armed robbery, burglary, residential burglary, burglary, possession of burglary tools, home invasion, unlawful use of a credit card, or forgery.	Additional provisions for felony charges are rendered when aggregate value exceeds $300 in a 1-year period.
New York, NY Penal Law § 155.25 (2022)	Petit larceny	≤$1,000	None.	When a person is arrested for stealing from a store where they have already been given a trespass notice, they can be charged with burglary in the third degree, a class D felony.
Pennsylvania, 18 Pa. C.S. § 3929 (2022)	Retail theft	<$150*	A third or subsequent offense is considered a felony offense regardless of the value of the merchandise.	Amounts can be aggregated across instances or stores when determining the grade of the charge.

*In Pennsylvania, retail theft is a (i) summary offense [considered less serious than a misdemeanor] when it is a first offense and value of the merchandise is less than $150. Retail theft constitutes a (ii) misdemeanor of the second degree when the offense is a second offense and value of the merchandise is less than $150 and (iii) misdemeanor of first degree when the offense is a first or second offense and value of the merchandise is $150 or more.

of criminal legal system involvement because of misdemeanor shoplifting charges. First, there is a broad range for the threshold value of stolen goods in deciding between misdemeanor and felony shoplifting charges. In Illinois, felony charges can be brought when the value of merchandise is $300. In New York, by contrast, felony charges can only be brought when the value of stolen goods exceeds $1,000. Other states have other thresholds, and there has been recent attention to changing felony theft thresholds to ensure that value-based penalties take inflation into account (Pew Charitable Trusts 2017). The state in which the theft occurs matters a great deal in terms of the value of merchandise stolen that can trigger felony charges.

Second, state statutes provide for escalating penalties based on a person's history. In Georgia, a conviction of a fourth or subsequent offense for shoplifting automatically results in a felony conviction regardless of the value of stolen merchandise (and is punishable by a prison sentence of up to 10 years). In New York, although there is no statutory language about escalating penalties for repeated misdemeanor shoplifting offenses, a person can be charged with burglary in the third degree (NY Penal Law § 140.20) if they have previously been issued a "trespass notice" by the retail store. In other words, someone who has been warned by a store that they don't have permission to shop there (via a trespass notice) and then returns and is caught attempting to steal something is now liable for a felony charge—"knowingly enter[ing] or remain[ing] unlawfully in a building with intent to commit a crime therein" (NY Penal Law § 140.20).

There is a history of case law that informs these statutes. In *United States v. Bean* (1971), the Superior Court for the District of Columbia held that a retail business establishment can exclude from its premises a particular member of the public solely on the grounds of his previous arrest for shoplifting and that criminal trespass statutes are applicable if the person refuses to leave (Duke Law Journal 1971). While common law suggests that business owners extend express or implied permission ("effective consent") to enter their business and can withdraw that permission at any time, the right to exclude is limited by certain constitutional and statutory provisions; for example, the Civil Rights Act of 1964 prevents exclusion based on race. However, the *Bean* ruling extended common law rights for property owners, allowing them to withdraw permission for entry based on a person's arrest record. Further, many state burglary statutes are written in such a way that once a person receives a notice from a store that they are no longer allowed on the premises (even if they do not receive a formal criminal trespass charge), such a notice constitutes a denial of "effective consent" to enter the property, and an act of shoplifting thus becomes a crime of burglary (Bailey 2010; Harwell 2016). (See Chapter 5, "Being in the Wrong Place," for a full discussion of the history of criminal trespass law and the authority of property owners to exclude people from spaces.) These issues, and the challenges that people with SMI, in particular, may face in understanding the relevant laws, are explored in more detail below in examining data from our study that assessed trajectories of people charged with retail theft or shoplifting.

Who Shoplifts, and Who Gets Accused of and Arrested for Shoplifting?

Despite the frequency of shoplifting in the United States, the literature on shoplifting is relatively limited. Rachel Shteir (2011) provided an overview of the history of shoplifting in her book *The Steal: A Cultural History of Shoplifting*. Shteir described how shoplifting "reflects our shifting moral code" (p. 10), tracing early attention to "lifters" in sixteenth century London and the development of laws making shoplifting punishable by hanging, to the coining of the word *kleptomania* in 1816, to the counterculture era of the 1960s when shoplifting was cast as revolution. "Shoplifting has been a sin, a crime, a confession of sexual repression, a howl of grief, a political yelp, a sign of depression, a badge of identity, and a back door to the American Dream," she wrote (p. 10). Since the 1960s, there have been several attempts to understand and classify "the shoplifter." Seminal studies include Cameron's (1964) work on "boosters" (professional thieves) and "snitches" (chronic shoplifters but otherwise "respectable" citizens), and Moore's (1984) typology of five different kinds of shoplifters ("impulse," "occasional," "episodic," "amateur," and "semi-professional").

Additional research has examined factors associated with shoplifting such as sex, age, race/ethnicity, and psychiatric disorder. Using data from the National Epidemiologic Survey on Alcohol and Related Conditions, Blanco et al. (2008) provided the most up-to-date understanding about the lifetime prevalence, correlates, and comorbidity of shoplifting among adults in the United States. At least five findings are noteworthy: 1) self-reported shoplifting was relatively common in the sample, with an overall lifetime prevalence of 11.3% (95% CI 10.6–12.1); 2) self-reported shoplifting was significantly higher in men than in women; 3) non-Hispanic White people had higher odds of shoplifting than Black, Hispanic, and Asian American people; 4) shoplifting was significantly more common among individuals with at least some college education and among those with individual incomes higher than $35,000 and family incomes higher than $70,000; and 5) the majority of individuals with a lifetime history of self-reported shoplifting (89.3%) had a lifetime history of at least one psychiatric diagnosis, compared with 49.5% in nonshoplifters. Among people with psychiatric disorders who shoplifted, the strongest associations were found for antisocial personality disorders and substance use disorders, as well as with other disorders associated with deficits in impulse control (e.g., bipolar disorder, pathological gambling).

Sex, Race, and Ethnicity

Research has been equivocal with respect to findings about race and sex and shoplifting behavior. For example, self-report and observational studies have found no significant differences along racial lines in shoplifting activity after controlling for socioeconomic status (Dabney et al. 2004; Gold 1970; Hindelang 1981). And while some studies suggest males have higher rates of shoplifting than females do (Bamfield 2012; Blanco et al. 2008), others demonstrate nearly equal rates for males and females (Marshal and He 2010).

Despite evidence that shoplifting behavior is likely similar across race and ethnicity, racial disparities exist in terms of who is accused of shoplifting and who is arrested for it, as well as what sentences people receive if convicted. There is a distinct literature on consumer racial profiling, more informally called "shopping while Black" (Dabney et al. 2006; Gabbidon 2003; Gabbidon and Higgins 2020; Harris 2003; Harris et al. 2005; Massey et al. 2022). Such literature describes situations in which suspicion of shoplifting in retail stores is frequently initiated by retail staff and disproportionately applied based on the customer's race. In these cases, racial profiling that starts in the community may then be compounded by additional discretionary decisions in the criminal legal system that are affected by racial bias (e.g., bias in decision-making around setting bail)—a type of "cumulative disadvantage" that adversely affects Black people charged with shoplifting (Kutateladze et al. 2014). In their study, Massey et al. (2022) found that Black men were more likely to be targets of "excess suspicion" insofar as they made up a significantly larger proportion of individuals who were initially suspected of larceny but who did not end up being arrested. In the same study, Black men were less likely than White men to be offered an Adjournment in Contemplation of Dismissal (ACD) for shoplifting. ACDs demonstrate some measure of leniency, since they are an agreement that allows for the eventual dismissal of charges against someone after a fixed period if the person is not arrested again during that time. Further, Black men convicted of larceny were 1.8 times more likely than White men convicted of larceny to receive a sentence that included incarceration (Massey et al. 2022). Findings from studies such as the one conducted by Massey et al. (2022) highlight the myriad ways that racial profiling permeates shoplifting cases, from the initial suspicions among retail staff to the consequences of that suspicion in terms of arrest and case outcomes; they also remind us that statistics on shoplifting arrest, convictions, and sentencing can reflect discriminatory suspicion and arrest patterns rather than any differences in actual shoplifting behavior.

Socioeconomic Status and Serious Mental Illness

As described above, epidemiologic survey data show that a history of shoplifting behavior is substantially associated with some behavioral health disorders, with the strongest associations found for antisocial personality disorders and substance use disorders (Blanco et al. 2008). The interaction between mental illness and socioeconomic status in relation to shoplifting behavior is less clear, however, and complicates an understanding of why people shoplift. The study by Blanco et al. (2008) found that shoplifting was more common among those with higher income and concluded that financial considerations are unlikely to be the main motivator for shoplifting in most cases. This focus on individual psychopathology rather than socioeconomic circumstances resonates with the literature on kleptomania and shoplifting as evidence of an impulse control disorder or OCD (Krasnovsky and Lane 1998; Shteir 2011). Conversely, several studies have found low income as a contributing factor to chronic shoplifting and economic disadvantage as a motivational factor in shoplifting cases (Krasnovsky and Lane 1998). In our research studies previously cited in Chapter 1 ("The System, the Process, and the Contexts"), shoplifting was among the most common charges in two samples of people with SMI. As the Georgia-based study described, among 240 patients recruited from three inpatient facilities, 39 individuals (6%) had been arrested for shoplifting, making it the fourth most common charge (behind criminal trespassing, willful obstruction of a law enforcement officer, and disorderly conduct) (Compton et al. 2022). In the New York–based study, petit larceny was the most common charge among all arrests in the state from 2010 through 2013, and the larceny theft uniform crime reporting (UCR) code was significantly more likely to be used in arrests involving individuals with an SMI indicator than in arrests involving those without the indicator

(16.3% vs. 13.6%) (Compton et al. 2023). These data suggest that people with SMI who also experience other criminogenic risks such as unemployment or underemployment, low education, and housing instability may be at high risk for behaviors such as shoplifting by virtue of their psychosocial circumstances rather than their mental illness per se. In the following sections, this dynamic between SMI and concurrent socioeconomic disadvantage is explored further by drawing on a case example and the perspectives of criminal legal system professionals who encounter and process shoplifting charges among people with SMI.

Case Example: Ms. George Arrested at a Bargain Store

Aleana George is a 31-year-old divorced Black woman who was living with her children in a hotel at the time of our interview with her. She was a client at a local mental health agency where she attended weekly appointments. She had a history of misdemeanor arrests, including for the charges of shoplifting, criminal trespass, and disorderly conduct. Ms. George described to us how her first arrest was for shoplifting an item worth about $25 from a bargain store and how it led to a long entanglement with the criminal legal system:

> Me and my sister were at [bargain store] and she was the one actually stealing. I don't steal. I wasn't stealing. But I was holding the purse, and I knew she was stealing. So, when we were walking out of [store], they stopped me and grabbed the purse, and my sister took off running. So, I was the one who took the fall for it basically. They made me go back to a room in [store] to see what I had. First, they told me I wouldn't go to jail because I was cooperating, and they would just write a ticket out. But because it was $25—[store's] policy I guess is if it's $25 or higher they have to prosecute and put you in jail. So, they ended up calling the police on me. That was my first time ever getting arrested. The police were actually nice to me. They weren't mean to me. They weren't rude. They weren't nasty. I got bailed out by my sister [after a few hours].

Although this initial interaction was relatively brief, Ms. George's criminal legal involvement was compounded in the coming months while she waited for her court case to proceed. As she described, "I had one court appearance and my brother told me to plead no contest. Then I skipped another court appearance, and I had a warrant out for my arrest." This missed court appearance proved to have serious consequences. After the warrant was issued, Ms. George got into an argument with her ex-husband about child custody concerns, and he called the police on her. When the police arrived, they ran a check and saw that she had a warrant; they arrested her immediately for her failure to appear in court and also added new charges for criminal trespass and disorderly conduct. Ms. George spent another 4 months in jail waiting for a new court date. She described how at that point her public defender wanted her to take a plea deal. "I ended up getting on probation. But then I broke my probation, and I did 45 days in jail." Her total stay in jail was approximately 5.5 months due to missing the court date and violating the probation stipulations—a cascade of criminal legal involvement that started with shoplifting a $25 T-shirt.

Criminal Legal System Professionals' Perspectives on Shoplifting Among People With Serious Mental Illness

Ms. George's arrest for shoplifting provides an opportunity for considering the perspectives of criminal justice professionals who are involved in some manner in the use and processing of this charge—from the police who respond to calls for service related to shoplifting to the prosecutors who bring shoplifting charges against defendants and the defenders who represent those facing such charges. In our study, professionals in each of these categories almost unanimously described shoplifting among people with mental illness as being a "crime of survival." Whether shoplifting items for daily personal use (e.g., food, soap) or items that could easily be resold on the street for money (e.g., razors, detergent), focus group participants described that items stolen were generally "very small dollar amounts." One police supervisor in Atlanta gave the following description:

> You think of shoplifting as somebody is gonna go in and steal a TV or something like that. And with these people, it's not always the case. They're going in to steal the things that you need on a daily basis to survive, you know, soap or food or a can of soup or whatever. And I would say 90%, maybe not that, about 80% of our shoplifting, that's what it is, little, small amounts, stuff like that.

The focus on stealing low-value, everyday items was supported by other professionals who talked about shoplifting among people with mental illnesses in the context of poverty. As one assistant district attorney (ADA) in New York remarked, "I'd say they're crimes of desperation. A lot of it is tied to poverty, and ... it's sometimes poverty related to mental illness." Some focus group participants also noted that shoplifting may be used to support drug use as a way of self-medicating—and that it could be difficult to untangle whether or how mental illness or substance use problems were driving shoplifting behavior.

Regardless of why a person is shoplifting—and even in the context of shoplifting items that are of low value—police described how their approach to shoplifting very much depends on what the store owner wants to do in any given scenario. "It goes on the complainant as well," remarked a Chicago officer. "I guess the dollar amount, how much they were stealing, whether the product was recovered.... And they [store owners] are like, 'Ok, well, it's on you guys [police], whatever you [police] want to do.' But it's actually on you—you're the complainant. What do you want? What do you want done?" Large chain stores and retail pharmacies often have loss prevention officers on site, and participants described such stores as being more likely to press charges. For smaller stores, although police described some store owners who "are adamant about locking somebody up for a bag of chips," they also noted that many store owners don't want to press charges. Rather, they just want a solution to prevent the individual from coming back to their store again. "They're tired of seeing that person and they want some kind of no-contact order...which is basically just a warning," noted a public defender in Chicago.

While issuing a warning for a first-time shoplifter might be considered a reasonable strategy for preventing the behavior in the future, criminal justice professionals described how shoplifting situations were especially complicated in cases where an individual has a mental illness because such individuals often "don't understand the risk" of repeated shoplifting incidents from a legal perspective. As shown in Table 6–1, states have escalating penalties for repeated shoplifting offenses. However, many stakeholders indicated that people do not always know about these escalating penalties, particularly if they have a mental illness. Had Ms. George been in New York, for example, and instead been given a trespass notice for her shoplifting incident, she might not have understood that any subsequent shoplifting incidents at the same store could be charged as a felony. Professionals spoke about people with mental illnesses returning to the same location to steal even after a warning because they didn't understand the risk of more serious consequences for repeated offenses. "The bottom line is [the store owners] want them to stay away for 3 to 6 months. Well, that's a creature of habit. This person is going to be there the next day," remarked a Chicago defense attorney. One prosecutor in Atlanta thought prosecutors bore some responsibility for helping all defendants, including those with mental illnesses, understand the severity of shoplifting very early on—perhaps by being less lenient on initial charges:

> I think in order to be fair to the person that's charged, if we're very lenient on the first three, so let's say, "Oh, we'll just give you time served for the night that you spent in jail." And the next time we say, "Oh, you'll spend the weekend," and then the next time we say, "We'll give you 2 weeks now." Well, now the fourth offense, that person is jumping from 2 weeks to a year in jail without being able to defer it, suspend it,

probate it, or anything like that…if they don't have some sense of how serious this is and what the consequences could be; there's some level of accountability that we have as prosecutors for that.

Alongside the risk of not fully comprehending how shoplifting charges may escalate, criminal justice professionals described how shoplifting is a charge that is commonly seen alongside more serious charges—especially for people with mental illnesses. That is, a shoplifting incident can escalate into situations where defendants face a series of charges. One Philadelphia defender reflected, "I find that I don't have any client that I can think of past, present, or probably future, who is severely mentally ill whose only charge is retail theft." He and his colleague described how what starts as stealing coffee at a convenience store can snowball:

> Public Defender 1: I mean, we're talking about, it could be a cup of coffee, and police end up getting called.
> Public Defender 2: Right. And then the coffee gets thrown into the police officer's face, and we have an aggravated assault.
> Public Defender 1: Unless they're a kleptomaniac, unless we're talking about that kind of mental illness. But I always see retail theft, it's usually a summary [charge], sometimes a misdemeanor charge with a robbery connected to it because they fight with the store security, or an assault because they throw the coffee. Those types of situations are very common. Also, we see that the person ends up in some kind of confrontation, and there's also frequently an aggravated assault charge on a police officer.

As the case of Ms. George demonstrates, once a person is arrested on a shoplifting charge (and, in some cases, additional charges stemming from the same incident), their resulting criminal legal system processing can lead to prolonged entanglement in the criminal legal system.

Ironically, some of the potential for this prolonged involvement stems from the pressure to resolve cases quickly. Prosecutors described the pressure for efficiency in the court system and how it results in offering plea deals of "time served" to defendants even when they think a defendant could benefit from a treatment plan integrated into the plea deal. "Trying to craft someone some sort of treatment plan that was part of a plea for someone with a serious mental illness is such a heavy lift that it just wasn't worth it, a lot of the times, for them, because they are so—they're a dime a dozen," reflected one Manhattan ADA. Prosecutors perceived that public defenders were often unwilling to consider mandated treatment as part of a plea deal since most shoplifting cases are resolved with time served. As described in depth in Chapter 4

("Common Themes and Tensions"), public defenders may be unwilling to accept treatment mandates for clients in part because they fear their client will fail out of the program and then face the consequences of such failure (i.e., rearrest or reincarceration). Further, defenders suggested that people with mental illnesses shouldn't have to face additional burdens such as treatment requirements when charged with a crime simply because of their mental illness.

Public defenders also acknowledged that they had an "ethical obligation" to present all offers to their client and that reducing time in the criminal legal system is always paramount. For this reason, one public defender reflected that he understood why other defenders advised their clients to plead guilty. However, this, too, creates challenges:

> They go to court. They offer time served, the client wants time served, right? The attorney has an ethical obligation to do their job.... Now the client's out of jail. We all know it's a setup, but that's their right. We can't not tell them they have a time served offer.... The state's like, time served. We're done. They're out. No meds, no plan, but they're in the legal system. We're not a hospital. We're not a social service organization, we're a jail and legal system. And when the legal case is done, we can just hope for the best. And that has been a hard pill for me to swallow my whole time there.

In this sense, the obligations of public defenders—and the fact that they aim to reduce the time a person is caught up in the legal system for any charge—does not mean they're satisfied with the outcomes. They may not want their clients to face onerous treatment mandates, but they likewise do not fully trust that systems of care are available in the community that will prevent their clients from future criminal legal involvement.

Criminal Legal System Reforms to Prevent Entanglement From Shoplifting Charges

The case of Ms. George and the perspectives of the professionals who interact with people with mental illnesses being arrested and charged for shoplifting make clear that resolving these sorts of low-level misdemeanors can be complex, given the variety of parties involved and the often-contradictory perspectives on the best solution. As described at length earlier in Chapter 3 and Chapter 4, multiple contexts and values shape the decision-making process for criminal legal system professionals at the point where they encounter someone with a mental illness. Decisions about whether, how, and when to enforce misdemeanor laws around retail theft are not simply automatic processes but rather entail a series of considerations that account for the law and policy environment, the location of the behavior, the expectations of stakeholders (in this case, store owners in particular), knowledge of mental illness, and access to community resources (Wood et al. 2023). So, too, do the different focal concerns of criminal legal system professionals and agencies animate decision-making and lead to different orientations to the agenda of reducing criminal legal contact among people with SMI. At the same time, there are opportunities for expanding relatively newer interventions that have promise for both reducing retail theft arrests among people with SMI and minimizing the collateral consequences for those who are arrested.

Individual Law Enforcement Officers

Individual law enforcement officers have considerable discretion in deciding whether to exercise their power of arrest, and they routinely make decisions not to arrest people. Historically, alternatives to invoking the criminal legal system have been relatively limited if police officers are unable to resolve the incident at the scene or do not think the person with mental illness will meet criteria for involuntary transport for psychiatric evaluation. Increasingly, however, jurisdictions are expanding pre-arrest diversion initiatives (also known as police-assisted diversion) that give police officers new options for resolving low-level misdemeanors such as shoplifting.

Philadelphia's Police-Assisted Diversion (PAD) program diverts individuals who might otherwise be charged with low-level, nonviolent drug, prostitution, and retail theft offenses (Anderson et al. 2022). Operating at the point of a police encounter, Philadelphia PAD offers an early point of diversion out of the criminal legal system and into supportive, peer-based social services (Wood et al. 2023). A similar program, the Policing Alternatives and Diversion Initiative (also known as PAD), operates in Atlanta and Fulton County, Georgia. Atlanta's PAD program is a Law Enforcement Assisted Diversion (LEAD) program site; the LEAD model has been replicated nationally as a strategy for reducing arrests for people whose unlawful behavior stems from unmet needs related to mental illnesses, substance use, or poverty. The diversion programs in both Philadelphia and Atlanta link individuals to community-based services that can assist them with basic needs (e.g., shelter, food) as well as care and treatment services. As Alexandra Natapoff (2015) described, these street-level diversion initiatives "go above and beyond the general commitment to 'community policing' …[they]

complicate the adversarial and punitive images of police and illustrate how even this quintessential law enforcement function may be taking on a more civil welfarist character" (p. 459).

Research on pre-arrest or police-assisted diversion programs is relatively limited given how new most programs are, but there is evidence of the promise of this approach. An evaluation of Seattle's LEAD program (the first large-scale adoption in the United States) demonstrated that LEAD participants experienced significant decreases in jail bookings, jail days, and prison incarceration, reducing criminal legal system utilization and associated costs (Collins et al. 2019). Participants were twice as likely to be sheltered in the 18 months after their referral (i.e., permanently housed or living in transitional housing, shelter, or a motel/hotel rather than sleeping on the streets or in abandoned buildings). They were also 33% more likely to be connected to income/benefits (e.g., wages, unemployment benefits, veterans' benefits, state and federal income assistance). Housing and employment obtained during LEAD involvement was associated with significantly less recidivism as measured by arrests (Clifasefi et al. 2017). A qualitative study of Philadelphia's PAD program also showed positive experiences for clients and support from police officers (Anderson et al. 2022).

This is not to say that implementation challenges were null. As documented in the Philadelphia study, police officers expressed some skepticism about service providers; restrictive eligibility criteria can limit referrals (e.g., clients are ineligible if they have an arrest warrant); and success depends on both client readiness to accept services and adequate service options (Anderson et al. 2022). For changes stemming from pre-arrest or pre-booking diversion programs to be sustainable, there will likely need to be far greater investment in social service systems than what currently exists. Even so, communities that do not currently leverage diversion opportunities at the point of police contact would do well to consider how such programs can be implemented and how they might be particularly appropriate to rely on when encountering people with SMI arrested on or at risk for arrest on low-level misdemeanors such as shoplifting.

Larger Criminal Legal System Reforms

Beyond giving police officers more discretion and tools to respond to people with mental illnesses who might otherwise be arrested for shoplifting, jurisdictions can contemplate strategies to lessen the consequences of an arrest or the possibility that an arrest leads to a protracted period of criminal legal system entanglement. Although pretrial (as opposed to pre-arrest) diversion programs and specialty courts are increasingly common across the country, they are not the focus of this chapter because of complicated trade-offs for defendants that such initiatives often entail. As described here and as elucidated in more depth in Chapter 4, encouraging diversion to a treatment program can reduce the immediate punitive impact of an arrest (e.g., the person spends no time or less time in jail) but also substitutes it for long periods of supervision for brief incarceration and therefore maintains and even extends control over people who have committed minor offenses.

Rather—returning to the case of Ms. George, who spent 4 months in jail for failing to appear in court and then another 45 days in jail for violating her probation—promising reforms could target specific policies and procedures that often get people caught up in the system. For example, some studies have estimated that as many as 25% of daily jail populations are people incarcerated on failure-to-appear charges (Bornstein et al. 2013). But evidence also suggests that providing court date reminders reduces the incidence of failure to appear in court and that effects are even larger when the people notified are those being charged with misdemeanors or violations rather than felonies (Zottola et al. 2023). If some failures to appear in court are the result of losing, forgetting, or not initially receiving the appropriate information about one's court date, then court reminders could save many people from the consequences of missing court. Although research is needed on what drives failure to appear among individuals with SMI and the impact of court reminder notifications among this population in particular, jurisdictions could easily implement such notification systems. Reducing incarceration for failing to attend a court date would also ensure that people with SMI stay connected to the community and treatment providers while proceeding through the judicial process.

Further reforms to probation, particularly those that reduce the use of incarceration for probation violations, are also needed. In 2021, nearly 3 million people were on probation in the United States, approximately one-third of whom were serving probation for misdemeanor offenses (Kaeble 2023). While probation is often considered an alternative to incarceration, revocations of probation are also one of the biggest drivers of incarceration. As the use of probation and the expansion of probation conditions have grown over the past several decades, so too have the numbers of people who violate the conditions of probation and are sent back to jail and prison (Jacobson et al. 2017). Such revocations are often for technical violations (e.g., missing a meeting with a probation officer, failing a drug test) rather than the commission of a new crime. Individuals who are sent to jail for a probation violation are exposed (or re-exposed) to the well-documented harms of jail incarceration such as job loss, housing instability, and family disruption (Pope et al. 2023). Evidence suggests, however, that agencies can reduce such harms and improve outcomes by decreasing the use of incarceration for supervision violations. Several studies have shown that incarceration is not better than noncustodial sanctions at reducing recidivism (Villettaz et al. 2015; Wodahl et al. 2015). As a result, at least 40 states now have statutes that authorize various forms of alternatives to incarceration, in many cases using graduated sanctions such as curfews, increased reporting, and removal of privileges to address violations (Pew Charitable Trusts 2020). Such approaches could have a meaningful impact on reducing the number of people with SMI who return to jail on probation violations for failing to comply with the often complex conditions of their probation.

Engaging Business Partners in Solutions

Finally, as it pertains to the charges of interest here, it is worth considering how criminal legal system professionals can partner with the business community to mobilize the community's own resources in providing solutions to shoplifting charges. Plentiful guidance already exists for store owners looking to reduce shoplifting: improving store layouts and displays, upgrading security, and posting warning signs on high-risk merchandise (see, for example, the Problem-Specific Guide Series feature on Shoplifting from the Office of Community Oriented Policing Services in the U.S. Department of Justice [Clarke and Petrossian 2013]). Chapter 3 also mentions the promise of problem-oriented policing approaches, but sometimes police may need to help elucidate the "institutional breakdowns" that lead to police responding to problems in the first place. David Thacher's (2022) work on "shrinking the police footprint" provides an example of responding to reports of theft from Walmart. Thacher explains the case of a Paducah (Kentucky) Walmart that was generating a crushing amount of police calls for service. What became clear on further review of the incidents was that Walmart had abdicated its own responsibility to control theft—removing door greeters, reducing the number of employees, and installing automatic checkouts. Over time, police used the knowledge they had developed about these incidents to force the Paducah Walmart to take more responsibility for managing its own problems and, in turn, to rely less on police. Thacher (2022) suggests that by focusing on fine-grained, context-specific categories such as low-value theft from Walmart, it is easier to devise nonpolice alternatives as solutions. A sustained commitment to such an approach could ultimately result in a large reduction in the police footprint in people's lives.

Mental Health System Reforms to Prevent Entanglement From Shoplifting Charges

Mental health providers also have a role to play in reducing entanglement for people with SMI who are at risk for being arrested for shoplifting, although perhaps not in the ways they might expect. It is unlikely that mental health treatment alone will stop shoplifting behaviors among people who are caught or arrested for such behavior. Shoplifting-specific treatment programs have emerged across the country, including Shoplifters Anonymous and other psychoeducational group counseling programs. However, there is little empirical evidence to support claims of success of these programs, with most studies showing that re-arrest rates for shoplifting are generally low and similar among people who receive treatment and those who do not (Krasnovsky and Lane 1998). Further, the notion that mental health treatment generally is the best way to stop people with mental illnesses from engaging in shoplifting rests on the tenuous assumption that mental illness is driving the behavior as opposed to the psychosocial circumstances created by the mental illness. There is increasing recognition that "first-generation" mental health interventions that rely on mental health treatment as the primary strategy for reducing criminal legal involvement among people with SMI are likely to fall short (Epperson et al. 2011, 2014). As described earlier and as supported by a growing body of research, the relationship between mental illness and crime is likely confounded by other factors such as poverty, homelessness, and substance use, and people with SMI encounter the criminal legal system for many of the same reasons as people without SMI (Draine et al. 2002; Epperson et al. 2014; Fisher et al. 2006)—they are just more likely to find themselves facing these reasons. In this sense, mental health providers need to think holistically about whether and how they can connect their clients to larger systems of social support that address the underlying needs not always managed by mental health treatment programs. For example, mental health professionals could ask their clients about their history of shoplifting charges and about shoplifting that didn't result in charges. They could ask their clients about basic needs that they don't have money for and strategize with them on how to obtain needed items lawfully without putting themselves at risk for charges.

Elsewhere, colleagues and I have also suggested that mental health providers have a role to play as strategic partners in helping clients understand the implications of and manage criminal legal system involvement if they are arrested (Pope et al. 2022). With reference to the problem of failure to appear, for example, mental health professionals could support clients by asking them about their criminal legal involvement and regularly following up about court dates and case outcomes. Supportive psychotherapy, case management, and other strategies can include person-centered approaches to keeping court appointments. Making such information exchange a routine part of the therapeutic encounter acknowledges the impact that legal cases can have on mental health and may lessen the stigma of criminal legal involvement.

KEY POINTS

- Shoplifting, or retail theft, is a very common charge in the United States for people with and without serious mental illness (SMI). What counts as misdemeanor retail theft is generally defined by threshold dollar values, and state statutes generally provide for escalating penalties for repeat shoplifting offenses (i.e., sentencing is based on an aggregate number of incidents or aggregate dollar value across incidents in a specific period).

- Studies have found no significant differences in shoplifting behavior along racial lines, but there are clear racial disparities in terms of who is accused of shoplifting, who is arrested for it, and what sentences people receive if convicted; literature on "shopping while Black" describes the consumer racial profiling that Black people experience.

- The relationship between socioeconomic status and shoplifting is not entirely clear, but some data suggest that people with SMI who also experience criminogenic risks such as unemployment/underemployment, low education, and housing instability may be at high risk for behaviors such as shoplifting by virtue of their psychosocial circumstances rather than their mental illness per se; this is further supported by criminal legal system professionals who describe shoplifting among people with SMI as a "crime of survival."

- Criminal legal system professionals balance multiple contexts and stakeholder concerns when responding to alleged shoplifting incidents, including the legitimate concerns of store owners, the pressure to resolve cases quickly, and the availability (or lack) of appropriate off-ramps from the criminal legal system.

• The entanglement caused by shoplifting arrests could be reduced through criminal legal reforms such as expansion of pre-arrest or police-assisted diversion opportunities, regular implementation of court date reminders, policy changes that limit the use of incarceration for probation violations, and collaboration with business owners.

• Mental health professionals can partner with their clients to understand their material needs and ability to pay for them, history of shoplifting, and extent of court involvement to prevent low-level misdemeanor charges such as shoplifting from becoming protracted periods of court involvement or jail time.

References

Anderson E, Shefner R, Koppel R, et al: Experiences with the Philadelphia Police Assisted Diversion program: a qualitative study. Int J Drug Policy 100:103521, 2022 34826788

Bailey DA: When did shoplifting a can of tuna become a felony: a critical examination of Arkansas's Breaking and Entering Statute. Ark Law Rev 63(2):269–282, 2010

Bamfield J: Shopping and Crime. London, Palgrave Macmillan, 2012

Blanco C, Grant J, Petry NM, et al: Prevalence and correlates of shoplifting in the United States: results from the National Epidemiologic Survey on Alcohol and Related Conditions (NESARC). Am J Psychiatry 165(7):905–913, 2008 18381900

Bornstein BH, Tomkins AJ, Neeley EM, et al: Reducing courts' failure-to-appear rate by written reminders. Psychol Public Policy Law 19:70–80, 2013

Cameron M: The Booster and the Snitch: Department Store Shoplifting. New York, Free Press of Glencoe, 1964

Center for Just Journalism: Retail Theft: What to Know and Where to Go. Washington, DC, Center for Just Journalism, 2023. Available at: https://just journalism.org/page/retail-theft. Accessed November 1, 2023.

Clarke RV, Petrossian G: Shoplifting, 2nd Edition. Problem-Oriented Guides for Police, Problem-Specific Guides Series, No. 11. Washington, DC, Center for Problem-Oriented Policing, U.S. Department of Justice, 2013. Available at: https://portal.cops.usdoj.gov/resourcecenter/content.ashx/cops-p030-pub.pdf. Accessed September 12, 2024.

Clifasefi SL, Lonczak HS, Collins SE: Seattle's Law Enforcement Assisted Diversion (LEAD) program: within-subjects changes on housing, employment, and income/benefits outcomes and associations with recidivism. Crime Delinq 63:429–445, 2017

Collins SE, Lonczak HS, Clifasefi SL: Seattle's Law Enforcement Assisted Diversion (LEAD): program effects on criminal justice and legal system utilization and costs. J Exp Criminol 15:201–211, 2019

Compton MT, Graves J, Zern A, et al: Characterizing arrests and charges among individuals with serious mental illnesses in public-sector treatment settings. Psychiatr Serv 73(10):1102–1108, 2022 35378991

Compton MT, Zern A, Pope LG, et al: Misdemeanor charges among individuals with serious mental illnesses: a statewide analysis of more than two million arrests. Psychiatr Serv 74(1):31–37, 2023 35795979

Criminal Justice Statistics Interagency Working Group of the National Science and Technology Council: Equity and Law Enforcement Data Collection, Use, and Transparency. Executive Office of the President of the United States, May 2023. Available at: https://www.whitehouse.gov/wp-content/uploads/2023/05/NSTC-Equity-and-Law-Enforcement-Data.pdf. Accessed November 2, 2023.

Dabney DA, Hollinger RC, Dugan L: Who actually steals? A study of covertly observed shoplifters. Justice Q 21:693–728, 2004

Dabney DA, Dugan L, Topalli V, et al: The impact of implicit stereotyping on offender profiling: unexpected results from an observational study of shoplifting. Crim Justice Behav 33:646–674, 2006

Draine J, Salzer MS, Culhane DP, et al: Role of social disadvantage in crime, joblessness, and homelessness among persons with serious mental illness. Psychiatr Serv 53(5):565–573, 2002 11986504

Duke Law Journal: Criminal law: customer's permanent exclusion from retail store due to prior shoplifting arrests held enforceable under criminal trespass statute. Duke Law J 5:995–1005, 1971

Epperson M, Wolff N, Morgan R, et al: The Next Generation of Behavioral Health and Criminal Justice Interventions: Improving Outcomes by Improving Interventions. New Brunswick, NJ, Rutgers University Center for Behavioral Health Services and Criminal Justice Research, 2011

Epperson MW, Wolff N, Morgan RD, et al: Envisioning the next generation of behavioral health and criminal justice interventions. Int J Law Psychiatry 37(5):427–438, 2014 24666731

Federal Bureau of Investigation: Crime in the United States, 2019. Washington, DC, U.S. Department of Justice, 2020. Available at: https://ucr.fbi.gov/crime-in-the-u.s/2019/crime-in-the-u.s.-2019. Accessed May 20, 2024.

Fisher WH, Roy-Bujnowski KM, Grudzinskas AJ Jr, et al: Patterns and prevalence of arrest in a statewide cohort of mental health care consumers. Psychiatr Serv 57(11):1623–1628, 2006 17085611

Gabbidon SL: Racial profiling by store clerks and security personnel in retail establishments: an exploration of "shopping while black." J Contemp Crim Justice 19:345–364, 2003

Gabbidon SL, Higgins GE: Shopping While Black: Consumer Racial Profiling in America. New York, NY, Routledge, 2020

Gold M: Delinquent Behavior in an American City. Belmont, CA, Brooks/Cole, 1970

Harris A-MG: Shopping while black: applying 42 U.S.C. § 1981 to cases of consumer racial profiling. Boston Coll Third World Law J 23:1, 2003

Harris A-MG, Henderson GR, Williams JD: Courting customers: assessing consumer racial profiling and other marketplace discrimination. J Public Policy Mark 24:163–171, 2005

Harwell J: Burglary at Wal-mart: innovative prosecutions of banned shoplifters under Tenn. Code Ann. 39–14–402. Tennessee Journal of Law and Policy 11(2):81–128, 2016

Hindelang MJ: Variations in sex-race-age-specific incidence rates of offending. Am Sociol Rev 46:461–474, 1981

Jacobson M, Schiraldi V, Daly R, et al: Less Is More: How Reducing Probation Populations Can Improve Outcomes. Cambridge, MA, Harvard Kennedy School, August 2017. Available at: https://www.hks.harvard.edu/sites/default/files/centers/wiener/programs/pcj/files/less_is_more_final.pdf. Accessed November 1, 2023.

Kaeble D: Probation and Parole in the United States, 2021 (NCJ 305589). Washington, DC, U.S. Department of Justice, Bureau of Justice Statistics, 2023

Krasnovsky T, Lane RC: Shoplifting. Aggress Violent Behav 3:219–235, 1998

Kutateladze BL, Andiloro NR, Johnson BD, et al: Cumulative disadvantage: examining racial and ethnic disparity in prosecution and sentencing. Criminology 52:514–551, 2014

Lewis N: What the Shoplifting Panic Reveals About U.S. Crime Policy. New York, The Marshall Project, 2023. Available from: https://www.themarshallproject.org/2023/02/27/shoplifting-retail-theft-lawmakers-response. Accessed January 26, 2024.

Lopez E, Boxerman R, Cundiff K: Shoplifting Trends: What You Need to Know. Washington, DC, Council on Criminal Justice, 2023. Available at: https://counciloncj.org/shoplifting-trends-what-you-need-to-know. Accessed January 26, 2024.

Marshal IH, He N: USA, in Juvenile Delinquency in Europe and Beyond: Results of the Second International Self-Report Delinquency Study. Edited by J Junger-Tas, IH Marshal, D Enzmann, et al. New York, Springer-Verlag, 2010, pp 139–157

Massey SG, Kauffman RA, Chen M-H, et al: Race, excess suspicion, and larceny in Upstate NY. Criminal Justice Studies 35:295–321, 2022

McCarthy C, Schnitzer K, Hogan B, et al: Shoplifting hit record highs last year: "We can't stop them." New York Post, February 10, 2023. Available at: https://nypost.com/2023/02/10/we-cant-stop-them-shoplifting-hit-record-highs-in-nyc-last-year. Accessed May 20, 2024.

Moore RH: Shoplifting in middle America: patterns and motivational correlates. Int J Offender Ther Comp Criminol 28:53–64, 1984

Natapoff A: Gideon's servants and the criminalization of poverty. Ohio State Journal of Criminal Law 12(2):445–464, 2015

National Association for Shoplifting Prevention: The Shoplifting Problem in the Nation. Huntington Station, NY, National Association for Shoplifting Prevention, 2021. Available at: https://www.shopliftingprevention.org/the-shoplifting-problem/. Accessed November 2, 2023.

National Retail Federation: National Retail Security Survey 2019. Washington, DC, National Retail Federation, 2019. Available at: https://nrf.com/research/national-retail-security-survey-2019. Accessed November 2, 2023.

National Retail Federation: National Retail Security Survey 2022. Washington, DC, National Retail Federation, September 14, 2022. Available at: https://nrf.com/research/national-retail-security-survey-2022. Accessed November 2, 2023.

Pew Charitable Trusts: The Effects of Changing Felony Theft Thresholds. Washington, DC, Pew Charitable Trusts, 2017. Available at: https://www.pewtrusts.org/~/media/assets/2017/04/pspp_the_effects_of_changing_felony_theft_thresholds.pdf. Accessed March 1, 2023.

Pew Charitable Trusts: Policy Reforms Can Strengthen Community Supervision: A Framework to Improve Probation and Parole. Washington, DC, Pew Charitable Trusts, 2020. Available at: https://www.pewtrusts.org/-/media/assets/2020/04/policyreform_communitysupervision_report_final.pdf. Accessed November 1, 2023.

Pope LG, Boswell T, Zern A, et al: Failure to appear: mental health professionals' role amidst pretrial justice reform. Psychiatr Serv 73(7):809–811, 2022 34704771

Pope LG, Pohl DJ, Ehntholt A, et al: New York State's Bail Elimination Act of 2019: a retrospective mental health impact assessment. Impact Assessment and Project Appraisal 41(6):430–443, 2023

Shteir R: The Steal: A Cultural History of Shoplifting. New York, Penguin Books, 2011

Thacher D: Shrinking the police footprint. Crim Justice Ethics 41:62–85, 2022

United States v. Bean, 443 F.2d 17 (5th Cir. 1971)

Villettaz P, Gillieron G, Killias M: The effects on re-offending of custodial vs. non-custodial sanctions: an updated systematic review of the state of knowledge. Campbell Systematic Reviews 11(1):1–92, 2015

Wodahl EJ, Boman JH, Garland BE: Responding to probation and parole violations: are jail sanctions more effective than community-based graduated sanctions? J Crim Justice 43:242–250, 2015

Wood JD, Watson AC, Pope L, et al: Contexts shaping misdemeanor system interventions among people with mental illnesses: qualitative findings from a multi-site system mapping exercise. Health Justice 11(1):20, 2023 37014478

Zottola SA, Crozier WE, Ariturk D, et al: Court date reminders reduce court nonappearance: a meta-analysis. Criminol Public Policy 22:97–123, 2023

7

Noncooperation With Officers and Using "Fighting Words"

Obstruction and Related Misdemeanor Charges and Criminal Legal System Entanglement

Brandon del Pozo, Ph.D., M.P.A., M.A.
Michael T. Compton, M.D., M.P.H.

Most professions must tolerate clients' poor behavior, even when clients obstruct the efficiency and effectiveness of a professional's work. Accountants, for example, must put up with clients who send in critical documents too close to the April 15 tax return deadline. Medical professionals must tolerate patients who are late for appointments, who miss them altogether, or who are noncompliant with their prescribed treatments. U.S. Postal Service drivers in the Northeast are frustrated when residents insufficiently shovel snow in front of their mailboxes after a snowstorm, making it impossible for them to carry out their appointed rounds. Restaurateurs must put up with late or missed reservations and impolite requests to make changes to a chef's well-crafted menu. Every profession meets frustrations, rudeness, refusals, and obstructions by their clients.

In one professional domain, however, such bad behavior may be considered a crime—a misdemeanor or even felony punishable by fines, probation, or imprisonment. Here, the professionals we are referring to are criminal legal system actors, police officers in particular. Among the populations the police interact with regularly, people with serious mental illness (SMI) are especially susceptible to being perceived as acting criminally when their behavior presents problems for officers—when they "obstruct" officers' work duties or "resist" officers' requests or demands.

In an important sense, these behaviors are unique among those that reflect noncooperation with police. Some people might resist officers because they are trying to evade apprehension for a crime. Others may not see the police as legitimate sources of authority, may not trust the police or the larger criminal legal system to treat them fairly or deliver the services they need (Shelby 2007), or may be engaging in a deliberate form of civil disobedience (Delmas 2018). A factor that makes encounters with people with SMI different is that the behaviors the police may perceive as criminal in nature may derive in part from a person's medical condition—it is the mental illness that drives the behavior more so than criminal intent or a series of deliberate choices. Additionally, the officer may not have the skills to foster compliance, which could escalate the situation—as such, the dynamic between the officer and the subject is as important. This raises essential questions about why and when criminal charges are appropriate during encounters with people with SMI, or what should be changed if the cause of the behavior is medical.

This chapter examines crimes such as resisting, obstructing, and using "fighting words," as well as related charges, in the specific context of SMI. We start by cataloging this family of charges and briefly outlining their history. We then describe how the challenges people with SMI face make them susceptible to these charges, and we illustrate their perspectives and those of criminal legal system professionals about these situations using case examples and the results of interviews and focus groups. We present the rationale police use for having these charges at their disposal to maintain order and ensure safe social cooperation in complex, dynamic environments but argue that they leave key underlying causes unaddressed and invariably yield highly inequitable outcomes according to race and socioeconomic status. Given the net harms and scant benefits criminal charges produce for people with SMI—for both patients and the public—we conclude by suggesting ways police and mental health professionals can safely and effectively reduce the incidence of these types of charges among people with SMI at individual and systems levels.

Criminal Charges Relating to Problematic Interactions With the Police

Broadly, three categories of criminal charges may apply when the interaction between a police officer and a subject is itself problematic—above and beyond any criminal behavior that prompted the encounter—with particular attention here to a person with an SMI (Table 7–1). The first directly concerns the police role and actions that interfere with the execution of police duties. These include charges such as resisting arrest, obstructing governmental administration, giving false information to a police officer, and filing false official reports. If obstructive behaviors escalate from noncooperation and passive resistance to acts of aggression or violence, they can culminate in a second category of charges, such as menacing and assault. A third category is when the police perceive a person's interaction with them to be disruptive enough to cause significant annoyance and alarm to the public in the vicinity of the incident, and police use this belief to make an arrest for a charge such as disorderly conduct. The nature of these charges suggests how encounters with people with SMI can result in misdemeanor arrests and criminal legal system entanglement.

Resisting arrest charges vary from state to state, but all of them include the use of force or physical resistance when a police officer is trying to take a person into custody. The criminal statute of Pennsylvania serves as an example:

18 PA. C.S. § 5104. RESISTING ARREST OR OTHER LAW ENFORCEMENT

A person commits a misdemeanor of the second degree if, with the intent of preventing a public servant from effecting a lawful arrest or discharging any other duty, the person creates a substantial risk of bodily injury to the public servant or anyone else or employs means justifying or requiring substantial force to overcome the resistance.

Obstruction broadens the scope of impeding police work from the time and place of arrest to the general performance of an officer's duties, and often extends the actors from police to public servants gener-

Table 7–1.   Three domains of the charges resulting from
                  problematic encounters between police and individuals
                  with serious mental illnesses

Types of actions that could result in charges during police encounters	Examples of charges	Victim
Actions interfering with police duties	Resisting arrest, obstructing governmental administration, giving false information, filing false reports	Government, acting on behalf of the public
Actions compromising officer safety	Menacing or criminal threats, assault	The officer
Actions potentially impacting public order	Disorderly conduct	The public

ally. For example, a person who prevents a city bus from moving along
its route or stops police from arresting someone else is acting in a way
that could merit the charge. In some contexts, simply refusing to give
your name can be charged as obstruction. New York State provides a
useful example of the statute concerned, notable for its breadth:

NY PENAL LAW § 195.05 OBSTRUCTING GOVERNMENTAL ADMINISTRATION IN THE SECOND DEGREE

A person is guilty of obstructing governmental administration when he intentionally obstructs, impairs or perverts the administration of law or other
governmental function or prevents or attempts to prevent a public servant
from performing an official function, by means of intimidation, physical
force or interference, or by means of any independently unlawful act.

Menacing, sometimes referred to as *criminal threats* or *intimidation*,
occurs when someone threatens to commit an act of violence against a
person in a way that appears credible and leads them to fear for their
safety. In New York State, menacing is a misdemeanor, but its character-
ization as a prelude to violence can lead states to classify it more seriously. This variation in classifications is a consistent theme across, and
within, states. Often the professional identity of the victim makes a difference, or one state simply categorizes a crime more seriously than another. In Illinois, for example, intimidation—its version of menacing—

is a Class 3 felony and becomes an even more serious charge when the victim is a police officer:

720 ILCS 5 / 12-6. INTIMIDATION

(a) A person commits intimidation when, with intent to cause another to perform or to omit the performance of any act, he or she communicates to another, directly or indirectly by any means, a threat to perform without lawful authority any of the following acts:
    (1) Inflict physical harm on the person threatened or any other person or on property; or
    (2) Subject any person to physical confinement or restraint; or
    (3) Commit a felony or Class A misdemeanor; or
    (4) Accuse any person of an offense; or
    (5) Expose any person to hatred, contempt or ridicule.

The case law concerning the related concept of *fighting words* either figures explicitly into the statutes under discussion here or embodies the principles that make verbal statements chargeable as menacing or, in some states, as forms of harassment or disorderly conduct (see later section on disorderly conduct). The laws vary from state to state, but all of them have a statute that allows officers to regulate speech that may not be a direct threat but that would unduly provoke a reasonable person. The use of fighting words could be motivated by sheer anger, poor impulse control, the stress and frustration of challenging life circumstances, or the influence of drugs and alcohol, as well as by features of an SMI itself. In practice, it is likely to be a combination of factors. The concept entered U.S. Law in the Supreme Court's decision in *Chaplinsky v. New Hampshire* (1942), which placed limits on First Amendment freedom of expression when the speech serves no purpose beyond threatening or inciting a person in their vicinity. In the case, Chaplinsky called a law enforcement officer a "damned fascist and a racketeer," which, at the time, was deemed to have met the threshold of being offensive and inciting. Courts have since become more permissive of speech generally, with the threshold for fighting words steadily rising as our tolerances shift with the times. As a result, simple profanity and insults no longer suffice; in Vermont, in *State v. Tracy* (2015), the court ruled that the speech must be "so inflammatory that it is akin to dropping a match into a pool of gasoline," and went on to affirm a conviction in which a suspect stood face to face with a Black police officer and used a well-known racial slur against him. Following a group of observant people in public while shouting religious slurs at them is similarly provocative and would support criminal charges in many states. It is important to remember that the purpose of such laws is to allow arrest for a speech act, rather than a physical one, that is provocative but not necessarily a direct threat. Physical *assault*, in which a person intends to cause physical injury or succeeds in doing so, is covered in Chapter 8 ("'That's Scary Because Now They're Showing Violence'").

Disorderly conduct consists of a wide range of behaviors that a reasonable person would find intolerably or dangerously disruptive, and the statutes that prohibit it have been used to police fighting words. State and federal case law imposes limits on what police can allege is disorderly (especially when it comes to speech), but even with these restrictions, police have broad discretion in interpreting the statute. In fact, it has been suggested that disorderly conduct laws are designed to prohibit an overly wide range of behaviors and confer too much discretion on law enforcement and private citizens to target individuals for behavioral regulation, physical removal, and community exclusion (Morgan 2021). As the officials who decide whether there is probable cause to believe a person's conduct is disorderly or not, officers can use the charge in response to behavior they find personally disruptive or disrespectful, provided they articulate that it was disruptive to bystanders as well. This prerogative is what empowers police to charge disorderly conduct during their own problematic encounters with people with SMI. The disorderly conduct statute in the New York State Penal Law is illustrative. It covers a wide range of conduct, from abusive speech to tumult and threatening behavior, as well as blocking foot or vehicle traffic, all of which are behaviors that can result when people with SMI encounter police:

NY PENAL LAW § 240.20. DISORDERLY CONDUCT

A person is guilty of *disorderly conduct* when, with intent to cause public inconvenience, annoyance or alarm, or recklessly creating a risk thereof:

1. He engages in fighting or in violent, tumultuous or threatening behavior; or
2. He makes unreasonable noise; or
3. In a public place, he uses abusive or obscene language, or makes an obscene gesture; or
4. Without lawful authority, he disturbs any lawful assembly or meeting of persons; or
5. He obstructs vehicular or pedestrian traffic; or
6. He congregates with other persons in a public place and refuses to comply with a lawful order of the police to disperse; or
7. He creates a hazardous or physically offensive condition by any act which serves no legitimate purpose.

In addition to these laws, spanning from resisting arrest to disorderly conduct, there are others that are fairly straightforward, and which we touch on briefly in this chapter. These include filing *false reports* and making *false statements*, especially concerning a person's identity. In Illinois, for example, providing a false identity to police (by either making one up or assuming someone else's) can be construed as the crime of obstructing identification, a hybrid of false reporting and obstructing an officer. These charges are meant to prevent people from derailing police investigations and wasting police resources by casting criminal suspicion on innocent people or from opening time- and resource-intensive investigations into acts that never occurred or that involve a suspect who cannot be reliably identified and processed.

Obstruction, Disorderly Conduct, and "Fighting Words": A Brief History

Many of these laws find their provenance in statutes that are intended to apply to all citizens and benefit the public in general, rather than just serve as tools to help officers manage interactions and conduct investigations. The fighting words doctrine, for example, is not simply a punitive response to poor behavior: it allows police to remove a person from a scene before their speech escalates to violence or escalates others to violence. Other laws, however, were created specifically to protect police and empower them to conduct their work safely and efficiently. They operate under the presumption that an officer has a legitimate goal in advancing public safety, is entitled to collect accurate information about people's identities to advance investigations and resolve conflicts, and cannot be subject to threats or intimidation in doing so or presented with deliberate lies and falsehoods in a person's attempt to thwart police work or avoid criminal responsibility. Underlying all of this is the presumption that the person who lies, obstructs, or threatens an officer does so as part of an ill-advised (albeit possibly spontaneous) plan. The laws therefore signal that such a plan has negative consequences, with the goal of deterring people from attempting such actions. Nowhere in this calculus, however, is the possibility that the person's actions stem from an SMI.

Disorderly conduct and resisting arrest can be charged together, and often are (Moran 2022). On their face, these charges suggest a person was significantly alarming members of the public, and when the officer decided to make the resulting arrest, they were met with resistance. Given the subjective nature of disorderly conduct, the breadth of the statutory definitions, and the officer's near-total discretion in deciding whether to level the charge, this combination of charges presents the risk that police will use disorderly conduct to "teach a lesson" to an argumentative person who challenges their authority (Morgan 2021), and when that person asserts their right to argue with the police and indignantly resists, the officer then adds the other charge to drive the point home (i.e., resisting arrest). If the officer believes the person interfered with some other goal the officer had such as dispersing a crowd, collecting evidence, or arresting a third party, obstruction can be an additional charge.

In criminal legal system parlance, these charges are colloquially referred to as "contempt of cop," with the implication that they can be a legally dubious, emotional reaction of an officer feeling challenged or slighted (Perras 2022). By extension, when a person's behavior stems from manifestations of an SMI, it may be the case that the officer perceives their behavior as rejecting their judgment and authority, rather than deriving from a psychiatric condition (and the power dynamic between officer and subject is also at play). In this way, it is possible for contempt of cop and criminal charges against people with SMI to go hand in hand.

Poor Interactions With the Police Are More Common Among Individuals With Mental Illness

As noted in Chapter 1 ("The System, the Process, and the Contexts") in an analysis involving 240 people with SMI being discharged from inpatient psychiatric stays in South Georgia (Compton et al. 2022), 171 (71%) had been previously arrested, and the second most common charge across all of their prior charges was willful obstruction of law enforcement officers. Although definitive data are lacking, it is likely that those with SMI are more likely to be in situations and display behaviors resulting in charges related to resisting, obstructing, menacing, and disorderly conduct for several reasons.

When one considers the behaviors described by these charges with an understanding of the challenges people with serious mental illness face, the reasons for this increased likelihood become clearer. For example, if a person is in an agitated state, their behavior or statements can be perceived as preassaultive or threatening and generate a charge of menacing. It is easy to see how a person in the midst of a mental health crisis could unleash a verbal onslaught against a police officer that would meet the fighting-words threshold, resulting in a charge of menacing or criminal threats. Someone who directs a loud, sustained outburst at a police officer, but does so in the presence of bystanders, can be charged with annoying and alarming the public. If a person with an SMI in a paranoid or fearful state resists being handcuffed, it will satisfy the requirements of the resisting charge in nearly every jurisdiction, and in many of them, so will the act of fleeing, which may or may not be covered by a separate charge. If the paranoia of a person with an SMI prevents them from properly identifying themselves to the government, in some states it could generate the corresponding obstruction charge. Furthermore, a person with an SMI may not be in a mental state to understand what making a false report implies; they may believe they are being persecuted by someone or had an offense committed against them that never actually occurred.

Taken in sum, the wide range of laws surveyed above can each be used to charge a person with an SMI with an offense owing to a problematic encounter with a police officer, albeit one potentially driven by a psychiatric condition, related psychosocial circumstances, or a low sense of procedural justice in the current interaction or past encounters, rather than genuine criminal intent. The situation faced by a man with an SMI as he contended with being off medication, hunger from religious fasting, and stress during a visit to a gas station is illustrative in the case example that follows.

Case Example: Mr. Gaston at a Busy Gas Station

Leon Gaston is a 43-year-old White man who resided in a group home three blocks from a very busy thoroughfare in a suburban area. He attended two weekly Wednesday morning groups at the local mental health center, along with monthly visits with his psychiatrist, where he was in treatment for schizophrenia. Mr. Gaston was unemployed, received Supplemental Security Income (SSI), and had very limited social interactions and few activities that others might consider productive or rewarding. He walked daily, regardless of the weather, from the group home to one or more of the various stores along the busy thoroughfare: two gas stations with food marts, a convenience store, a relatively small grocery store, three fast food outlets, and a pet supply store. He did not have a pet but enjoyed looking at the fish, birds, and rodents for sale. Mr. Gaston usually visited one of the gas stations or the convenience store daily, to purchase sodas and snacks with his very limited personal funds (as most of his SSI check went to the group home), along with one of the other stores where he liked to "browse" and think about possible purchases for when his check arrived on the first of the month.

Mr. Gaston rarely missed a group or appointment at the mental health clinic, although his providers there had not been able to convince him to regularly attend primary care appointments in the adjacent federally qualified health center; this despite concerns about both prehypertension and prediabetes. He was generally agreeable at the group home, where six others with mental illnesses lived, and staff viewed him as the second most calm and cooperative patient of the group. Mr. Gaston did, however, tend to become defensive and at times argumentative over perceived invasions of his privacy. Having been at the group home for more than 3 years, he was one of three residents who had earned the privilege of his own private room (the remaining four shared double rooms). Mr. Gaston nearly always adhered with his medications: benztropine 1 mg nightly, valproate 1,000 mg nightly, and a monthly long-acting injectable antipsychotic. Although his auditory hallucinations (voices of "prophets") and mood instability were largely controlled, he had persistent delusional content that had been refractory to treatment but was minimally impairing. He tended to be very focused on righteousness, the Ten Commandments, and several Old Testament prophets. Much of his thinking revolved around these themes.

The group home and mental health center provided Mr. Gaston with stability. He was less alienated from family, for example, usually attending a church service and lunch monthly with his mother and aunt. They had hopes that the church attendance would "normalize" his thinking about religion and the Old Testament. Mr. Gaston was also stable—over the past 18 months, at least—from a criminal legal system perspective. About 18 months earlier, he completed an 8-month stint on probation, which had followed his seventh detention in the county jail. His prior arrests had included shoplifting at the ages of 26 and 40, criminal trespass at the ages of 27 and 32 (the second of those including a resisting arrest charge), misdemeanor "theft by taking" at the age of 36, simple battery at 39, and disorderly conduct and willful obstruction of a law enforcement officer at 41.

During the week leading up to Passover, Mr. Gaston decided to take a 4-day fast. He discontinued his benztropine and valproate, as instructions on the pill bottles indicated that they should be taken with food. On the last day of the fast, Mr. Gaston was undoubtedly preoccupied by hunger and had gone several days without the benefit of his medications. Under these stressful circumstances, a trip to the gas station three blocks away resulted in his eighth arrest, this time for two misdemeanor charges: disorderly conduct and willful obstruction of a law enforcement officer. The first, for disorderly behavior, was likely driven by his mental illness, and the second for impeding the officer's work, in part related to previous negative experiences with law enforcement and the criminal legal system.

Situations that end like Mr. Gaston's happen with great frequency. First, people with SMI commonly have police contacts, which set the stage for police contact-related charges. A systematic review of 48 studies (Livingston 2016) documented that ~12% of people with mental illnesses have police involved in their pathway to mental health care, although the 18 studies from the United States had a rate of 29%. Additionally, some 25% of people with mental illnesses had histories of police arrest (from 21 studies). Second, prior contacts with police may not have gone well or may even have been perceived as frightening or lacking in procedural justice (Watson and Angell 2007)—the latter construct including participation (having a voice, or the opportunity to present one's own side of the situation and be heard), dignity (being treated with respect and politeness and having one's rights acknowledged), and trust that the authority is concerned with one's welfare. Previous encounters lacking in perceived procedural justice may further set the stage for less-than-ideal subsequent interactions with police, which could escalate verbally or even physically. Third, features of some mental illnesses—from cognitive impairments to psychotic symptoms such as paranoia and hallucinations—could increase risk for uncooperative behavior or what might appear as uncooperative behavior. A sampling of these is given in Table 7–2.

Patients' Perspectives on Obstruction-Related Charges

Although there is much we wouldn't know about Mr. Gaston's own perspective, we have done some research with people with lived experiences that is instructive. In a series of qualitative interviews for a study on misdemeanor arrests (see Chapter 1), several individuals in treatment for SMI recounted their own prior experiences with willful obstruction of a law enforcement officer charges. A 43-year-old Black man described an obstruction charge as one charge among several others during a traffic stop:

> I was driving and the officer said he spotted me go across the center line, so he got behind me and pulled me over. And when he pulled me over, he asked for my license and, um, registration. I had the registration to show him, but, of course, I told him that I had no license. So then, um, he saw an open container of alcohol in my car, so he asked me when's the last time I drank. I told him the last time I drank was earlier that morning. So, he asked me to get out of the vehicle, but during that time, I had gout in both feet. He asked me if I could do a sobriety test. I told him, no, that I wasn't going to do a sobriety test because my feet were hurting. And I also hadn't eaten anything, so I told him that my blood sugar was dropping. We swapped words, and he asked me if I was gonna do the test. I told him no, and I gave the reason why. Even though it was a medical condition, he wouldn't listen, so that's how I ended up getting the obstruction charge, because I refused. I said, "I'm not going

---

Table 7–2.   Features of some mental illnesses that could increase
risk for uncooperative behavior, or what might appear
as uncooperative behavior

Cognitive impairment, including inattention, poor executive function,
    impaired abstract thinking, and verbal working memory impairments
Excitement-related symptoms, such as anxiety, hypervigilance, excessive
    energy, hyperactivity, irritability, agitation, and hostility
Formal thought disorder or conceptual disorganization, such as loosening
    of associations, flight of ideas, or thought blocking
Intoxication on or withdrawal from substances
Negative symptoms, such as alogia, amotivation, anhedonia, and
    psychomotor retardation
Poor impulse control
Psychotic symptoms, including paranoia and auditory hallucinations

---

to do it. You're just going to have to take me to jail." The officer could
have been more professional. And then, by the time he called a second
officer up, which was a Black officer, you know, I was already placed in
the back of the car. When you can see somebody that's physically in
pain, and you're still trying to get them to do an exercise, I think that's
wrong because if someone's telling you that they're in pain, and that
they need to eat, you need to let them get something to eat and then let
them get comfortable so that you can do your job right.... The charges
were obstruction tied to, uh, failure to maintain lanes, an open container,
and driving with no license, and, uh, "DUI less safe," which means they
don't have a breathalyzer test.

A 29-year-old Black woman described a domestic dispute that resulted in an obstruction charge, and her experience with the criminal legal system processes that followed:

I was at my mother's house. I'm separated from my husband, so I live
with her. My mother called the police because we were packing, and I
broke some dishes. My mom called the police—we were packing to
move to the place where we stay now, and they gave me trespassing,
and the officer gave me obstruction of law enforcement and so, my
mom's trying to do everything, but they say once it's in the state's hands
there is nothing you can do. I live there so it wasn't trespassing, but I
have a trespassing and obstruction on the one case. He said I obstructed
him from whatever when I was just like, I mean I live here. I stay there,
and my mail comes there, and I live there so it can't be trespassing when
that's the place where I live. They said it was out of my mom's hand at
that moment. I was in [jail] for 30 days, and they gave me a bond and
my best friend got me out. I had a public defender.... The prosecutors
and judges? I mean, they weren't rude, but it was just like, you know,
they don't want to hear what you gotta say. Prosecutors around here get

you and add stuff on [i.e., additional charges] and so I, I don't trust prosecutors. It's their job to win as many cases as they can. The prosecutors, I mean, they're just trying to win everything they can even when they know they can't prove anything. She was just like, "Well if we go to court with this, I'm gonna charge you on four charges." It's very aggressive. No dignity. No respect. It was just like, "This is what I'm gonna come at you with. We'll charge you with four." Because she added on two more.

A 45-year-old White woman described her felony obstruction experience that resulted in five years of probation, with employment consequences:

Well, I had a psychotic break, so some of it I can't remember. I was with my father and aunt. They were on the casino machines, and I was just visiting with them. They asked me to go order them a soda at the bar. The only other person at the bar was an undercover cop. The bartender knows me and has never liked me—she had it out for me. So, I didn't do anything wrong. I promise I did nothing wrong. My purse was hanging from the next bar stool and when I went to get my wallet, the bar stool fell down. The cop just grabbed me, threw the handcuffs on me, and said she was arresting me. She said, "That's enough, I'm taking you to jail. You're under arrest." And I didn't know what the heck was going on, so I fought her. I was like, "What are you doing? You can't just take me. I didn't do anything wrong." Then they tried to say that I threw furniture, and they were afraid for their lives. And then three more cops came in. So, they handcuffed me and, apparently, I had a psychotic break. I kicked one of them and hit one in the face, while I was handcuffed during all of this. They tased me. My father was screaming, telling them, "You need an ambulance, not police officers." There were several charges, but they dropped all of them except for the felony obstruction. I got five years of probation.... I have a felony. I can't even get a job. I've only got another 33 hours to finish my degree and then I cannot get a job, even after my degree because I can't get this felony off me. I have to hire a lawyer to try to get early release off probation, and then it'll come off my record if the judge will approve it. I already paid all my fines off.

Criminal Legal System Professionals' Perspectives on Obstruction-Related Charges

In our four-city (Atlanta, Chicago, Manhattan, and Philadelphia) study of misdemeanors, which included focus groups with criminal legal system professionals, in one of the cities, focus group participants (police officers, police supervisors, prosecutors, judges, and public defenders) were prompted to discuss the use and processing of obstruction charges.

In general, officers did not view the charges as indicative of a serious transgression or as critical for a community's public safety, but rather as charges used to address situations that they felt might otherwise be intractable or would require nonpolice mental health resources that were not available to them at the scene, or where inaction might leave them open to criticism from the public that they left a problem unaddressed.

Police officers gave examples of individuals with mental illnesses receiving misdemeanor obstruction charges. One officer described a subject—a homeless veteran who had been taken repeatedly to the Veterans Affairs medical center by officers—who would always refuse to speak or give officers needed information. The officer noted, "He's in such a state that he doesn't communicate with you. You can be having a conversation with him for five minutes, and he'll never respond to you. He'll be looking out and just talking on his own." The situation is complicated when the person is on someone else's property, as described by a police officer:

> We want them to leave. We've explained to them that the homeowner or the property owner or the business wants them to leave, but they don't want to leave. We've explained to them, or even just trying to get their identification, uh, the misdemeanor obstruction on that is that you're required to provide information, you're required to let us know name, date of birth, address, phone number. That's required by law when we have articulable suspicion or probable cause.

Another officer noted that there is both a city ordinance for obstruction, for which a ticket can be written, and a state charge. That officer also noted that other obstruction-related charges often pertain to giving false information (as opposed to refusing to give information), and resisting arrest:

> What I've seen mostly with mental health people is they will either give us a false name or date of birth. I have this one guy, talks to you just fine. But as soon as the handcuffs come out, he'll fight you. I've had multiple encounters with him, and that's been [the situation] every single time. So, it's kind of like a trigger, I feel.

Another officer described how the charge is often secondary to other charges, or may arise from behaviors driven by previous experiences with law enforcement:

> A lot of ours [are] in conjunction with criminal trespass or disorderly conduct. The only time that really may not be is if you're encountering somebody that just simply is afraid of the uniform. They see the uni-

form; they've had bad experiences before with the uniform. You could have a rapport with this person, but the second they see the uniform, it's like "I've got to run, I've got to run. The last three times I've dealt with a person in uniform, they've taken me to jail." Even though you're walking up to them with a real relaxed demeanor and everything like that. There is a case of ... an individual for years I'd dealt with, uh, next to the interstate. Every time I dealt with him, I'd show up and he immediately took off running.... Um, and that is part of misdemeanor obstruction, just taking off and running from us when we may have a reason to be there. But most of the willful obstruction is in conjunction with a [separate] criminal charge.

In a focus group with police supervisors, one discussed a prototypical case in which a person was sleeping in front of a grocery store that had recently closed. The supervisor made the distinction between misdemeanor and felony obstruction:

They're out in the sight of public and somebody called. So it looks like we don't do our job if we don't go up there and kind of at least get them, you know, to go somewhere else instead of sitting in that same spot. So he genuinely didn't think he did anything wrong. He was refusing to give his name and his birthdate, um, which refusing to give your name and your birthdate is another way to get the obstruction charge. But I think a lot of times these people don't think they actually have done anything wrong. They're just more or less refusing to cooperate than they are offering harm or violence to police. Unless you get seriously hurt, you know, in an obstruction charge, you're not gonna get a felony obstruction. I mean, our, our judges won't sign it anyway.

Another police supervisor recalled a recent event in which possible substance use led to confusion and fighting behavior:

Well, I just had an incident last week where I approached a gentleman thinking that he needed medical assistance. He was laid out on the middle of the [subway] platform. I'm trying to see if he needed an ambulance, and he immediately jumped up—I guess he was on substances or whatever—and he just started fighting us. So the fight was on. He did end up getting an obstruction charge, but while we're processing him, he kept saying that he was attacked, and it all came out of nowhere. So he does not recall any of the medical questions. He doesn't recall any type of assistance nor anything, like he only remembers that, or like he kept saying that he was just attacked. So I think the way that they respond ... is what causes them to get obstruction charges because they're not really in the moment to know what's going on.

In another focus group, a prosecutor noted how obstruction may be a secondary charge, and in some instances the obstruction behavior itself may result in another charge being given that would not have been had there been no oppositional behavior:

> We will get an obstruction that stands alone, but a lot of times it accompanies with something. Like let's say it's a criminal trespass. A lot of times, officers, I believe, are not trying to arrest somebody for criminal trespass, generally.... They're showing up, "Hey, mister or missus such and such, the owner wants you to leave, will you leave?" And that person's like, "No." And they're like, "Come on, please, you gotta go." And then when they're finally like, "Okay, now I have to place you under arrest," then the person attempts to run or they kind of pull away when they're trying to put them in handcuffs.... If they're struggling, like, "I'll kill you," or they reach out to punch the officer, then that makes it a felony. So normally, an obstruction comes from the officer having to encounter them about something, and they don't like it, so they wanna run.

In the focus group with judges, several noted feeling that the charge is overused in their state, that it often relates to running (or walking) away, and that in some communities it is understandable why one would want to leave when law enforcement arrives: "I really do think it's a much-overused charge. You can run from the police, you can fail to give them some information, or just be kind of obstreperous, and they can use that charge." Another judge commented, completing the thought: "And many times it's because the officer is upset ... because he had to run and catch you." Another judge concurred and expanded:

> In our community when the police show up, everybody runs. Even if I've not done anything, I'm gonna start walking away. So when [officers or attorneys] come in and say they left, that's what people do in communities where [the police] show up. And so I have those charges, unless you've pulled, you know, pulled a knife or kicked him—walking away, not bringing your hands up to them saying, cuff me, not helping them to lock the key on you. So, it's a catch-all that they use.

In another focus group at that site, with public defenders and service providers who work closely with them, the tone toward the use of misdemeanor willful obstruction of a law enforcement officer was much harsher. One defender began the discussion with, "I literally had a cop tell me one time that it is basically just pissing off the po-po." Another participant said, "We get it a lot as like an additional charge with the disorderly conduct because he was resistant in some way, shape, or form." And another, "When there's a serious injury, we understand that; that's how it becomes a felony obstruction." One noted how behaviors resulting in felony obstruction, however, may come about by improper de-escalation—or actual escalation—of a situation:

Herein lies the problem with the mentally ill, right? The inability to control themselves when they're having an episode, when a law enforcement officer is called out. A phone call comes in from the mom, "My son has schizophrenia. He's having an incident. Can somebody come over and help." The cop gets there, but they will not wait for [EMS]. [EMS] is on their way. They will not wait for [EMS]. The client is sitting on his, um, on the couch, eating a banana. The cop starts ordering him instead of leaving it be for a little while, and she escalates the situation. She grabs him and he goes nuts. And you know, for me, that's the issue that we have with the wrong people being called at the wrong time.... It starts as a parent calling for help or the client themselves calling for help, or somebody else calling for help ... and it turns into something where the cop ends up getting hurt or hurting the client.

One defender noted that "even though [the obstruction charge] grows out of something else, they sometimes don't charge the initial one," resulting in a single charge of obstruction:

They don't charge him with anything else but the felony obstruction. And sometimes the defense is about the lawful right to resist an unlawful arrest. Or sometimes [the County] won't indict the underlying, like what got them into the scene, especially for a felony obstruction, they just find it more of a waste of time and they just move forward with a single count of the felony obstruction. So, if I [as the public defender] was to put up the criminal trespass and the felony obstruction in front of a jury and the jury wanted to figure out something—they don't want the client to just walk, but they don't want this more serious charge—they're going to give them criminal trespass, right? But now they only have one option [the felony obstruction].

Finally, it was noted that prior experiences between the same officer and client may result in an obstruction charge related as much to the past as to the current situation:

This client and this cop had been seeing each other for years. They know each other. So they've had interactions. So when that cop rolls up, the client's already like, "Bump you. You've already arrested me 10 times. I'm not talking to you. You sent me to the ground last time." So it could be just a past history where they're like, "nah, dude, I'm not showing you my ID." Or the cop doesn't like this guy because he's always on the corner. So there is a history of personal interaction—they know each other. It's the same cop on the same corner with the same homeless guy. And they're both sick of each other.

These accounts across criminal legal system professionals suggest that: 1) officers report that they sometimes need to rely on these types of charges to resolve situations for which they have few solutions;

2) context matters in officers' using the charges, such as previous encounters, potentially even between the same officer and subject; 3) such charges are often secondary to other charges (e.g., criminal trespass) related to situations or behaviors that initiated the encounter; 4) situations of multiple charges can influence the processing of each of them; and 5) defenders and even judges may view the charges as overused.

Rationale for the Existence of Obstruction-Related Charges to Support Police Work

Although the constellation of public order and obstruction laws discussed in this chapter pose problems and challenges during police encounters with people with SMI, law enforcement stakeholders contend that they can be viewed as critical for effective police work and as tools for maintaining public safety. Some legal scholars have called for the elimination of disorderly conduct statutes under the rationale that such laws are too often used inappropriately, especially in ways that are racially discriminatory (Moran 2022; Morgan 2021). One of the challenges with doing so, however, may be that the police need broad, somewhat nonspecific laws that they can enforce at their discretion to solve the public order problems typical of complex communities and dense urban areas (del Pozo 2022b). They need to be able to enforce laws that keep sidewalks passable and roadways drivable, and that disassemble escalating situations and simmering crowds before they become truly violent or go on to disrupt the public sphere. At the same time, on New Year's Eve in Times Square or in the aftermath of momentous political and cultural events—or when people respond quickly and respectfully to police instructions to cease their behaviors—officers need the ability to make exceptions to enforcement. Sometimes a situation can be resolved without enforcement—such as by ordering a rowdy group to leave a corner or moving a protest from the street back onto the sidewalk—but to do so, the police need the underlying force of law in the first place.

If taking away police discretion in enforcing these more minor offenses would transform these statutes from problem-solving tools to intolerably harsh laws, then repealing the laws wholesale would leave police powerless to broker and enforce the fair terms of order and social cooperation in public spaces, which is a core function of the government. The actions covered by laws such as disorderly conduct aren't inherently immoral or even uniformly prohibited: an experience of disorder on a Sunday morning in the suburbs would come off as extraordinary calm on Bourbon Street in New Orleans during Mardi Gras, a city where drinking alcohol in public is lawful. This subjectivity is precisely why the police would argue they need both broad laws and broad discretion to thoughtfully preserve a sense of public order that is inherently context dependent.

The rationale for obstruction and related charges, and the discretion inherent in enforcing them, follows a similar line of thinking. It may be natural for people facing arrest to want to deceive the police or resist their efforts, but following the instructions issued by officers and supplying them with truthful information about one's identity are key elements of the good order and efficiency of law enforcement and public safety. It is one thing to remain silent or selectively withhold damning statements by invoking the Fifth Amendment, which is everyone's right, but it is another to break silence by providing police with deliberately misleading or false information. By comparison, these state-level laws are not as serious as making deliberately false statements of any kind to an FBI agent conducting an official investigation. Giving such deliberatively false statements is not a misdemeanor but a felony punishable by up to 5 years in prison.

With this understanding, it is natural to see the jeopardy these state laws create for people with SMI. If we expect police to use these laws to maintain order, ensure their safety, and conduct their work efficiently, then a key element of these charges is therefore intentionality, or the mental state of the person the police are interacting with. If the person would not have engaged in obstruction but for their mental illness (and but for the officers' inability to recognize it and accommodate the interaction accordingly), then it is unclear what enforcing these laws might accomplish. The range of circumstances in which these charges could be leveled, combined with an officer's near-total discretion in doing so, are an acknowledgment that no single police approach to the behaviors these laws address will provide a satisfactory one-size-fits-all solution. In the case of addressing the behaviors of those with SMI, even if the laws are what nominally empower the police to act, using them to level criminal charges isn't likely to be a useful solution in either the immediate case or the long term. In this way, the discussion here mirrors the concerns brought up in Chapter 5 ("Being in the Wrong Place") about the use of trespass charges. An arrest isn't necessary for police to act *in situ* during an encounter with a person with an SMI and is unlikely to change the person's behavior in the future unless they are effectively treated for their condition. Yet, criminally charging a person with an SMI for actions they took resulting from their psychiatric condition entangles them in a criminal legal system that has been shown, time and again, to be ill equipped to deliver the interventions they need to improve their mental health.

Risk of Racial Inequities in Issuing Obstruction-Related Charges

Law enforcement in the United States remains heavily characterized by racial inequity. From disparities in the people who are stopped and searched by police, to arrest rates, criminal convictions, and resulting fines and incarceration, the most coercive outcomes of policing and the criminal legal system are significantly more likely to be levied on minority populations. This includes persistent disparities in the use of deadly force (Nix and Shjarback 2021), including in cases where the people killed by police were unarmed (Ross et al. 2021). Criminal charges against people with SMI as the result of problematic encounters with the police are no exception.

There are several reasons for these disparities in addition to the underlying causes of structural racism and the elevated levels of stigma that minority people with SMI contend with. Some of them manifest as outcomes based on rural/urban divides and corresponding access to care. Behaviors that are likely to be disruptive in public are less likely to come to the attention of police in rural areas. Other causes are related to socioeconomic status and the ways in which structural racism exacerbates its disparities. Affluent people—who are more likely to be White—have the private spaces and financial resources that allow mental health crises to play out beyond public view and often beyond the reach of the police (del Pozo 2022b). Insofar as trauma, elevated exposure to the comorbidities of addiction and homelessness, and the consequences of inadequate social and economic supports cause or exacerbate SMI, minority populations remain at elevated risk of both SMI and the problematic encounters with police that can result (del Pozo 2022a; Laniyonu and Goff 2021).

This increased exposure to policing and enforcement makes the corresponding criminal legal system reforms a matter of not only general health equity, but also racial justice. When people pursue innovation and reform in mental health service delivery, they should be attuned to prioritizing the intersection of race, SMI, and policing. If they do, they will find themselves engaging with the needs of especially vulnerable communities, as well as improving the systems that they are most likely to touch or be thrust into. If racial equity is a goal, it is therefore not enough to simply expand and improve the public mental health systems that treat SMI; we also need to provide strong, well-trusted linkages between these systems and communities of color. Additionally, given that the criminal legal system remains one of the most common points of contact between minority populations and their government, the public mental health system must work to provide opportunities for diversion at every point or "intercept" along the criminal legal continuum, and emphasize the earliest off-ramps.

Policing and Criminal Legal System Reforms to Reduce Obstruction Charges Among People With Serious Mental Illness

An effective public health response to SMI requires that police distinguish between the legitimate use of myriad charges related to obstruction and resisting or assaulting police officers versus those that further entangle people with SMI in a criminal legal system that is unlikely to address their behavioral health needs. The criminal legal system is not designed to improve the factors that lead to problematic encounters between the police and people with SMI because it fails to account for the origin and nature of the behavior that leads to interactions and charges. Some reforms are possible, however, at the levels of both the individual officer and the larger criminal legal system.

Individual Law Enforcement Officers

In encounters with people with SMI, police officers should look beyond the law as a coarse means to remove a person from the scene of a disruption or to teach them a lesson. Instead, officers should take a problem-solving approach to each call that operates on two time horizons: one that does what it will take to safely resolve the situation at hand, and a second that will prevent the condition of a person with SMI from getting worse and harder to treat, which will only perpetuate the cycle of problematic police encounters. People with SMI are contending with symptoms, psychosocial adversities like poverty and marginalization, and the related potential crises that can yield uncooperative behavior, and in their most acute moments, they can be significantly disruptive.

Crisis Intervention Team (CIT) training and de-escalation training in its various forms strive for safe, practical resolutions to encounters with people with SMI. Effective curricula acknowledge the limits of threats of force and the limited usefulness of criminal charges when a person's mental state leaves them unresponsive to reasoning and deterrence. Patience, time, distance, and good tactics enable officers to resolve situations that would require force and criminal charges if the only goal is to resolve the situation as quickly as possible or if the officer is at least partially motivated by a desire to teach the person a lesson for being argumentative and disrespectful. Police officers should not only develop and practice the skills that allow them to negotiate problematic encounters with people with SMI safely for all involved, but also reorient their basic approach. If the goal is to prevent recurrence, criminal charges are unlikely to be the solution. Mental health professionals can be active participants in local efforts embedded within the criminal legal system, such as CIT programs within their own communities, to help with training and to provide officers with support.

The Larger Criminal Legal System

At the agency level and beyond, police need reassurances that when the actions taken to resolve a situation involving a person with an SMI do not result in an arrest, those actions will not result in civil liability or departmental discipline. While officers have near-complete discretion in their decision to make an arrest under most circumstances, it can manifest as doing nothing beyond giving a warning. In the case of people with SMI, however, it can mean police sometimes use a modicum of force to restrain or move a person or protect themselves from assault, and then opt not to charge. Police officers are concerned that if they use any force to resolve a situation with a person with an SMI, an arrest is required to properly document the encounter to avoid both liability and discipline. Similarly, if officers allow a disruptive person with an SMI to avoid arrest and do nothing beyond issue a warning, and that person then commits a crime in the aftermath, they worry they will be liable for not taking the person into custody when they had the opportunity to do so. The underlying belief in both cases is that an arrest is proof that an officer followed procedure, that they did all they were empowered to do, and that their actions and decisions were supported by law.

The criminal legal system should take steps to ensure that this is unnecessary. Documenting that a person's actions derived from manifestations of an SMI and the person's mental state precluded criminal liability should suffice to avert an arrest, and a linkage to care should hold just as much weight as any other outcome. Prosecutors and other criminal legal system officials are well situated to help bring about such a shift in other jurisdictions. As a person in custody moves through the criminal legal system, their condition should be screened by detention officials, who can flag individuals screening positive for symptoms of SMI and notify the police chain of command that a detainee may have a mental health condition that contributed to their behavior. Prosecutors should be thorough in determining if a defendant's mental state supports the charges they are facing and reduce or drop charges when a person lacked *mens rea* (i.e., criminal intent or knowledge of wrongdoing) by virtue of the presence of an SMI. When they do, they should notify the arresting agency of the reason for the outcome.

Beyond correcting the course with these checks and balances, the criminal legal system needs to partner with the health and treatment sector to do two things: 1) expand treatment capacity for those with SMI and 2) establish linkages that place a referral to effective treatment on par with making arrests. A police encounter with someone with an SMI that results in linkage to treatment rather than arrest should be considered a performance outcome as acceptable as criminal charges and as efficient a process as bringing a person to court for arraignment.

At present, this is rarely the case. The means to arrest a person and bring them to court are omnipresent across the nation, whereas the means to bring that same person to treatment for an SMI is often strained, inefficient, or simply unavailable, especially on nights and weekends. The alternative, which is most often a trip to a local emergency department, places undue strains on police resources and, in effect, asks emergency medical physicians to handle a condition that clearly requires referral to a specialist. It is a stopgap at best. We can implore police to make fewer arrests when they have problematic encounters with people with SMI, but it will be difficult to demand it of them until the health system and its partners provide truly feasible alternatives.

Mental Health Reforms to Reduce Obstruction Charges Among People With Serious Mental Illness

Just as changes can be made within the criminal legal system, mental health professionals and the larger mental health system could make changes to ensure that people with SMI are not inappropriately entangled by these types of misdemeanor charges.

Individual Mental Health Professionals

Given that a number of mental illness symptoms and impairments could increase the risk of "fighting words" and other behaviors resulting in obstruction-related charges, addressing and ameliorating those symptoms to the largest extent possible is mandatory. This likely entails both pharmacological and psychotherapeutic approaches. Beyond the optimal treatment of symptoms, asking about previous police contacts and strategizing with clients about advanced planning for future contacts is not outside the clinical purview if a goal is to help clients reduce their entanglement in the criminal legal system. This might include motivational approaches, role-playing, and the like, especially for those with prior police contacts and in particular for those with prior poor contacts or related charges.

Clinicians should take thorough histories in the area of prior police contacts and previous criminal legal system involvement. Because past behaviors and events predict future ones, knowing about a client's past experiences—and then planning and strategizing accordingly using a shared decision-making approach—could help clients reduce their risk of legal system involvement for the misdemeanors (or even felonies) discussed in this chapter. Clinicians should also take thorough histories of the various social determinants of health and psychosocial adversities, which clearly impact risk for police contacts.

The Larger Mental Health System

As noted, the police can only make fewer arrests when they have problematic encounters with people with SMI if the health system and its partners provide feasible alternatives. All elements of the crisis response system must be strengthened, including crisis centers that welcome referrals from (or immediate drop-off by) law enforcement officers. The larger mental health community can also partner with law enforcement with CIT programs and CIT training, which would include efforts to improve interactions through building rapport, focusing on procedural justice, and enhancing verbal de-escalation skills.

KEY POINTS

- A number of criminal charges—mostly misdemeanors—can arise directly from one's interaction with a law enforcement officer, including resisting arrest, obstructing a law enforcement officer, giving false information, menacing, and disorderly conduct.
- These types of charges are founded in part in case law on "fighting words," which allows police to remove a person from a scene before their speech escalates to violence or escalates others to violence.

- Public order and obstruction laws are critical for effective police work and can be used as tools for maintaining public safety; yet measures should be in place to reduce entanglement in the criminal legal system among individuals with mental illnesses for resisting- and obstructing-related charges when possible and appropriate.

- Individuals with mental illness, especially serious mental illness (SMI), may be at increased risk for interactions with police that could result in resisting- and obstructing-related charges. The increased risk may, in part, result from features of their illness (e.g., cognitive impairment, excitement-related symptoms, poor impulse control, psychotic symptoms), as well as prior negative experiences with the criminal legal system (e.g., poor perceived procedural justice).

- Whereas the various criminal legal system professionals may view such charges as needed to solve situations, as often secondary to other charges (e.g., criminal trespass), and as potentially overused, people with SMI facing such charges often view them as unfair and not representing the actual situation.

- Mental health professionals should take thorough legal histories, and when indicated, plan and strategize with clients, using a shared decision-making approach, around measures to reduce their risk for these types of charges.

References

Chaplinsky v. New Hampshire, 315 U.S. 568, 62 S. Ct. 766 (1942)

Compton MT, Graves J, Zern A, et al: Characterizing arrests and charges among individuals with serious mental illnesses in public-sector treatment settings. Psychiatr Serv 73(10):1102–1108, 2022 35378991

del Pozo B: "Arrest all street mendicants and beggars:" homelessness, social cooperation, and the commitments of democratic policing. Am Crim Law Rev 54(4):1681–1696, 2022a 35663245

del Pozo B: The Police and The State: Security, Social Cooperation, and the Public Good. Cambridge, U.K., Cambridge University Press, 2022b

Delmas C: A Duty to Resist: When Disobedience Should Be Uncivil. New York, Oxford University Press, 2018

Laniyonu A, Goff PA: Measuring disparities in police use of force and injury among persons with serious mental illness. BMC Psychiatry 21(1):500, 2021 34641794

Livingston JD: Contact between police and people with mental disorders: a review of rates. Psychiatr Serv 67(8):850–857, 2016 27079990

Moran R: Doing away with disorderly conduct. Boston Coll Law Rev 63(1):65–122, 2022

Morgan JN: Rethinking disorderly conduct. Calif Law Rev 109:1637–1702, 2021

Nix J, Shjarback JA: Factors associated with police shooting mortality: a focus on race and a plea for more comprehensive data. PLoS One 16(11):e0259024, 2021 34758026

Perras CJ: Prosecuting First Amendment retaliation. Department of Justice Journal of Federal Law and Practice 70(2):95–113, 2022

Ross CT, Winterhalder B, McElreath R: Racial disparities in police use of deadly force against unarmed individuals persist after appropriately benchmarking shooting data on violent crime rates. Soc Psychol Personal Sci 12(3):323–332, 2021

Shelby T: Justice, deviance, and the dark ghetto. Philos Public Aff 35(2):126–160, 2007

State v. Tracy, 130 A.3d 196, 2015 Vt. 111 (Vt. 2015)

Watson AC, Angell B: Applying procedural justice theory to law enforcement's response to persons with mental illness. Psychiatr Serv 58(6):787–793, 2007 17535938

"That's Scary Because Now They're Showing Violence"

Simple Assault Charges and Criminal Legal System Entanglement

Amy C. Watson, Ph.D.
Elisabeth E. Jackson, M.A.

The terms *assault* and *battery* are often used interchangeably. However, according to *Black's Law Dictionary* (Black and Garner 1999), *assault* refers to the threat of force or imminent harmful contact, while *battery* refers to actual contact in the form of nonconsensual physical violence or constraint inflicted on another person. At the federal level and in some states, assault encompasses both "an unlawful physical attack or threat of attack" (Bureau of Justice Statistics 2023). Assaults range in severity from minor verbal threats to physical attacks causing potentially life-threatening injuries. State legal codes vary in their approaches to assault and battery, in terms of whether there are separate statutes for domestic and nondomestic offenses and also what criteria are applied to distinguish a misdemeanor from a felony. However, overall, these terms refer to threats or actual violence against another person.

This chapter explores misdemeanor assault and battery offenses that lead to system entanglement for people with serious mental illness (SMI). We begin by exploring what is known about the frequency of violent crime generally, the characteristics of perpetrators/arrestees of these offenses, and the involvement of people with mental illness in violent crimes. We then explore the specific charge definitions in the home states of our four study sites, Georgia, Illinois, New York, and Pennsylvania, with attention to how each state handles domestic versus nondomestic offenses. The remainder of the chapter draws from our work exploring the perspectives of criminal legal system stakeholders in Atlanta, Chicago, Manhattan, and Philadelphia about how they approach assault and battery offenses committed by people with SMI.

Scope of the Problem: Violent Crime in the United States

Violent crime is the focus of significant media and policy attention, with recent attention focused on violent crime perceived to be committed by people with SMI. In New York City, for example, concern about unprovoked attacks on the subway have led to *New York Post* headlines such as "The subways are an insane asylum on wheels—we must get the mentally ill off the trains" (Cuozzo 2023) and Mayor Eric Adams stating, "When you do an analysis of the subway crimes we are seeing, you are seeing it is driven by people with mental health issues" (Feldman 2022), a claim that has been disputed. While the more serious and sensational acts of violence receive the most attention, lower-level assaults, the focus of this chapter, are far more common, comprising ~80% of all assaults nationwide (Thompson and Tapp 2023).

Existing national-level data do not allow us to determine what percentage of assaults are committed by people with SMI. However, data from the Bureau of Justice Statistics (BJS) National Crime Victimization Survey (NCVS) provide some context on general rates of violent victimization (Thompson and Tapp 2023). In 2022, the rate of any violent victimization (rape or sexual assault, robbery, aggravated assault, and simple assault) was 23.5 victimizations per 1,000 people, or 6.6 million victimizations. Included in this figure are simple assaults, which accounted for 13.7 victimizations per 1,000 people or roughly 3.86 million victimizations. Approximately 21% of all violent victimizations were domestic violence, and 45.1% were stranger violence, and less than half (41.5%) of all violent victimizations were reported to police. These numbers represent a significant decline in total violent victimizations from a high of 79.8 per 1,000 in 1993. The FBI's Uniform Crime Reporting (UCR) Program gathers data on arrests for violent crime but is limited to four felony charges: murder and nonnegligent manslaughter, rape, robbery, and aggravated assault. For those crimes, the rate was 3.69 per 1,000 people in 2018, which represents a 14.6% decrease from 2009 (Federal Bureau of Investigation 2019).

Predictors of Violent Crime Among People With (and Without) Serious Mental Illness

It is important to note that most people with SMI are not violent. As a broad group, however, they are at a modestly increased risk of committing violence against others (Fazel et al. 2009, 2010). Research has identified few specific clinical factors associated with increased violence risk other than threat/control-override delusions (delusional beliefs that cause the person to believe they are under threat coupled with intrusive thoughts that override impulse control) (Harris and Teasdale 2021) and treatment nonadherence (Elbogen et al. 2006). Rather, research indicates that violence is multiply determined and that risk factors for violence among people with SMI are generally the same as those for people without SMI (Elbogen et al. 2016; Silver and Teasdale 2005).

Factors at the individual, dispositional, situational, and community levels all play a role in violence risk for people with (and without) SMI. Individual-level factors increasing risk include male sex, younger age, substance use, psychopathy, and a history of victimization (Fazel et al. 2017; Skeem and Mulvey 2001; Swanson et al. 2002). Dispositional factors increasing risk include anger and perceived threat. Situational factors include impaired social relationships and stressful life events (disruptions or changes in employment, relationships, and living situations). Community-level factors such as violence in the surrounding environment also contribute to increased violence risk (Markowitz 2011). There is evidence that these factors largely, or entirely, mediate the relationship between SMI and violence (Elbogen et al. 2016). Put simply, SMI places people at higher risk of substance use, victimization, impaired social relationships, stressful life events, and living in neighborhoods with higher rates of violence and crime, all factors that increase their risk of violence.

Half of all violent acts committed by people with SMI are against family members (Estroff et al. 1998; Monahan et al. 2001), with ~20% of family members of people with SMI reporting they have experienced physical violence from their family member in the past year (Labrum and Solomon 2017). A review of the literature on violence by people with SMI toward family members indicates that the risk factors for family violence are similar for people with and without SMI. They include offender-victim co-residence, younger age, unemployment, substance use, and a history of violence (Labrum et al. 2021). Risk factors specific to those with SMI include nonadherence to medication or mental health treatment; reliance on family members for support; limits set by family members and the presence of criticism; and hostility and verbal aggression from the family member (Labrum et al. 2021). Research suggests that although people with SMI are modestly more likely to be offenders in adult child-parent incidents with police involvement, they are less likely to use nongun weapons and inflict injuries requiring medical attention (Labrum and Solomon 2022).

Arrests for Assault and Battery Among People With Serious Mental Illness

While NCVS and UCR provide information—however imperfect—about the rates of violent crimes, they do not include information on the mental health status of alleged perpetrators. Several studies have combined arrest and public mental health system data to examine arrests among people with SMI. Fisher et al. (2011) compared arrest rates of public mental health service recipients categorized as living with SMI and the general public across a broad range of offenses in Massachusetts in 1991 and 1992. They found that 32.8% of the cohort with SMI were arrested, making them nearly two-thirds more likely (OR 1.62) to have any arrest during the 12-month period. When looking specifically at crimes against persons, however, people with SMI were more than three times more likely (OR 3.17) to be arrested for a felony, more than four times more likely (OR 4.22) to be arrested for a misdemeanor, and nearly six times more likely (OR 5.96) to be arrested for assault and battery of a police officer.

As described in Chapter 1 ("The System, the Process, and the Contexts"), our analysis of all arrests in New York State from 2010 through 2013 found that simple assault was among the most common charges of arrestees with an SMI indicator, comprising 14% of arrests, versus 14.9% for arrestees without an SMI indicator (Compton et al. 2023). This differed from Fisher et al.'s (2011) earlier finding that people with SMI were significantly more likely to have been arrested for misdemeanor crimes against persons. However, it is consistent with a study examining self-reported criminal legal system involvement among individuals with schizophrenia being treated with antipsychotic medications, which found that among those reporting any criminal legal system encounters (at baseline or during the study period), 13% reported they had been arrested for assault (Ascher-Svanum et al. 2010).

Substance use has consistently been found to increase the risk of violence and arrest for violent crimes among people with SMI. Swartz and Lurigio (2007) analyzed data from the National Survey on Drug Use and Health and found a relationship between psychiatric disorder and past-year arrest for nonviolent crime that was entirely mediated by substance use. This means that psychiatric disorder is associated with nonviolent crime arrests primarily because the disorder increases the risk of substance use. When looking at arrests for violent crime, however, they found the relationship between psychiatric disorders and past-year arrest to be only partially mediated by substance use, suggesting that SMI had both an indirect effect (via substance use) and an independent effect on likelihood of arrest for violent crimes.

The reliance on police to respond to mental health crisis situations may also increase the risk of arrest for violent crime for people with SMI. A recent study found that 8.9% of all arrests for assault and battery of a law enforcement officer in Virginia over a 10-year period were filed against individuals with a recent mental health commitment order history (Agee et al. 2019). Based on this temporal association, the authors surmised that a subgroup of these charges is likely directly due to acute crisis and apprehension, related to emergency commitment orders.

Criminal Charges Relating to Threats and Violence

In this chapter, we focus on misdemeanor assault and battery charges, or what is often referred to as simple assault. In general, this term refers to verbal or physical attacks that do not involve weapons and result in no injury, minor injury (e.g., bruises, cuts, swelling), or an injury necessitating <2 days of hospitalization. It also includes attempted assaults without the use of a weapon. In comparison, aggravated assault (a felony charge) signifies a more severe attack, not simply a threat. It encompasses the use of weapons, regardless of whether the victim sustains injuries, as well as assaults without a weapon that cause serious injury.

States vary regarding the terms and definitions of specific charges related to threats of violence and actual violent acts. Some states, such as Pennsylvania, use the term *simple assault* for threats and low-level violent contact, whereas other states, such as Illinois, define assault as a threat and battery as a completed assault with actual physical contact. Table 8–1 provides relevant statutes for assault- and battery-related charges in Georgia, Illinois, New York, and Pennsylvania, where our four study sites are located.

All four states distinguish incidents between family or household members as domestic or family violence, and three treat repeat domestic offenses as more serious than repeat violence between strangers. Georgia, for example, escalates domestic battery charges to felonies after the second offense instead of the third, which is the threshold for nondomestic violence (Ga. Code § 16–5–23.1). In New York, an assault (the state's term for battery) is charged as a felony if it is against a household member and the defendant has been convicted (not merely charged) of a similar assault or battery in the past (NY Penal Law § 120.00). Illinois approaches things quite similarly—if the defendant batters a family or household member while also having been convicted of a similar offense in the past, the charge is upgraded to a Class 4 felony (720 ILCS 5/12–3.2). Pennsylvania, however, makes no distinction between offenses committed against family members versus strangers or acquaintances, in terms of how the offense is charged (18 Pa. C.S. § 2701). Two of our study sites—Chicago (Cook County) and Atlanta (Fulton County)—have separate courts for handling domestic violence cases.

Case Example: Ms. Ruiz

Lisa Ruiz is a 59-year-old Latina woman diagnosed with schizoaffective disorder. She lived with her mother until her mother's death 2 years ago. When her mother was alive, Ms. Ruiz was engaged in services at the local community mental health agency, had a part-time job at a local thrift store, and assisted her mother around the house. After her mother's death, she had been staying with her younger brother's family, but she did not get along with her brother's wife. Several months ago, the police were called, and she was arrested for domestic battery. No one was injured, but her brother's wife insisted that she not be allowed to return. Since then, she has been homeless, alternating between sleeping under a footpath bridge and in a public park. She lost the paperwork she was given after she was arrested, including the information with her court date. Thus, she missed her court date, and a failure-to-appear warrant was issued. It was November, the weather was getting colder, and she needed to find someplace warmer to sleep. She located an apartment building vestibule that had a broken door lock and slept there for a couple of nights. During the day, she spent her time near the building, sometimes pacing on the sidewalk mumbling to herself. Sometimes she thought the people going in and out of the building were staring and planning to harm her. In fact, they were alarmed by her presence and

Table 8–1. State assault and battery statutes

Item	Georgia	Illinois	New York	Pennsylvania
Statute	Ga. Code §16–5–20; Ga. Code §16–5–23.1	720 ILCS 5/12–1; 720 ILCS 5/12–3; 720 ILCS 5/12–3.2	NY Penal Law § 120.00; NY Penal Law § 240.75	18 Pa. C.S. § 2701
Offense	Simple assault, battery	Assault, battery, domestic battery	Assault in the third degree (no separate battery statute)	Simple assault (no separate battery statute)
Domestic offense	Family violence battery—same as assault and battery charge, but against household member	Domestic battery—bodily harm to family/household member, insulting or provoking contact	Domestic violence—no separate statute, but the term applies to violence between household members	Domestic violence—no separate offense, but term applies to violence between household members
Threshold for felony	Three or more offenses against same victim; two if intrafamilial; two if prior "forcible felony"; aggravated assault/battery	Class 3 felony if "aggravated battery"; Class 4 felony if against household member and defendant has similar prior conviction	Class E felony if against household member and defendant has similar prior conviction (aggravated family offense)	First- or second-degree felony if aggravated (no distinction for household members)
Grading	Misdemeanor (for assault, battery, family violence battery)*	Class A misdemeanor (for assault, battery, and domestic battery)	Class A misdemeanor	Second-degree misdemeanor
Notes	*Assault* = threat of violence; *battery* = physical harm from violence. Violence between household members is treated as more egregious and escalates to felony sooner.	*Assault* = threat or risk of battery; *battery* = actual harm inflicted. A repeat offense of domestic battery against a family/household member is a Class 4 felony.	The basic requirement for any assault conviction is that the defendant causes physical injury.	Battery, while not a separate charge, is essentially a completed assault. There is no distinction or additional escalation for family/household members.

*Georgia does not have degrees or classes of misdemeanors; simple assault is either "misdemeanor" or "misdemeanor of a high and aggravated nature."
Source. Illinois Compiled Statutes Criminal Code 2022; New York Penal Law 2022; Official Code of Georgia Annotated 2022; Pennsylvania Consolidated Statutes 2022.

were talking to each other about whether they should call the building manager or the police. When a man who lived in the building walked past and asked her what she was doing there, Ms. Ruiz felt threatened, pushed the man to the ground, and yelled "I know what you are up to, leave me alone!" At that point, another resident called the police, and Ms. Ruiz was arrested on misdemeanor battery charges and a failure-to-appear warrant for her domestic battery case. This time she was taken to the county jail.

Before her first court appearance, Ms. Ruiz met with her public defender and a case manager from the Certified Community Behavioral Health Clinic (CCBHC) program that works with court-involved clients. They put together a plan to reconnect her to services but explained that the judge may not release her because she had no place to live, a history of missing court dates, and now two cases involving violent crimes.

Criminal Legal System Stakeholders' Perspectives on Assault-Related Charges

Our four-city study (Atlanta, Chicago, Manhattan, and Philadelphia) encompassed focus groups with professionals within the criminal legal system, including police officers, police supervisors, prosecutors, judges, and public defenders—as well as a focus group with people with lived experience of mental illnesses and criminal legal system involvement. One area of questioning was the use and handling of assault and battery charges. Before exploring the perspectives of professional stakeholders, we consider how people with mental illnesses experience arrests for assault-related charges and their resulting criminal legal system involvement.

Lived Experience Perspectives

During our focus group with people with lived experience, participants described feeling unfairly arrested, helpless and overwhelmed in court, and poorly treated in jail. One participant discussed being arrested for third-degree assault after he hit a person with an umbrella on the side of the arm in self-defense during an argument:

> I don't have the right to put my hands on anybody else unless it's to help them or to protect myself. So if I'm gonna be protecting myself and, you know, I hit somebody with an umbrella, and for them to take that and turn it around and say, "This is assault with a deadly weapon"?

Another participant related the story of her arrest for assault, following an accusation from another person staying at a shelter:

> I walked into the shelter, and they arrested me, the DHS [Department of Homeless Services] police. And it didn't matter what I said that, you know, I wasn't even around there that day.... There's nothing on my hands. I was, you know, just because she said it, they actually made me go struggle the whole night [in lock-up] through [until] court, [then] took me into the hospital. They [police] treated me like shit. They wouldn't even let me sit down on like the chair.

Charges were later dropped because the participant was not at the shelter the day the alleged assault occurred, but she still faced collateral consequences:

> But then I was not allowed to go back to that shelter. So I ended up on the street.... I lost everything I owned, and just, you know, and because the prosecutor wanted me to go to jail and wanted the $1,500 bail, because a girl said that I hit her, and [I] never touched her.

Thus, even when charges are dropped, the negative consequences of an arrest can be particularly devastating for a person with an SMI living with very limited social supports.

Criminal Legal System Professionals' Perspectives

Professionals working in or with the criminal legal system discussed typical simple assault scenarios, how the situations are approached by first responders, and the subsequent processing and dispositions of these charges. Overall, they indicated that assault-related charges are common among the people with SMI who they see coming into the system. When asked about the typical scenarios that result in misdemeanor assault-related charges, they discussed domestic assault cases involving members of the same household, as well as cases involving non-related individuals that include acquaintances, police officers, and complete strangers. We begin with descriptions of the different types of simple assault cases, and then examine considerations and concerns of criminal legal professionals in their handling of these cases.

DOMESTIC ASSAULT

The stakeholders in our study described how domestic assault cases involving people with SMI typically involve an adult living with a parent, most often their mother, who is struggling to manage their adult child's behavior. As a Chicago-based community mental health professional discussed, the lack of resources often leaves families with limited options when they do not feel safe with the person in their home:

> A lot of the times, the family members don't want that person to be in jail, but they don't feel safe. And so, like as we mentioned, there aren't a lot of resources, there aren't housing or facilities. There's not support for people with severe mental illness and substance use problems. So, if they're having these issues and they're the victim of violence, the only thing that they can think of to do is call the police, even though they're not interested in having their son or their sister or whatever, sit in jail for 90 days or a year. So, it's pretty sad.

Public defenders indicated that sometimes family members call the police because they simply "want a break" from their adult child with an SMI or because they are at a loss for how to effectively diffuse an escalating or potentially violent situation.

NONDOMESTIC ASSAULT

Stakeholders described a variety of nondomestic misdemeanor assault and battery offenses involving people with SMI, including those committed against acquaintances, police officers, and complete strangers. According to a Philadelphia prosecutor, acquaintance assaults often are the result of altercations with neighbors:

> That happens often with neighbors because, unfortunately, people with mental illnesses sometimes act out, they're loud … we often have people that bang against walls, something of that nature. And then the neighbor confronts them about that, and that can turn into assault, threat, something of that nature.

A Manhattan prosecutor explained his impression that when mental illness is not a factor, acquaintance assaults are generally one-time events, with no further interaction between the people involved, whereas assaults involving a person with an SMI sometimes involve continued contact or stalking. A different Manhattan prosecutor explained it as follows:

> So maybe there'll be issues between acquaintances, particularly, there will be instances of continued contact, whether it be on the phone, on text message, on other mediums, showing up at their place of residence that either escalates into assaultive conduct or starts with assaultive conduct and then continues one way or the other.

Several participants indicated that they commonly see cases of assaults on police officers by people with SMI, often related to another charge. Sometimes these are the result of an officer on patrol engaging with a person they see trespassing.

A Chicago mental health professional also provided insight into how situations sometimes escalate when a person with an SMI is being arrested:

> Yeah, because if someone's getting arrested for something else and they're experiencing symptoms or they're, I don't know, just like in the middle of something like that, then they're getting escalated and escalated and then there's not someone there who can help de-escalate, or it's just automatically pretty traumatizing and horrible to get arrested, so that's not going to calm them down. So it just contributes to the situation.

The category of assault that generated the most concern in our discussions was seemingly random attacks on strangers. Prosecutors indicated that this type of assault is a flag for mental illness. As one Manhattan prosecutor indicated, "You know it's generally when you see you have a pattern of those cases, really, there's some mental health issues here. But then, you know, we have competing concerns—we want, you know, long story short, we want them to stop attacking people on the street."

In addition to recognizing a pattern, sometimes the victim identifies a potential mental health issue. As a Chicago prosecutor explained, "The [complaining witnesses] in those instances are telling us, like, I think something's not right here. And that's kind of how we are flagging those cases."

Participants provided examples of these types of assaults that included a person walking around the neighborhood punching people in the face, shoving someone on a public transit platform, or punching someone they perceive to be making fun of them or a panhandler threatening or hitting a person who does not give them money. Stranger assaults were of particular concern for stakeholders in Manhattan, as one prosecutor explained: "There's not one prototypical case. What I would say is it usually centers around something that sets off the defendant and makes them angry, and their reaction is to punch somebody in the face. And that's scary because now they're showing violence."

OPTIONS AND CONSIDERATIONS AT THE POINT OF POLICE CONTACT

Police officers have several options for handling situations involving simple assault that vary depending on whether the case is domestic or nondomestic. Options that participants discussed included custodial arrest, citations, and taking the person to the hospital with or without charges. They noted that police officers must strike a delicate balance between victim preferences and safety. Discussing domestic violence–related assaults specifically, Chicago officers explained that they consider the preferences of the victim, the severity of the situation, and whether the battery was a direct result of the person's mental illness. In general, unless there is a weapon involved, they prefer to take the person to the hospital. As one officer indicated, "I can't speak for the whole city, but I don't know of any officer where I work that would rather take them to jail than go sign them into the hospital."

Even in cases where the family initially wants an arrest, they often change their minds once the police arrive. As one police officer in Chicago explained:

> In the heat of the moment, [the family is] going to sign anything to everything just so that person goes to jail. But within 10 to 15 minutes, you talk some sense, and they're like, "Yeah, you know what, you're right. Yeah, get him to a hospital." Because you've got to remember, they're the ones that just received a beating or whatever.

Criminal legal options for nondomestic simple assaults varied across our study cities. Specifically, in Manhattan and Philadelphia, when officers decide to address a nondomestic assault as a crime, they are directed to issue desk appearance tickets (DATs) or citations in lieu of arrests for nondomestic misdemeanor assault cases. This is frustrating for the officers who must explain to victims why they're not making a custodial arrest. As a Philadelphia officer stated, "So you mean to tell me you're not going to lock him up? That's exactly what I'm telling you. That's our policy."

A Manhattan prosecutor expressed concern about DATs and the escalation of violent behavior, citing a case in which a person assaulted a random person on the subway and was given a DAT: "But guess what, they give this defendant a desk appearance ticket and guess what happens, a few weeks later, that defendant pushes somebody in front of a subway." In these situations, officers in Philadelphia indicated that they may be able to take a perpetrator with an SMI to the hospital on a 302 petition (involuntary psychiatric commitment) and charge them later, but that the process is very time consuming and, in their view, not very productive, as prosecutors often do not follow up and go through with charges. Although Chicago officers were encouraged to issue citations for low-level offenses in the height of the pandemic, they no longer are so encouraged and can make custodial arrests for misdemeanor domestic and nondomestic assault and battery offenses.

In discussing assaults on police officers, Philadelphia officers expressed frustration and indicated they often do not bother to charge people with assault on an officer or resisting, "Because we know it's not going anywhere." They further explained that assaults against them rarely get upgraded to aggravated assault (a felony). Prosecutors in Chicago explained that although minor assaults on officers can be charged as felonies, they have some leeway in charging depending on the level of injury to the officer. Usually, officers are agreeable to charging at the misdemeanor level. However, as one prosecutor explained, "It's the breaking the skin and the spitting where the leniency is gone."

CHALLENGES WITH EXISTING POST-ARREST OPTIONS

In cases in which officers do make an arrest for misdemeanor simple assault, options tend to be more limited than they are for nonviolent offenses and vary by site and type of assault. Stakeholders discussed challenges with the available options related to the need to consider victim preference and public safety, the impact of housing instability and lack of housing on considerations of noncustodial options, the onerous requirements that are difficult for people with SMI to successfully navigate, and the lack of good mental health treatment options.

Concern about public safety was paramount in the minds of criminal legal professionals, as well as the need to balance this concern with victim preferences. In discussing Atlanta's domestic violence diversion program, judges stated that they reserve these programs for less serious domestic violence assaults in which there are no severe physical injuries ("It has to be—you can't have any black eyes, any tooth missing"). The underlying concern is the safety of the family members and the public. Prosecutors in Atlanta indicated, however, that with more serious offenses, they have an advantage because they can offer a short initial jail sentence that provides time to get the person into treatment, with the threat of a longer jail sentence if the person does not follow through with treatment:

> So the only reason we go forward on those cases [is] if we see an immediate ability to impact public safety in our court. So it may be through incapacitation, because we can give up to 180 days in jail, instead of the year that you can get on this charge. We can leverage that jail time to get treatment for somebody to go [to] a mental health outpatient or an inpatient facility.... So there's an opportunity for an immediate impact on correcting people's behavior.

Although prosecutors generally indicated that they try to honor the victim's preferences, they also described persuading victims who either wanted the case to be dismissed or wanted the defendant to be sentenced to the maximum amount of jail time that the best option from a public safety perspective would be a mental health treatment plan supervised by the court. A Philadelphia prosecutor explained:

> We're kind of that middle ground and say listen, I want to keep this here for a while, have them engage in treatment, come back to you, and you know, at the end of the day, we all get what we want, where hopefully, this person will be in a better place and will continue to take their medication and, at the same time, not have a criminal record as a result. So people, our victims, the ones that want the case ... like I said, they don't want to see the person prosecuted, they don't see them with a record, they don't want to see them in jail. When they have this option, they're more willing to let the case remain open.

Emphasizing how seriously they take random stranger assaults, a Manhattan prosecutor stated, "Those are horrifying and terrifying and those escalate very quickly, and we see people who subsequently get arrested for very tragic charges after that." The concern about the potential for escalating violent behavior makes these cases top priority for prosecutors in her office. Random stranger assaults are also a concern for judges, as a Chicago public defender pointed out:

> You know, there was like a pregnant woman walking down the street and the guy like tackled her from behind. I mean, it's just nonsensical. And that's—the judges are very disturbed by that.... Well, with my judge, who was obviously about getting help for the client, but protecting the public [too], they don't want their name in the newspaper for this guy going out and tackling the pregnant woman again.

Public defenders and mental health professionals discussed how not having housing led to people with SMI spending more time in jail on simple assault charges. A Philadelphia defense attorney explained that if the person has a place to live, they can line up services and present a plan to the judge. However, if the person does not have a place to live or cannot return to where they were previously living, they may be stuck in jail for a while:

> Judges are very, very cautious about letting people in custody go to the shelter system or the streets, especially with people with SMI. They want more structure. The shelters are dangerous, they are not structured. And living on the streets is not an option. So therefore, if we have the client who is in jail on an assault charge who wants to get out and has no place to live, they're going to be in jail for a while.

In domestic assault cases, judges may be hesitant to release people with SMI if they do not have somewhere besides the victim's home to live, even if the family wants to drop the charges. As a Chicago-based community mental health professional indicated, "It's sort of the same thing we were talking about earlier with criminal trespassing is they'll want there to be a different housing plan in place, which we typically can't provide. And so, again, people get stuck in jail."

Onerous court requirements were another concern of stakeholders. These requirements can come into play early in the process, at the point of arraignment. Judges may be willing to release a person with an SMI while their simple assault case is pending but may place extra conditions that can further entangle a client. A public defender in Manhattan explained that it's not always a good strategy to bring up their client's mental illness at the arraignment hearing:

> So one thing that's really hard about assault three cases [assault in the third degree], in particular for people who have serious mental illness or any mental illness, is that bringing that up at arraignment, it's such a trap. Because it's often needed to explain why someone has a record that they do, especially failures to appear or like why they need to be home to stay connected to their services. But then the judge hears: "Oh, he has schizophrenia, like, and this is an allegation of violence, like, those are related. What this person needs in this case is supervised release." And I feel like that's often the thing of like, you need to bring it up for a judge to even entertain the argument, and then they're put under more conditions.

Stakeholders also discussed how often the requirements of diversion programs are difficult for people with SMI to navigate, which may set them up to fail. For example, Philadelphia has a diversion program for low-level domestic violence charges. However, Philadelphia defenders noted that this option is not always appropriate for arrestees with SMI who are too acutely symptomatic to participate in the program. In Chicago, the Domestic Violence Court does not offer any post-arrest diversion options. Moreover, the standard requirements of domestic violence courts are often steeper and potentially challenging for people with SMI to navigate. As a supervisor in the Domestic Violence Court in Chicago put it:

> Usually, there's mandatory treatment or anger management or whatever [the courts] want to mandate, and orders of protection to be entered. So, there's a lot more compliance issues. And then when you talk about somebody that's on meds, you know medication—or if they should be—compliance, just in life, is difficult. But then [they're] deal-

ing with those issues or a whole other list of requirements, just to stay out of jail.

Finally, participants expressed frustration that the lack of mental health services in the community is another barrier for clients trying to navigate court requirements. A Chicago public defender indicated that victims, prosecutors, and judges are generally amenable to a mental health service plan but expressed concern that the lack of mental health resources may set clients up for failure.

> I think you can usually get most victims on board with treatment and judges on board with treatment and the state, if there is some evidence that it will be effective. But the courts are so underresourced to provide meaningful mental health treatment that keeps people accountable that … a lot of times when you try to get people help, the resources are so few that you're setting them up for failure and perhaps a worse outcome down the road. So, I think it's hard. Like, we all know what we would like to see happen, but the resources don't exist for that to happen.

Thus, even in situations in which the person with SMI avoids jail initially, they may struggle to satisfy court requirements, which may prolong their entanglement. Let's return to Ms. Ruiz's battery case.

Case Example, continued: Ms. Ruiz's Battery Case

When her public defender presented the plan to reconnect her with mental health services to the judge, the judge immediately asked if Ms. Ruiz had a place to live. The public defender explained that she did not, but a case manager from the CCBHC was working on finding her housing. The judge replied, "Great, once they find her a place to stay, we can talk about supervised release. She can get treatment at the jail while she waits."

In the week that followed, the victim called the prosecutor's office to say he only suffered a minor abrasion and really did not have time to go to court and pursue the case. He did not feel it made sense for Ms. Ruiz to be prosecuted and jailed, as long as she stayed away from the apartment building. Plus, the building manager finally fixed the lock on the vestibule door. Concerned about potential future violent behavior, the prosecutor persuaded the victim that prosecuting the case would be best for Ms. Ruiz and for public safety in general, because they could ensure she followed the treatment plan for a while. By the next court date, the case manager had located temporary housing for Ms. Ruiz, and the prosecutor and public defender negotiated a plea agreement for her cases that required her to report to probation every 2 weeks and follow a treatment plan, along with a number of other conditions, for 12 months. Although Ms. Ruiz was not sure she could keep track of all of the court requirements, she was happy to get out of jail. She was hopeful that with housing and the support of her case manager, she would be able to avoid going back to jail.

Criminal Legal System Reforms to Reduce Entanglement of People With Serious Mental Illness on Misdemeanor Assault Charges

Simple assault cases carry public safety concerns that are more pronounced than those associated with most other misdemeanor offenses common among people with SMI entangled in the criminal legal system. This added complexity is reflected in the perspectives of professional stakeholders as well as the story of Ms. Ruiz. While they were all working to prevent further violent behavior and criminal legal system involvement, professionals in different roles varied in their perspectives, or *focal concerns* (see Chapter 4, "Common Themes and Tensions"). For example, prosecutors worked to keep people under the supervision of the court, whereas public defenders preferred to assist people in connecting to services but to get them out from under court requirements and monitoring as quickly as possible. As with shoplifting and trespass charges, decisions about pursuing and processing simple assault charges were influenced by the law and policy environment (e.g., policy related to DATs), where the behavior occurred (e.g., public transit), the preferences of victims, the availability of community resources (housing in particular), and knowledge of mental illnesses (Wood et al. 2023). Understanding the concerns of stakeholders and the complexity of the decision-making environment (see Chapter 3, "Decision-Making Contexts of Misdemeanor Charges") suggests multiple levers of reform in the criminal legal and mental health systems that have potential to reduce the entanglement of people with SMI on misdemeanor assault charges.

Policing Reforms

As discussed earlier in the chapter, recent criminal legal system reforms in New York City and Philadelphia direct police to issue DATs or citations in lieu of arrest for nondomestic simple assaults. Although this policy frustrates officers' and prosecutors' efforts to maintain public safety, it keeps people out of jail and may prevent disruption in housing and services for people with SMI. However, as in Ms. Ruiz's story, people with SMI, particularly those with unstable housing, may have difficulty keeping track of their court dates and end up with failure-to-appear warrants when they miss court dates. These warrants set them up for additional police contacts that carry a risk of escalating to resisting arrest or assault on a police officer. Although they are not "policing reforms," strategies to ensure people make their court dates could mitigate this risk. Several jurisdictions, including New York City, have experimented with court date reminder calls and found the approach effective for reducing failures to appear (Ferri 2022).

A variety of approaches to improve how police respond to calls involving people with SMI show potential for reducing arrests and getting people connected to mental health care. They may also reduce the likelihood of encounters escalating and the person with mental illness being charged with an assault on an officer. Probably the most well-known, the Crisis Intervention Team (CIT) model, was first developed in 1988 following the fatal shooting of a Black man with an SMI by a Memphis police officer. The core components of the model include partnerships between police, mental health service providers, and advocates; specialized training for officers; and an identified receiving center where officers can take people in need of immediate psychiatric care. While there is significant variation in how communities are implementing the model, the evidence is strong that CIT implementation increases linkages to mental health services (Compton et al. 2014; Kubiak et al. 2017; Watson et al. 2021). Although less robust, the evidence also shows that CIT can likely reduce arrests and uses of force (Compton et al. 2014; Morabito et al. 2012; Steadman et al. 2000). Another model growing in popularity is the co-responder model, in which clinicians respond to mental health crisis calls alongside officers. The available evidence suggests that these co-response teams may reduce unnecessary emergency room transports and effectively connect people to care. As with CIT, the evidence that they may reduce arrests is limited (Bailey et al. 2022), and one study found co-response to be associated with reduced use of force in suicide threat/attempt calls (Blais and Brisebois 2021).

In the aftermath of the murder of George Floyd, calls to reduce the footprint of law enforcement, particularly in communities of color, have been vocal and many. Communities across the country are now building the capacity to send unarmed, non-law-enforcement community responder teams to locations of 911 calls. Depending on the community, these teams may respond to mental health crisis calls, welfare check calls, minor disputes, and calls related to homelessness and social vulnerability. Operating out of the Whitebird Clinic since 1988, Crisis Assistance Helping Out On The Streets (CAHOOTS) teams are dispatched via the Eugene, Oregon, emergency communications center. Comprising a crisis counselor and a medic, CAHOOTS teams provide crisis intervention services that include crisis counseling, conflict resolution, and housing assistance. Recent research on Denver's community response team, Support Team Assisted Response (STAR) program, suggests that in the first 6 months of STAR pilot implementation, reports of low-level misdemeanor crime (trespass, resisting arrest, public disorder) decreased 34% (Dee and Pyne 2022). Although in general, community response teams do not respond to crime-related calls, they provide nonpolice options in other types of situations. These options could reduce opportunities for assault on a police officer and resisting arrest charges. By providing crisis support, conflict mediation, and housing assistance, such teams have the potential to address the underlying situations that sometimes lead to simple assaults. Imagine if the apartment building residents concerned about Ms. Ruiz's presence had the option of accessing a community responder team that engaged and assisted in finding her somewhere else to sleep and spend her time. Perhaps the interaction between Ms. Ruiz and the building resident (and resulting battery charges) could have been avoided altogether.

Larger Criminal Legal System Reform

Moving beyond the initial police contact, a variety of specialized mental health court and community supervision programs, designed to serve people with SMI, are in place. These programs typically require compliance with treatment requirements and regular monitoring over a period of 12 months or more. Successful program completion may allow the defendant to avoid a conviction or time in jail or prison. Some do not accept defendants charged with violent crimes, whereas others will with the consent of the victim. Although there is some evidence that mental health court programs may have a small effect on reducing recidivism compared with normal court processing (Lowder et al. 2018), concerns have been raised about such programs widening the net of who is brought into the system and prolonging the entanglement of people with mental illness who struggle to comply with program requirements and enhanced monitoring.

The Cook County (Illinois) Fitness Diversion Program discussed by our Chicago stakeholders (see Chapter 2, "Using System Maps to Understand Entanglement and Guide Change") offers a promising approach that connects misdemeanor defendants with SMI to care and monitors their engagement with treatment for up to 90 days before disposing cases. This may avoid lengthy fitness evaluation and restoration processes (i.e., those related to competency) or longer-term entanglement in mental health court programs, while ensuring that defendants are connected to care. To be eligible, however, defendants cannot have a violent background. Although acceptance decisions are made on a case-by-case basis, individuals charged with misdemeanor assault and battery may not qualify. As programs such as this grow, however, there may be opportunities to expand eligibility to a broader set of misdemeanor charges.

Some people assessed by Cook County's Fitness Diversion Court are transferred to civil court for assisted outpatient treatment (AOT) orders. Hoge and Bonnie (2021) have recently proposed this pathway as a new form of civil commitment that would divert defendants with SMI into treatment provided under civil rather than criminal court supervision. Unlike criminal-system diversion programs that require voluntary entry, this pathway could be initiated by various parties and would not require consent of the defendant. The process they propose would differ from the usual civil commitment process by considering criminal legal factors (e.g., likelihood of reoffending), including more restrictions, and placing greater emphasis on public safety and maintaining compliance. The intensity of court involvement in this new form of civil commitment would be high and perhaps more appropriate for those who have committed more serious violent offenses. However, although there is some evidence that standard AOT orders, paired with comprehensive services over an adequate period of time, may reduce low-level violent behavior, no evidence suggests that it reduces more serious acts of violence (Swartz et al. 2017). Ensuring the availability of comprehensive services and supports, which often are not easily accessible, could improve many outcomes for people with SMI at risk for low-level violent behavior and criminal legal system entanglement. Rather than legal system reforms, that would require mental health system reforms.

Mental Health System Reforms to Reduce Entanglement of People With Serious Mental Illness on Misdemeanor Assault Charges

As discussed earlier, violence risk factors for people with SMI are generally the same as for people without SMI (Elbogen et al. 2016; Silver and Teasdale 2005). However, the psychosocial circumstances often associated with having an SMI increase exposure to violence risk factors. Thus, mental health system efforts seeking to reduce entanglement of people with SMI would be wise to address psychosocial risks related to substance use; situational factors such as impaired social relationships and stressful life events (disruptions or changes in living situations, employment, and relationships); and living in neighborhoods with high crime rates and disadvantage.

Addressing housing issues, in particular, has the potential to mitigate risk factors for violence by reducing disruptions in the living situations of people with SMI. Programs using the Housing First model provide low-barrier, permanent supportive housing for people experiencing chronic homelessness. The largest randomized trial of Housing First, the Canadian At Home/Chez Soi Demonstration Project, found positive outcomes related to achieving and maintaining stable housing, quality of life, and community functioning (Aubry et al. 2015). Interview data from that study indicated that having stable housing and positive and supportive social contacts were key to positive life outcomes. Studies looking at the impact of Housing First interventions on criminal legal system involvement have shown mixed results. Several studies have found reductions in criminal legal system involvement associated with Housing First interventions, although they do not differentiate types of crime (Ellsworth 2022; Kriegel et al. 2016). However, two randomized studies specifically looking at arrests found that those enrolled in Housing First programs did not experience fewer arrests (Aubry et al. 2015; Stergiopoulos et al. 2015). From the perspectives of the criminal legal professionals in our study, housing is an important factor in decisions to release people with SMI from jail while their case is pending and in developing plans for disposing cases. In Ms. Ruiz's case, low-barrier supportive housing might have prevented her contact with police in the battery case.

The mental health system and mental health professionals also have a role in addressing violence against family members, which makes up half of all violent offenses committed by people with SMI (Estroff et al. 1998; Monahan et al. 2001). Risk factors for family-related violence are increased when the person with an SMI is financially dependent on the family member, particularly when that family member is the payee for the person's Social Security benefits (Elbogen et al. 2005; Labrum and Solomon 2016). Furthermore, in several studies, families have reported that efforts at setting limits or insisting their relative with mental illness take medications preceded the acts of family violence (Labrum and Solomon 2016; Straznickas et al. 1993; Varghese et al. 2016). Promising strategies to reduce violence toward family members may include strengthening support services for people with SMI so that they are less financially dependent on family members, improving strategies to engage people in treatment, and enhancing family members' abilities to prevent and manage conflict (Labrum et al. 2021). Considering Ms. Ruiz's story, such interventions would have been indicated early on when she was having conflicts while living with her brother's family.

Finally, current efforts at the state and federal levels to support the creation of responsive crisis service systems (see Chapter 10, "Reform in an Era of Mental Health and Crisis Services Innovation") hold promise for providing support to people with SMI without engaging the criminal legal system. These efforts include the expansion of mobile crisis team capacity, which may reduce the reliance on police as responders to mental health crises and, as with community responder teams, reduce the opportunities for situations that result in charges related to assaults on officers. These efforts also include crisis stabilization centers, or somewhere besides hospital emergency departments and jails, for people to go when experiencing a crisis. In cases in which police are involved, they may be more willing to forgo an arrest if they have a mobile crisis team to call or a crisis stabilization center to take a person in crisis to. Further, crisis respite facilities or other forms of short-term housing, where people can stay for a few days to several weeks, provide an option when family tensions are high or caregivers have reached the limits of their ability to support a loved one in crisis.

KEY POINTS

- Most people with serious mental illness (SMI) are not violent. Risk factors for violence among people with SMI are generally the same as for people without SMI.

- Across professional stakeholders, public safety and reducing the risk of subsequent violent offenses by people with SMI—whether they are against family members, acquaintances, or complete strangers—is of paramount importance, particularly in the context of media and public concern about violent crime.

- Prosecutors viewed pursuing charges and keeping cases open in the system as a mechanism to leverage mental health treatment participation, and as a result, improve public safety. Public defenders expressed concerns that adding more conditions of release and community supervision due to a defendant's mental illness alone are a trap that sets up their clients for failure and long-term entanglement in the criminal legal system.

- Public defenders and mental health professionals noted the lack of mental health and social service system resources, and housing in particular, as factors that make it nearly impossible for their clients with SMI to be disentangled.
- Crisis Intervention Teams, co-responder teams, and community responder teams show potential for reducing client entanglement at the point of initial police contact. Larger criminal legal system efforts to address the needs of people with SMI include mental health courts and fitness diversion programs (deferred prosecution).
- State and federal efforts to develop crisis services have potential to provide support to people with SMI without engaging the criminal legal system. Furthermore, addressing housing issues has the potential to mitigate risk factors for violence by reducing disruptions in the living situations of people with SMI.

References

Agee ER, Zelle H, Kelley S, Moore SJ: Marshaling administrative data to study the prevalence of mental illness in assault on law enforcement cases. Behav Sci Law 37(6):636–649, 2019 31957089

Ascher-Svanum H, Nyhuis AW, Faries DE, et al: Involvement in the US criminal justice system and cost implications for persons treated for schizophrenia. BMC Psychiatry 10(1):11, 2010 20109170

Aubry T, Nelson G, Tsemberis S: Housing first for people with severe mental illness who are homeless: a review of the research and findings from the at home-chez soi demonstration project. Can J Psychiatry 60(11):467–474, 2015 26720504

Bailey K, Lowder EM, Grommon E, et al: Evaluation of a police–mental health co-response team relative to traditional police response in Indianapolis. Psychiatr Serv 73(4):366–373, 2022 34433289

Black HC, Garner BA: Black's Law Dictionary, 7th Edition. St. Paul,?West Group, 1999

Blais E, Brisebois D: Improving police responses to suicide-related emergencies: new evidence on the effectiveness of co-response police-mental health programs. Suicide Life Threat Behav 51(6):1095–1105, 2021 34254702

Bureau of Justice Statistics: Violent Crime. Washington, DC, Bureau of Justice Statistics, 2023. Available at: https://bjs.ojp.gov/topics/crime/violent-crime. Accessed November 2, 2023.

Compton MT, Bakeman R, Broussard B, et al: The police-based Crisis Intervention Team (CIT) model: II. Effects on level of force and resolution, referral, and arrest. Psychiatr Serv 65(4):523–529, 2014 24382643

Compton MT, Zern A, Pope LG, et al: Misdemeanor charges among individuals with SMI: a statewide analysis of more than two million arrests. Psychiatr Serv 74(1):31–37, 2023 35795979

Cuozzo S: The subways are an insane asylum on wheels—we must get the mentally ill off the trains. New York Post, July 24, 2023. Available at: https://nypost.com/2023/07/23/we-must-get-mentally ill-off-subways-for-our-safety-and-theirs. Accessed November 2, 2023.

Dee TS, Pyne J: A community response approach to mental health and substance abuse crises reduced crime. Sci Adv 8(23):eabm2106, 2022 35675395

Feldman E: Adams says mental illness leads to crime. The data is not so clear. Spectrum News NY1, December 6, 2022. Available at: https://www.ny1.com/nyc/all-boroughs/transit/2022/12/06/adams-says-mental-illness-leads-to-crime—the-data-is-not-so-clear-#:~:text=%E2%80%9CWhen%20you%20do%20an%20analysis,inevitably%20commit%20a%20violent%20act. Accessed January 17, 2024.

Elbogen EB, Swanson JW, Swartz MS, et al: Family representative payeeship and violence risk in severe mental illness. Law Hum Behav 29(5):563–574, 2005 16254743

Elbogen EB, Van Dorn RA, Swanson JW, et al: Treatment engagement and violence risk in mental disorders. Br J Psychiatry 189:354–360, 2006 17012659

Elbogen EB, Dennis PA, Johnson SC: Beyond mental illness: targeting stronger and more direct pathways to violence. Clin Psychol Sci 4(5):747–759, 2016

Ellsworth JT: Housing and criminality: the effect of housing placement on arrests among chronically homeless adults. J Soc Distress Homeless 31(2):130–141, 2022

Estroff SE, Swanson JW, Lachicotte WS, et al: Risk reconsidered: targets of violence in the social networks of people with serious psychiatric disorders. Soc Psychiatry Psychiatr Epidemiol 33(Suppl 1):S95–S101, 1998 9857786

Fazel S, Långström N, Hjern A, et al: Schizophrenia, substance abuse, and violent crime. JAMA 301(19):2016–2023, 2009 19454640

Fazel S, Lichtenstein P, Grann M, et al: Bipolar disorder and violent crime: new evidence from population-based longitudinal studies and systematic review. Arch Gen Psychiatry 67(9):931–938, 2010 20819987

Fazel S, Wolf A, Larsson H, et al: Identification of low risk of violent crime in severe mental illness with a clinical prediction tool (Oxford Mental Illness and Violence tool [OxMIV]): a derivation and validation study. Lancet Psychiatry 4(6):461–468, 2017 28479143

Federal Bureau of Investigation: Crime in the United States, 2018. U.S. Department of Justice Uniform Crime Reports. Washington, DC, U.S. Department of Justice, 2019. Available at: https://ucr.fbi.gov/crime-in-the-u.s/2018/crime-in-the-u.s.-2018/topic-pages/violent-crime.pdf. Accessed November 2, 2023.

Ferri R: The benefits of live court date reminder phone calls during pretrial case processing. J Exp Criminol 18(1):149–169, 2022

Fisher WH, Simon L, Roy-Bujnowski K, et al: Risk of arrest among public mental health services recipients and the general public. Psychiatr Serv 62(1):67–72, 2011 21209302

Harris MN, Teasdale B: The prediction of repeated violence among individuals with serious mental disorders: situational versus dispositional factors. J Interpers Violence 36(1–2):691–721, 2021 29294909

Hoge SK, Bonnie RJ: Expedited diversion of criminal defendants to court-ordered treatment. J Am Acad Psychiatry Law 49(4):517–525, 2021 34610969

Illinois Compiled Statutes, Chapter 720, 5/12–1, 12–3, 12–3.2, Assault, Battery, Domestic Battery. (2022). Available at: https://law.justia.com/codes/illinois/2022/chapter-720/act-720-ilcs-5/title-iii/. Accessed September 12, 2024.

Kriegel LS, Henwood BF, Gilmer TP: Implementation and outcomes of forensic housing first programs. Community Ment Health J 52(1):46–55, 2016 26438288

Kubiak S, Comartin E, Milanovic E, et al: Countywide implementation of Crisis Intervention Teams: multiple methods, measures and sustained outcomes. Behav Sci Law 35(5–6):456–469, 2017 28983959

Labrum T, Solomon PL: Factors associated with family violence by persons with psychiatric disorders. Psychiatry Res 244:171–178, 2016 27479109

Labrum T, Solomon PL: Rates of victimization of violence committed by relatives with psychiatric disorders. J Interpers Violence 32(19):2955–2974, 2017 26231334

Labrum T, Solomon P: Serious mental illness and incidents between adult children and parents responded to by police. Psychol Med 52(1):102–111, 2022 32662365

Labrum T, Zingman MA, Nossel I, et al: Violence by persons with serious mental illness toward family caregivers and other relatives: a review. Harv Rev Psychiatry 29(1):10–19, 2021 33417373

Lowder EM, Rade CB, Desmarais SL: Effectiveness of mental health courts in reducing recidivism: a meta-analysis. Psychiatr Serv 69(1):15–22, 2018 28806894

Markowitz FE: Mental illness, crime, and violence: risk, context, and social control. Aggress Violent Behav 16(1):36–44, 2011

Monahan J, Steadman HJ, Silver E, et al: Rethinking Risk Assessment: The Macarthur Study of Mental Disorder and Violence. New York, Oxford University Press, 2001

Morabito MS, Kerr AN, Watson A, et al: Crisis Intervention Teams and people with mental illness: exploring the factors that influence the use of force. Crime Delinq 58(1):57–77, 2012

New York Penal Law, §§ 120.00, 240.75. Assault in the Third Degree, Aggravated Family Offense. (2022). Available at: https://law.justia.com/codes/new-york/2022/pen/part-3/title-h/article-120/120-00/ and https://law.justia.com/codes/new-york/2022/pen/part-3/title-n/article-240/240-75/. Accessed September 12, 2024.

Official Code of Georgia Annotated § 16–5–20, 23.1, Simple Assault, Battery. (2022). Available at: https://law.justia.com/codes/georgia/2022/title-16/chapter-5/article-2/section-16-5-20/ and https://law.justia.com/codes/georgia/2022/title-16/chapter-5/article-2/section-16-5-23-1/. Accessed September 12, 2024.

Pennsylvania Consolidated Statutes, § 2701, Simple Assault. (2022). Available at: https://law.justia.com/codes/pennsylvania/2022/title-18/chapter-27/section-2701. Accessed September 12, 2024.

Silver E, Teasdale B: Mental disorder and violence: an examination of stressful life events and impaired social support. Soc Probl 52:62–78, 2005

Skeem JL, Mulvey EP: Psychopathy and community violence among civil psychiatric patients: results from the MacArthur Violence Risk Assessment Study. J Consult Clin Psychol 69(3):358–374, 2001 11495166

Steadman HJ, Deane MW, Borum R, et al: Comparing outcomes of major models of police responses to mental health emergencies. Psychiatr Serv 51(5):645–649, 2000 10783184

Stergiopoulos V, Hwang SW, Gozdzik A, et al: Effect of scattered-site housing using rent supplements and intensive case management on housing stability among homeless adults with mental illness: a randomized trial. JAMA 313(9):905–915, 2015 25734732

Straznickas KA, McNiel DE, Binder RL: Violence toward family caregivers by mentally ill relatives. Hosp Community Psychiatry 44(4):385–387, 1993 8462950

Swanson JW, Swartz MS, Essock SM, et al: The social-environmental context of violent behavior in persons treated for severe mental illness. Am J Public Health 92(9):1523–1531, 2002 12197987

Swartz JA, Lurigio AJ: Serious mental illness and arrest: the generalized mediating effect of substance use. Crime Delinq 53(4):581–604, 2007

Swartz MS, Bhattacharya S, Robertson AG, et al: Involuntary outpatient commitment and the elusive pursuit of violence prevention. Can J Psychiatry 62(2):102–108, 2017 27777274

Thompson A, Tapp SN: Criminal Victimization, 2022 (NCJ 307089). Washington, DC, Bureau of Justice Statistics, Office of Justice Programs. U.S. Department of Justice, 2023

Varghese A, Khakha DC, Chadda RK: Pattern and type of aggressive behavior in patients with severe mental illness as perceived by the caregivers and the coping strategies used by them in a tertiary care hospital. Arch Psychiatr Nurs 30(1):62–69, 2016 26804503

Watson AC, Owens LK, Wood J, et al: The impact of Crisis Intervention Team response, dispatch coding, and location on the outcomes of police encounters with individuals with mental illnesses in Chicago. Policing (Oxf) 15(3):1948–1962, 2021 34659453

Wood JD, Watson AC, Pope L, et al: Contexts shaping misdemeanor system interventions among people with mental illnesses: qualitative findings from a multi-site system mapping exercise. Health Justice 11(1):20, 2023 37014478

Part 3

Toward Reform and System Improvements

9

The Current Era of Multifaceted Criminal Legal System Reform

Athena Kheibari, Ph.D.
Megan Hicks, Ph.D.
Erin Comartin, Ph.D., L.M.S.W.
Hosanna Fukuzawa, B.A.
Leonard Swanson, M.S.W.

Case Example: Ms. Johnston

The leader of the Eastside assertive community treatment (ACT) team, Ms. Charlaine Johnston, participated in the county's Stepping Up Initiative, which strives to reduce the overincarceration of people with men-

The authors thank Sheryl Kubiak, Ph.D., for her mentorship and leadership at the Center for Behavioral Health and Justice in the School of Social Work at Wayne State University, Detroit, Michigan.

tal illnesses. The county's Stepping Up planning commission included elected county commissioners and various administrators representing community mental health, two substance abuse treatment providers, two social and human services providers, the county sheriff's office, the Eastside and Westside city police departments, the district court's mental health court staff, the president of the local chapter of the National Alliance on Mental Illness (NAMI), and a peer support specialist at the local peer agency. Through the course of her work, Ms. Johnston also developed connections with the local public defense offices to learn about the ways attorneys and social workers support their clients' legal and nonlegal needs. At one of the first meetings, Ms. Johnston presented the significant criminal legal profile of her team's caseload and discussed current policy and programmatic strengths, weaknesses, and gaps within the county.

Ms. Johnston noted that a key strength of their community is the number of Crisis Intervention Team (CIT) officers that can be dispatched to calls involving someone having a mental health crisis. She reported an instance in which a CIT officer contacted her directly after they de-escalated a crisis situation and learned that the individual was previously connected to the Eastside ACT team. After that event, Ms. Johnston re-engaged the individual in services in hopes of preventing future crisis events and further entanglement in the criminal legal system.

Ms. Johnston noted that many of her team's clients who have current charges could benefit from the mental health court program, but there is a long waitlist. She told the planning commission that individuals with mental illnesses who are in the jail or going through traditional court proceedings should have a direct referral pathway to a mental health court that can meet the demand. She pointed out that the mental health of many people in jail or involved in the court goes unnoticed, and therefore, a screening instrument should be used that flags this need and assesses eligibility for a diversion or mental health court program. Furthermore, she highlighted the benefits of holistic defense practices, in which public defenders work in interdisciplinary teams to identify the behavioral health and social support needs of their clients; develop strategies to work with court staff to consider the circumstances leading to the individual's charges and potential for rehabilitation; and use treatment interventions to lessen the severity of the court case outcomes. Successful completion of these court programs or holistic defense advocacy efforts by defense teams can result in a clean criminal record, which allows the individual with a mental illness to engage in social supports, employment, and education services that would have been hindered by a criminal record.

Last, Ms. Johnston advocated for more mental health services in the jail that facilitate early release for individuals with mental illness, when possible. She noted the importance of early release, as she has seen many of her clients significantly decompensate while in the facility. She noted that mental health workers could also help prepare individuals for discharge, with their needed medications in hand, connection to a mental health case manager, and housing supports that are ready as soon as they return to the community. She also highlighted the critical need for services that address risks for individuals with co-occurring mental illness and substance use disorders. This could include training for staff in the criminal legal and service provider systems that breaks down the stigma associated with the health care rights and needs of this population. She suggested that more attention could be placed on interventions for members of this population, as they are often high users of health care and crisis services in the community.

Imagine a fishing boat with a captain who is in charge of making all the decisions about boat operations and a crew that assists with casting the fishing net and retrieving the fish for processing. A key factor in this fishing process is the size and shape of the net's mesh holes. A net with small mesh holes will capture a greater variety of fish, whereas a net with large mesh holes will capture larger fish while allowing smaller fish to swim out of the mesh, reducing the burden of overfishing on the population. The captain and crew also have the discretion to release fish back into the waters rather than keeping them on the boat to take back to the market.

The fishing boat operations can be a metaphor for the criminal legal system and the ways that individuals, including those with serious mental illness (SMI), get unnecessarily caught up in the system. The captain represents the court decision-makers (law enforcement officers, judges, prosecutors, jurors, and probation officers). The fishing net represents the criminal legal system, which determines the offenses captured by the system's design. The boat represents the jails where captured people are detained. The boat crew represents law enforcement that casts the large net and retrieves those who are captured. And finally, the release of some fish back into the waters refers to the diversion of some individuals out of the system. The current design of the U.S. criminal legal system has small holes: it captures a large number of individuals, including many that law enforcement should never have captured, and far too few are diverted out of the system by court decision-makers.

Efforts to reduce unnecessary system involvement and increase the number of diversions—essentially widening the mesh holes in the net—began in the 1990s with growing concern about mass incarceration; those with SMI have been the target of some of these efforts. Individuals involved in the criminal legal system are disproportionately affected by SMI, have low incomes, are chronically ill, and often receive health care services through Medicaid (Bronson and Berzofsky 2017; Harper et al. 2021).

This chapter discusses program interventions to divert individuals with SMI at each intercept of the criminal legal system and ends with a review of federal and state policy ideas to improve crisis response and criminal legal interventions for individuals with SMI. The Sequential Intercept Model (Munetz and Griffin 2006) is a framework used to consider the mechanisms and opportunities for interventions to divert individuals with SMI away from the criminal legal system and into treatment when possible (see Figure 9–1). There are six different points across this model: Intercept 0—Community Services, Intercept 1—Law Enforcement, Intercept 2—Initial Detention, Intercept 3—Jails/Courts, Intercept 4—Reentry, and Intercept 5—Community Corrections.

Law Enforcement Reform

In response to the growing frustration with and urgency to reform problematic law enforcement response to mental health crises, many municipalities have attempted reforms within law enforcement departments as well as reforms to community crisis responses (see Chapter 2, "Using System Maps to Understand Entanglement and Guide Change"). Reforms at intercepts 0 and 1 include a focus on interventions in the community and law enforcement—before the individual is formally charged, convicted of any charges, or sentenced to confinement. If we refer back to the fishing boat metaphor, the interventions at these intercepts represent changes in the way the fishing crew operates and the net they cast to capture individuals into the criminal legal system which, in the United States, has historically entangled (Bronson and Berzofsky 2017) too many and resulted in the deaths (Fuller et al. 2015) of a disproportionate number of people with mental illness. In the next two sections, we describe two such interventions: the CIT model and Law Enforcement Assisted Diversion (LEAD). Other law enforcement interventions, such as co-response teams, are discussed in Chapter 10.

Crisis Intervention Team Model

STRUCTURE AND PURPOSE

The CIT model is a law enforcement response to mental health crises, calling for specialized training for officers, accessibility of mental health services, and partnerships between law enforcement, mental health services, and advocacy (Dupont and Cochran 2002). The original Memphis model requires 40-hour training for officers, interdisciplinary advisory committees, linking those in crisis to psychiatric care, and other key community-level services. However, the CIT model has not been consistently implemented across the country (Watson et al. 2017). Some communities focus on the training; others emphasize the holistic, inter-

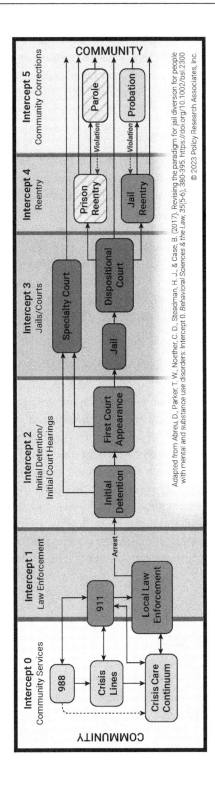

Figure 9–1. Sequential intercept model.

Source. Adapted from Abreu, D., Parker, T. W., Noether, C. D., et al. (2017). Revising the paradigm for jail diversion for people with mental and substance use disorders: Intercept 0. *Behavioral Sciences and the Law,* 35(5–6), 380–395. https://doi.org/10.1002/bsl.2300
© 2023 Policy Research Associates, Inc.

disciplinary nature of the original model's intention. Similarly, the percentage of officers within a department who are trained in CIT varies. The original model maintained that CIT officers should volunteer and be vetted as well suited for the specialist role, but some departments mandate CIT training for all officers.

EXAMPLES AND OUTCOMES

CIT is one of the most prevalent models of mental health crisis response in the past 20 years, and as such, it has been studied more than recent clinician-involved models. Studies have shown improvements in officer-level cognitive and attitudinal outcomes, certain officer-level behavioral outcomes such as use of force and officer injury, and some transportation outcomes to mental health resources (Comartin et al. 2019; Kubiak et al. 2017; Watson et al. 2017). Evidence is mixed in the academic literature about whether CIT training reduces arrests, with some studies finding a decrease in arrests (Compton et al. 2014) and others finding no impact on arrest (Watson et al. 2010).

LIMITATIONS

Although CIT has shown officer-level improvements, to date, there has been scant research on subject-level outcomes, and we have little information about the program's effect on people with mental illness who interact with law enforcement (Watson et al. 2017). Some critics of the CIT model advocate for the removal of law enforcement presence from mental health crises altogether, given the risk of arrest and potentially fatal encounters when they are present. However, not even the most progressive community responder models are designed to respond to calls involving weapons or active violence incidents, and some mental health crises are indeed violent and dangerous. Because of this potential risk, mental health professionals or crisis response teams may fear for their own safety when responding to crisis events without the presence of law enforcement.

Law Enforcement Assisted Diversion

STRUCTURE AND PURPOSE

In 2011, an interdisciplinary group of first responders, harm reduction agencies, and courts created the first LEAD program to divert individuals with low-level offenses—such as drug possession or engaging in sex work—away from the criminal legal system and to community-based, harm-reduction intervention services. As law enforcement officers engage with individuals with behavioral health needs in the community, they use their discretionary authority to refer them to an intensive case management program in lieu of charging them with an offense. The intensive case management covers a wide range of services that are designed to serve the specific needs of each individual in domains including housing, medical care, employment, and more (LEAD Support Bureau 2024). Participating in services and abstinence are not required to remain in the program, as the harm reduction approach taken by LEAD focuses on meeting individuals "where they are" to ensure long-term outcomes (Collins et al. 2017). With programs such as LEAD, the structure of the fishing net is changed to capture fewer individuals into the criminal legal system.

EXAMPLES AND OUTCOMES

LEAD has been implemented in >50 sites across the United States, and more are being developed internationally. Results from the LEAD program in Seattle showed decreased recidivism, increased employment, and stabilized housing (Clifasefi et al. 2016; Collins et al. 2017). In the first 5 years of the program, participants had significantly fewer jail bookings and were less likely to be charged with a felony than those who did not participate in the program (Collins et al. 2017). Additionally, Clifasefi et al. (2016) found that participants in the program were twice as likely to be sheltered (e.g., permanent housing, temporary housing, emergency shelter, or motel/hotel) and 89% more likely to obtain permanent housing during an 18-month follow-up period compared with a control group.

LIMITATIONS

When the LEAD program was launched in New Haven, Connecticut, during the first 9 months, only two arrests were diverted (Joudrey et al. 2021). Joudrey et al. (2021) identified barriers to implementation as including the procedural complexity of diversion, the stigma of substance use disorders, concerns about reduced penalties for substance use, and the perceived punitive role of policing by law enforcement officers. It may be difficult to replicate the success of Seattle's LEAD program at scale unless a jurisdiction has a broad interdisciplinary consensus about diverting low-level criminal activity toward harm reduction or treatment approaches.

Court Reform

If community crisis management efforts and policing practices (i.e., the ship crew) do not prevent an individual with SMI from being captured in the fishing net of the criminal legal system, then the next opportunity for system diversion for misdemeanor offenses is at the court intercept. The chance for "catch and release" at this point in the process falls at the discretion of the ship's captain—in other words, the decision-makers in the court (i.e., judges, prosecutors, jurors). In the next section, we review reforms at intercepts 2 and 3 and describe current court strategies, such as treatment court and alternative sentencing programs, to divert individuals away from the criminal legal system. Some of these efforts are supported by holistic defense teams who present information to court decision-makers and advocate on behalf of individuals for fairer outcomes. Diversion efforts at the court intercept can apply to prosecutors who agree to drop or refrain from filing criminal charges in favor of an alternative solution, such as community-based support services and treatment. They may also take the form of a judge reducing a jail sentence for an individual based on a sentencing mitigation report provided by a holistic defense team that advocates for the rehabilitation of an individual with an SMI.

Not discussed in this chapter are attempts to reform competency to stand trial practices, particularly when applied to individuals charged with misdemeanors. Concern is growing that individuals with mental illness experience increased symptomatology while awaiting this evaluation, leading to further decompensation when they could be diverted to treatment in the community (National Center for State Courts 2022).

Mental Health Courts and Other Treatment Courts

STRUCTURE AND PURPOSE

Mental health courts (MHCs) were established as an alternative to incarceration in the 1990s (Boothroyd et al. 2003). These courts were designed with the recognition that individuals with mental illness may have different needs than those without mental illness, and that traditional court processes were not adequately addressing the underlying mental health issues. Other treatment courts may also serve individuals with mental illness, including co-occurring mental health and substance abuse courts and veterans' courts. These specialized court programs aim to divert individuals with SMI from the traditional criminal legal system and into treatment and support programs.

MHCs are typically structured as a collaborative effort between criminal legal (i.e., judge, prosecutor, defense attorney, probation officers, and court staff) and mental health (i.e., clinicians, case managers) professionals (Council of State Governments Justice Center 2007). The goal of MHCs is to provide treatment and support to individuals with mental illnesses who have been accused of committing certain types of crimes, including both misdemeanor and felony offenses. Generally, individuals accused of specific offenses (homicide, sex offenses) or with extensive criminal histories are ineligible. Participants are required to comply with conditions of the court, such as regular attendance at treatment sessions, drug and alcohol testing, and regular court appearances.

EXAMPLES AND OUTCOMES

MHC participation can lead to improved mental health outcomes, such as engagement in treatment and increased access to social services and supports (Sarteschi et al. 2011). Additionally, MHCs lower the cost to the criminal legal system and show improvements in public safety via reductions in recidivism (Kubiak et al. 2015).

LIMITATIONS

MHCs are available to only a small subset of individuals accused of crimes based on eligibility criteria (Comartin et al. 2021b). This is unfortunate, given the evidence showing MHCs to be equally effective for individuals with felony charges, particularly for those who successfully complete the program (Ray et al. 2015). Additionally, individuals with felony charges showed a reduced number of postprogram days spent in jail, whereas individuals with misdemeanor charges showed an increased number of days spent in jail after the MHC program. These findings beckon the risk-needs-responsivity model (Bonta and Andrews 2007), in that the treatment dosage and court monitoring often involved in this intervention may be best suited for the risk and needs of individuals with felonies as opposed to individuals with misdemeanor charges. Some have raised concerns that MHCs can even widen the criminal justice net because the legal imposition of mandated treatment can present more difficulties than traditional sentencing would (Cooper 2017). Individuals may prefer to face traditional misdemeanor charges than face potentially lengthier MHC treatment requirements. Furthermore, Seltzer (2005) argues that MHCs pose a risk to various civil rights (e.g., procedural concerns regarding voluntary participation, right to withdraw) and are inherently flawed because they signal an acceptance of involving individuals with mental illnesses in the legal system.

Holistic Defense

STRUCTURE AND PURPOSE

Another strategy to divert individuals from the criminal legal system at the court intercept is holistic defense. All low-income individuals facing criminal charges have had the right to court-appointed legal counsel since the landmark 1963 U.S. Supreme Court case *Gideon v. Wainwright*. However, the practice of public defense generally reflects a narrow focus on the legal issues of a criminal case, with little consideration of the client's underlying nonlegal issues that may contribute to their involvement with the legal system. In the late 1990s, a new movement emerged that changed the way public defenders viewed their clients and broadened the scope of their work.

The Bronx Defenders of New York pioneered a holistic defense approach that centers the needs of the individuals impacted by the system, reflecting a recognition that high-caliber lawyering alone was not enough to achieve justice and lasting change for clients (Steinberg and Keeney 2016). By combining legal advocacy with interdisciplinary teamwork, the goal of holistic defense is to reduce or eliminate jail and prison sentences and increase collaboration between the partners in the criminal legal system and social service providers to offer community-based alternatives to incarceration. The holistic approach is applicable across different categories of criminal charges, including misdemeanor charges.

FOUR PILLARS OF HOLISTIC DEFENSE

Holistic defense includes a broad range of practices and services, and the implementation of this approach varies across public defender agencies. Four core pillars guide the approach: 1) access to legal and social support services; 2) interdisciplinary teamwork and communication; 3) enhanced client-centered, interdisciplinary skillsets; and 4) connection to the community served (see Figure 9–2) (Steinberg and Keeney 2016).

Access to Services. To identify the appropriate social services, a holistic defender office must perform a comprehensive needs assessment of the client and their community, because each individual has their own unique challenges that contribute to their involvement in the criminal legal system. A one-size-fits-all model is inadequate. Clients are more likely to benefit from these social services when the access is "seamless"—reducing the burden of complicated administrative procedures (i.e., exhaustive intake and eligibility processes required by each service provider). Therefore, once an office has identified those services, the holistic defender office is responsible for handling the administrative complexities of connecting clients to them, through community partnerships with social service providers, if necessary, but sometimes through in-house provision.

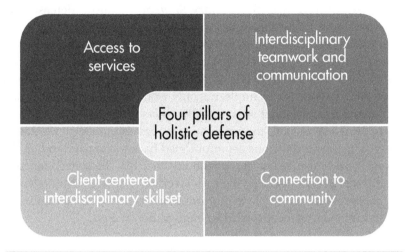

Figure 9–2. Four pillars of holistic defense.

Interdisciplinary Teamwork and Communication. Unlike traditional models of defense that tend to be siloed, a holistic defense approach provides clients support through an interdisciplinary team consisting of criminal defense and civil lawyers, social workers (or other mental health professionals who have background training in systems and human behavior), investigators, and other social service advocates. Social workers complete an intake and psychosocial assessments with the client, coordinate services in the community, recommend evaluations by expert witnesses, gather relevant documentation from the client's background, and interview relevant witnesses (e.g., client's family, friends). This process facilitates the production of client-centered sentencing mitigation reports, which inform the court decision-makers about the biopsychosocial history of the client, the context of the client's SMI, and the potential for rehabilitation. Open, dynamic, and nonhierarchical communication among all members of the holistic defense team and the client is necessary so that the team grasps the big picture of the client's life and can identify effective strategies for support. For example, an LGBTQ+ client preparing to reenter the community from jail may lack social support and the resources to obtain stable housing and may struggle with mental health—all issues that could affect their ability to meet their probation conditions and increase likelihood of continued contact with the system. A holistic defense team would address these issues by drawing on an interdisciplinary exchange of ideas and information and reduce the burden on the client to address these complex issues alone.

Client-Centered Interdisciplinary Skillset. Holistic defense representation translates to a commitment from each team member to develop an interdisciplinary knowledge base and specific skillsets that are client-centered. That means that each team member is aware of the function of the other team members and practices in ways that support each other's work. For example, not only would the lawyer on the team be knowledgeable about what social workers can do, they would also have gained some skills to spot some of the common signs of mental illness, which would then be communicated back to the team so that the social worker can assess the possibility that the client needs mental health services. Conversely, the social worker will be aware of relevant legal processes and be able to perform basic screenings for potential legal issues, such as those related to immigration status.

Connection to Community. The final pillar of holistic defense is community understanding and engagement. If the goal of holistic defense is to reduce incarceration, facilitate successful reentry, and lower recidivism rates, the holistic defense team must be community oriented, because communities also have a vested interest in preventing and reducing crime. Fostering ties with community members, allied groups, and social service providers builds trust and respect, which can be instrumental in supporting clients. Leveraging these community connections can also contribute to grassroot coalitions that advocate on behalf of clients to achieve systems-level change. Holistic defense practitioners who have spent time in the client's community and have built rapport with members of their community will have a more authentic understanding of the client. Engaging with clients' families, neighbors, and other community members also facilitates a community-based support network.

EXAMPLES AND OUTCOMES

An increasing number of public defender offices across the United States are utilizing in-house social workers (or other mental health professionals who can perform the same functions) and other advocates to practice holistic defense along a spectrum. For example, in 2016, the Michigan Indigent Defense Commission partnered with the Urban Institute to develop the Social Worker Defender Project, which sought to implement and measure the outcomes of social worker involvement in holistic public defense teams (Kramer et al. 2020). A large-scale study conducted by Anderson et al. (2019) found that although holistic representation did not affect conviction rates, it was associated with a 16% and 24% reduction in probability of custodial sentences and expected sentence length, respectively. Holistic defense teams are successful at obtaining charge downgrades and reduced incarceration time, and these impacts are substantial for those charged with low-level offenses, such as larceny or drug offenses. Individuals who receive holistic representation are no more or less likely to receive a conviction and no more or less likely to get re-arrested (up through 10 years post-arraignment) (Anderson et al. 2019).

LIMITATIONS

One of the limitations of holistic representation is that it may result in cases taking longer to resolve (9% increase in amount of time, as reported by Anderson et al. 2019). One possible reason is that the process of providing holistic care may require more extensive screening processes. Another major limitation is that holistic defense requires additional funding and resources to support the implementation of the interdisciplinary team-based approach, such as funding for in-house social workers. Many public defender offices are underfunded, particularly in rural areas, making it difficult to provide clients with this type of representation.

Alternative Sentencing and Other Programs

STRUCTURE AND PURPOSE

Alternative sentencing programs are remedial programs or plans that divert cases from the court system and redirect individuals from detainment to community-based alternatives. The goal of alternative sentencing is to decrease or eliminate jail and prison sentences, reduce the burden of court dockets, and provide individuals with opportunities for rehabilitation. These programs are not uniform across jurisdictions and may be delivered through different mechanisms. Some alternative sentencing programs are housed in public defender offices, whereas others are delivered through the court system.

EXAMPLES AND OUTCOMES

Kentucky has a nationally recognized Alternative Sentencing Worker Program (ASWP) that aims to redirect individuals with substance use disorders or SMI from incarceration to community-based treatment and rehabilitation (Kentucky Department of Public Advocacy 2024). This ASWP is housed in Kentucky's Department of Public Advocacy and employs more than 50 alternative sentencing workers, with at least one at each public defender field office. ASWP workers collaborate with lawyers to identify and assess individuals' risks and needs. The ASWP workers then meet with the individual to develop a comprehensive alternative sentencing plan that will promote positive outcomes for the client and, therefore, the community. The plan is presented to the court in hopes of obtaining an outcome other than incarceration. Although Kentucky's ASWP works hand-in-hand with public defenders, it constitutes a separate activity from that performed by the individual's holistic defense team, because ASWP workers exclusively develop sentencing recommendations, whereas a holistic defense team may perform a broader range of functions with different goals. For example, a public defender working on a misdemeanor case may identify that their client is eligible for alternative sentencing and would then work with the ASWP worker to develop a sentencing recommendation that is an alternative to incarceration, such as probation and a commitment to participate in mental health or substance use treatment. This would be different from a holistic defense team that would utilize the social worker on the team to, for example, conduct multiple interviews with the client and their family, gather official records, and identify expert witnesses to testify at trial to explain to the court how the client's SMI contributed to their involvement in a crime (Buchanan and Nooe 2017; Kheibari et al. 2019). Holistic defense can be applied to a wider range of cases, such as capital murder cases, whereas ASWP workers would only work on cases involving lower-level offenses.

In some court-based approaches to alternative sentencing, a client-centered approach is not used, meaning that the client is not an *equal collaborator* in developing the sentencing plan. Therefore, sentencing plans may be developed for clients by some courts without considering the person's unique needs and without efforts to "meet the person where they are." The District of New Jersey's Pretrial Services Agency has a pretrial diversion program in which eligible individuals avoid prosecution altogether and receive no record of criminal charges. These pretrial services entail a risk assessment of the individual to evaluate a variety of factors, including housing, employment, mental health, and substance use history. If deemed eligible, the individual may be required to participate in targeted programs such as mandatory drug testing, substance use treatment, and court supervision (e.g., court call reminders, check-ins, GPS monitoring) (Bradford 2012). Not all jurisdictions use pretrial services, but among programs in Montgomery County, Maryland; Washington, District of Columbia; and five counties in California, pretrial services were shown to result in improved court appearance rates and stable or reduced rates of re-arrests (i.e., pretrial services and early release did not result in increased re-arrest) (Aungst 2012; Chung 2012; Cohen and Reaves 2007; Neal 2012; Pretrial Detention Reform Workgroup 2017; Pretrial Justice Institute 2012).

In Michigan, various actors in government, law enforcement, education, and mental health services and advocacy groups came together in 2018 to establish the Wayne County Jail Mental Health Initiative. As a result, in 2021, the Wayne County Probate Court launched the Behavioral Health Unit pilot project, which set out to connect nonviolent individuals with SMI and substance use disorders to appropriate treatment services as an alternative to going through the criminal legal system (Michigan Courts 2022).

LIMITATIONS

Alternative sentencing programs are not standardized across jurisdictions or systems, resulting in considerable variability in how they are structured and operate. This diversity in approaches to alternative sentencing makes it difficult to measure outcomes and identify what works and what does not. Furthermore, programs that are operated through courts or sheriff offices—as opposed to ones operated through public defender offices—may lack the client-centered approach taken by many public defender offices, particularly those that are holistic minded. It is important for individuals with SMI to have a voice in their sentencing plans so that the courts can meet people where they are and have a better chance of successfully meeting their goals.

Jail Reform

Reforms at intercepts 2 and 3 occur within the jail setting, and they focus on the operations of the boat in our fishing analogy. Strategies at the jail level include the treatment services offered to individuals with SMI while incarcerated, opportunities for early release and diversion to treatment, and discharge planning and community-based follow-up care (see Figure 9–3).

For those who cannot be diverted away from incarceration by law enforcement during initial court hearings or during initial jail detention (intercepts 0, 1, and 2), some policy and program interventions attempt to ease the conditions of a jail stay for those with SMI, with continued access to treatment in jail and upon reentry to the community. Another critical area of intervention to reduce recidivism and reform the current criminal legal system is jail-based mental health treatment.

Jail-Based Mental Health Treatment

STRUCTURE AND PURPOSE

Jail-based mental health services were created in response to the number of incarcerated individuals in jails with SMI, and jails are federally mandated to provide mental health treatment (*Estelle v. Gamble* 1976). In

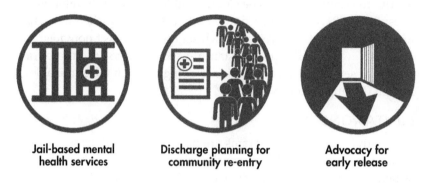

| Jail-based mental health services | Discharge planning for community re-entry | Advocacy for early release |

Figure 9–3. Reforms for individuals with serious mental illness in jails.

line with the sequential intercept model, jail-based mental health services are a crucial step to assist in the transition back into the community and to reduce recidivism. Unfortunately, these services are very limited, and standards of care vary by county (Comartin et al. 2022).

EXAMPLES AND OUTCOMES

Jail-based programs may differ in their eligibility requirements, program structure, and options for alternative sentencing activities. In 2015–2016, New York City funded a collaboration between the Department of Health and Mental Hygiene, the oversight agency for jail health care contracts, and the Department of Correction to create Program for Accelerating Clinical Effectiveness (PACE) units (Ford et al. 2020). PACE units are therapeutic environments comprising mental health professionals and specially trained correctional staff. The PACE units specialize in jail-based treatment focused on reducing psychiatric hospitalizations, clinical decompensation in jail (medication nonadherence, social isolation, and not engaging in daily living activities), and psychiatric assessments. Referrals to the PACE units are received through Correctional Health Services or hospital clinical staff. Evaluation showed decreased rates of violent injury and improved rates of medication adherence for patients who engaged in the PACE units compared with patients who did not engage with the PACE units.

In Colorado, the Arapahoe County Sheriff's Office offers a free jail-based multilevel developmental program for offenders with mental illness called Arapahoe Diverts the Mentally Ill for Treatment (ADMIT). Participants of the program are identified as having stayed longer in the Arapahoe County Detention Facility, consumed more resources during the stay, and returned more frequently to the detention facility. In the three-step program, participants start with a high frequency of contact with trained staff and program intervention. Individuals move through the levels based on achieving their treatment goals and remain in the program based on the level of their judicial sentence. Upon completion of their judicial sentence, participants of the program graduate from ADMIT, or they are discharged and connected to community mental health treatment options (Arapahoe County Sheriff n.d.).

Empirical studies of jail-based mental health services often draw on small sample sizes, single-site designs, and nonrandomized controlled trials (Comartin et al. 2022). Also, few programs address both clinical and public safety outcomes or provide an evaluation of their effectiveness. It is even difficult, based on information currently available, to assess what services jail-based mental health interventions include across the nation.

Those studies that exist suggest that jail-based mental health services have positive results. Specifically, they tend to reduce jail stays and recidivism as well as increase treatment engagement after release (Case et al. 2009; Lange et al. 2011; Sirotich 2009). Research also shows that positive outcomes of successful jail-based mental health treatment depend on treatment modality, service delivery by nonprofit providers, availability of community resources, and whether the program is mandated (Broner et al. 2005; Comartin et al. 2021a; Ryan et al. 2010; Scott et al. 2013).

LIMITATIONS

Epperson et al. (2014) called for jail-based mental health services that assess contextual risk factors that place individuals with SMI at elevated risk for criminal legal contact; for example, housing, food security, social support, and other psychosocial issues. Addressing risk factors and improving the implementation of jail-based mental health services may be effective in improving diversion from the criminal legal system among individuals with SMI.

Mental Health Advocacy for Early Release

STRUCTURE AND PURPOSE

Despite the limitations of jail-based mental health services, in some cases they may stabilize an individual who was prone to criminal behaviors, such that continued incarceration provides no benefit to public safety. In such cases, early release is advisable. Research shows that community organizations are better equipped to holistically address the needs of incarcerated individuals with SMI than jail-based services. Further, research has shown that early release from jail allows individuals to engage with community-based services more quickly and connects individuals with SMI with providers who can address their mental health needs (Comartin et al. 2022; Hicks et al. 2022).

EXAMPLES AND OUTCOMES

States have begun to make pathways for early release. Since 2020, Kentucky has allowed individuals to receive credit on their sentence if they receive a high school equivalency diploma or college degree or complete an educational or vocational program, a drug treatment program, or work for time credit (Commonwealth of Kentucky 2020). Additionally, Vermont passed legislation in 2020 that increases opportunities for vulnerable inmates to reduce their sentences and removes requirements for inmates to participate in correctional programming to be able to earn good time. Also, this act requires state actors to draft recommendations regarding the availability of mental health assessments and how these assessments affect individual case plans (National Alliance on Mental Illness 2022).

Mental Health Re-entry Planning

STRUCTURE AND PURPOSE

To complement early release for individuals with SMI, transition planning before release should occur. Research has shown that transition planning pre-release is crucial for reducing recidivism, especially for individuals with SMI (Hamilton and Belenko 2016; Substance Abuse and Mental Health Services Administration 2017). Such planning has multiple dimensions. For example, on release, a person may not have proper identification, a housing plan, or appointments for health care services, and it may be difficult for them to transition back to daily life or integrate into family routines. Jails have implemented reentry job and resource fairs to address these needs (Altmann and Myrick 2021). In many cases, correctional agencies and community agencies work together to provide resources (Altmann and Myrick 2021). Reentry job fairs can be the product of such partnerships, providing legal assistance for reestablishing a life in the community, employment assistance, social services, health insurance information, food assistance, and job opportunities. However, transition planning is the least offered mental health service within jail settings (Substance Abuse and Mental Health Services Administration 2017).

EXAMPLES AND OUTCOMES

Indiana has made many strides in reentry programming from jails (Silva 2021). Hampton (2021) highlighted a specific effort by the Indiana Office of Public Health and Safety implemented in 2020, a Re-entry Job and Resource Fair. It provided reentry job and resource fairs to incarcerated people, with preference given to individuals with SMI and substance use issues and implemented recommendations from a state-funded study on a comprehensive reentry approach. Another effort in Indiana is the Marion County Reentry Court, which was created to help individuals not recidivate to jails. This program provides individuals who are eligible for early release with rehabilitation and treatment services, drug screenings, housing, and employment assistance. Hampton (2021) recommended that jails and communities work together to provide person-centered care, comprehensive mental health assessments, comprehensive services and support to meet the needs of the individual, and integrated collaboration between the criminal legal systems and community providers. Additionally, they reported the importance of involving families and other allies of the incarcerated individuals. The comprehensive services that are needed for the individuals should be community based, client driven, culturally responsive, and evidence based, and should use peer supports and mentoring. In Chicago, the Cook County Reconnect program provides rental assistance (100% of rent for the first 3 months, 30% of income for the remainder of the lease) for eligible referred adults returning from the Illinois Department of Corrections. Cook County Reconnect program residents are also eligible for holistic wraparound services, including behavioral health care, employment services, and job training.

Policy Reform

Although program interventions have expanded across the criminal legal system, policy barriers exist that impede successful implementation and outcomes of individuals with SMI who are involved in the criminal legal system. Thus, the federal government, states, and localities have introduced significant pieces of legislation to assist communities in their efforts to divert away from criminal legal involvement and into treatment in the mental health system. Reforms at intercept 1 (law enforcement) include those focused on improving de-escalation techniques, co-responding with mental health professionals, triaging 911 calls to crisis lines, and using citations in lieu of arrest, whereas reforms at intercept 2 (courts and jails) include legislation related to restrictions on setting cash bail.

One focus of reform has been limiting use of force by law enforcement officers. State bills have been introduced that prohibit the use of chokeholds, carotid holds, and no-knock warrants; some require annual reporting on use of force incidents. Other states have sought to implement more de-escalation training, as well as increased use of and requirements to maintain body-worn cameras (National Alliance on Mental Illness 2022).

Another reform opportunity at intercept 1 is the increased use of citations by law enforcement in lieu of arrest and detention. Law enforcement officers can issue a citation, or directive, to a person that notes the charges against them (most often a misdemeanor or civil infraction) and gives the individual the date and time they must appear in court. The individual then signs the citation, promising to appear in court. Citations are used by a majority of law enforcement agencies across the country, but limitations exist on the types of offenses that are eligible for citation, and the culture of most law enforcement agencies favors arrest over citation (International Association of Chiefs of Police 2016). Recent studies investigating the outcomes of new citation policies show a significant reduction in jail bookings (Baumer and Adams 2006) and that increases in failure to appear at court did not ensue (Vaske 2020).

A focus of policy reform at intercept 2 is related to cash bail (the financial payment amount required before a defendant is allowed to be released from custody, set by the court on an individual basis and paid directly by the defendant or their family). Although these changes do not focus solely on individuals with mental illnesses, the cash bail system disproportionately leaves individuals in poverty in jail longer, and many individuals with SMI live in poverty (Substance Abuse and Mental Health Services Administration 2020). In the United States, a person's access to monetary funds is one of the most important determining factors in whether they are detained in jail while awaiting trial. The cash bail system was intended to serve as collateral to guarantee that an individual abides by court terms, such as showing up to court appearances and avoiding re-arrest. If the individual successfully meets the court terms, they are refunded the bail amount minus administrative and processing fees. A small percentage of individuals awaiting trial get denied cash bail because the court deems them to be a "flight risk" or danger to the community. However, a sizeable portion of those eligible for pretrial release are unable to pay the cash bail and may continue being detained primarily because of their inability to pay (Reaves 2013). Not only do these individuals struggle with affording the bail fees, but they also continue to lose income or opportunities to generate income when they are detained. Thus, the U.S. cash bail system contributes to a vicious circle of jail time and poverty for low-income individuals who cannot afford to post bond (a financial surety to appear in court, paid on the defendant's behalf by a third party such as a bail bond agency, who assumes responsibility for payment and court appearance) (Rabuy and Kopf 2016). The disparities are even greater for low-income individuals who struggle with SMI and are from communities of color (Lam 2014). The Center for Justice Innovation in New York has a bail reform strategy to influence laws and policies (Center for Justice Innovation 2024). In 2019, New York State passed sweeping bail reforms that rule out monetary bail for most misdemeanor and nonviolent felony charges. If a bail is set, these reforms require that the judge consider the individual's economic status before determining the bail amount and provide individuals at least three options for making bail so that it is less burdensome (New York City Comptroller 2022).

Conclusion

Reforming the criminal legal system to reduce the number of individuals with SMI who become entangled in the system requires an "all-hands-on-deck" approach. The current approach to how laws, policing, and decision-making in courts are practiced has resulted in a system that is unjust and ensnares a disproportionate number of people with mental illness. Returning to the metaphor of the fishing boat operation that overfishes and destroys the aquatic community by casting too fine a net and indiscriminantly retaining those that are captured, our criminal legal system requires an overhaul to change the density of the netting. These efforts have been supported by interdisciplinary advocates, policymakers, and practitioners at federal, state, and local levels and give hope to the idea that a new wave of change is on the horizon—one that has the backing of all parties involved.

Many challenges remain in this goal to overhaul the system. One of these challenges is that criminal legal systems are predominantly organized at local, city, or county levels; as such, many of these interventions can only be accomplished one jurisdiction at a time. As noted in Chapter 3 ("Decision-Making Contexts of Misdemeanor Charges"), variability is rampant across criminal legal systems and criminal legal decision-making. It will take patience, unwavering commitment, and strong enthusiasm from all partners in this work—law enforcement, prosecutors, public defenders, and community members—to succeed in implementing promising and evidence-based policies and practices across every municipality in the United States. Of course, federal- and state-level policies financially supporting mental health treatment services (beyond Medicaid funding) would enable broader opportunities for successful diversion. Nonetheless, we must still appreciate that progress, even at the rate of one jurisdiction at a time, can make a world of difference for many individuals struggling with SMI, and that is something worth fighting for.

KEY POINTS

- Since the establishment of mental health courts, many diversion programs have been implemented to redirect individuals with mental illnesses away from the criminal legal system toward treatment; however, these are not standardized or widely available in many communities in the United States.
- Historically siloed behavioral health and criminal legal systems must have shared goals and effective collaboration for prevention and intervention programs to be successful in their diversion efforts.
- Public defense teams that practice holistic defense seek to address their clients' mental health needs and factors that led to their involvement with the criminal legal system to mitigate case outcomes and reduce recidivism.
- Increased jail reform strategies are needed for individuals with serious mental illness (SMI). Strategies that have been implemented include jail-based mental health services, discharge planning, and advocacy for early release.
- Expanded policy reform has assisted in diversion of individuals with SMI. Limited use of force by law enforcement officers, increased use of citations instead of arrest or detention, and reforms to the cash bail system are a few policy changes that have reduced the number of individuals with SMI in the legal system.

References

Altmann N, Myrick P: From incarceration to community: criminal justice reform for people affected by mental illness in Minnesota. MSW Program Policy Advocacy Briefs, Mankato, MN, Minnesota State University, March 2021. Available at: https://cornerstone.lib.mnsu.edu/msw-student-policy-advocacy-briefs/31. Accessed January 19, 2024.

Anderson JM, Buenaventura M, Heaton P: The effects of holistic defense on criminal justice outcomes. Harv Law Rev 132(3):819–893, 2019

Arapahoe County Sheriff: Arapahoe Diverts the Mentally Ill for Treatment (ADMIT). Arapahoe County Sheriff's Office, Detention Services Bureau. Centennial, CO, n.d. Available at: https://files.arapahoeco.gov/Sheriffs%20Office/Bureaus/Detective%20Services%20Bureau/ADMIT%20outline%20program%20description.pdf. Accessed January 19, 2024.

Aungst S: Pretrial Detention and Community Supervision Best Practices and Resources for California Counties. Sacramento, CA, CA Fwd: Partnership for Community Excellence, 2012. Available at: https://www.courts.ca.gov/partners/documents/pdr-cal-cpfc_pretrial_detention_and_community_supervision.pdf. Accessed January 19, 2024.

Baumer T, Adams K: Controlling a jail population by partially closing the front door: an evaluation of a summons in lieu of arrest policy. Prison J 86(3):386–402, 2006

Bonta J, Andrews DA: Risk-Need-Responsivity Model for Offender Assessment and Treatment (User Report No. 2007–06). Ottawa, ON, Public Safety Canada, 2007

Boothroyd RA, Poythress NG, McGaha A, et al: The Broward Mental Health Court: process, outcomes, and service utilization. Int J Law Psychiatry 26(1):55–71, 2003 12554000

Bradford S: For Better or for Profit: How the Bail Bond Industry Stands in the Way of Fair and Effective Pretrial Justice. Washington, DC, Justice Policy Institute, 2012. Available at: http://www.justicepolicy.org/research/4388. Accessed May 21, 2024.

Broner N, Mayrl DW, Landsberg G: Outcomes of mandated and nonmandated New York City jail diversion for offenders with alcohol, drug, and mental disorders. Prison J 85(1):18–49, 2005

Bronson J, Berzofsky M: Indicators of Mental Health Problems Reported by Prisoners and Jail Inmates, 2011–12. Washington, DC, Bureau of Justice Statistics, June 2017. Available at: https://www.bjs.gov/content/pub/pdf/imhprpji1112.pdf. Accessed May 1, 2023.

Buchanan S, Nooe RM: Defining social work within holistic public defense: challenges and implications for practice. Soc Work 62(4):333–339, 2017 28957575

Case B, Steadman HJ, Dupuis SA, et al: Who succeeds in jail diversion programs for persons with mental illness? A multi-site study. Behav Sci Law 27(5):661–674, 2009 19557758

Center for Justice Innovation: Bail reform, in Areas of Focus. New York, Center for Justice Innovation, 2024. Available at: https://www.innovatingjustice.org/areas-of-focus/bail-reform. Accessed May 1, 2023.

Chung J: Bailing on Baltimore: Voices From the Front Lines of the Justice System. Washington, DC, Justice Policy Institute, September 2012. Available at: http://www.justicepolicy.org/research/4412. Accessed May 1, 2023.

Clifasefi SL, Lonczak HS, Collins SE: LEAD Program Evaluation: The Impact of LEAD on Housing, Employment and Income/Benefits. Seattle, WA, Harm Reduction Research and Treatment Center, 2016. Available at: https://static1.1.sqspcdn.com/static/f/1185392/27047605/1464389327667/housing_employment_evaluation_final.PDF. Accessed May 1, 2023.

Cohen T, Reaves B: Pretrial Release of Felony Defendants in State Courts (NCJ No 214994). Washington, DC, U.S. Department of Justice, 2007. Available at: https://bjs.ojp.gov/content/pub/pdf/prfdsc.pdf. Accessed May 1, 2023.

Collins SE, Lonczak HS, Clifasefi SL: Seattle's Law Enforcement Assisted Diversion (LEAD): program effects on recidivism outcomes. Eval Program Plann 64:49–56, 2017 28531654

Comartin E, Swanson L, Kubiak S: Mental health crisis location and police transportation decisions: the impact of Crisis Intervention Team training on crisis center utilization. J Contemp Crim Justice 35(2):241–260, 2019

Comartin E, Nelson V, Hambrick N, et al: Comparing for-profit and nonprofit mental health services in county jails. J Behav Health Serv Res 48(2):320–329, 2021a 32914286

Comartin E, Nelson V, Smith S, et al: The criminal/legal experiences of individuals with mental illness along the sequential intercept model: an eight site study. Crim Just Behav 48(1):76–95, 2021b

Comartin E, Burgess-Proctor A, Hicks M, et al: A state-wide evaluation of jail-based mental health interventions. Psychol Public Policy Law 28(3):433–445, 2022

Commonwealth of Kentucky: Probation program credit: CPP30.4, in Kentucky Corrections Policies and Procedures. Frankfort, KY, Commonwealth of Kentucky Department of Corrections, 2020. Available at: https://corrections.ky.gov/About/cpp/Documents/30/CPP%2030.4%20Probation%20Program%20Credit%20.pdf. Accessed May 1, 2023.

Compton MT, Bakeman R, Broussard B, et al: The police-based Crisis Intervention Team (CIT) model: II. Effects on level of force and resolution, referral, and arrest. Psychiatr Serv 65(4):523–529, 2014 24382643

Cooper J: Trapped: the limits of care in California's mental health courts. Soc Justice 44(1):121–141, 2017

Council of State Governments Justice Center: Improving Responses to People With Mental Illnesses: The Essential Elements of a Mental Health Court. Washington, DC, Bureau of Justice Assistance, 2007. Available at: https://bja.ojp.gov/sites/g/files/xyckuh186/files/Publications/MHC_Essential_Elements.pdf. Accessed May 1, 2023.

Dupont R, Cochran C: The Memphis CIT Model, in Serving Mentally Ill Offenders: Challenges and Opportunities for Mental Health Professionals. Edited by Landsberg G, Rack M, Berg L. New York, Springer, 2002, pp 59–69

Epperson MW, Wolff N, Morgan RD, et al: Envisioning the next generation of behavioral health and criminal justice interventions. Int J Law Psychiatry 37(5):427–438, 2014 24666731

Estelle v. Gamble, 429 U.S. 97, 97 S. Ct. 285 (1976)

Ford EB, Silverman KD, Solimo A, et al: Clinical outcomes of specialized treatment units for patients with serious mental illness in the New York City jail system. Psychiatr Serv 71(6):547–554, 2020 32041509

Fuller D, Lamb R, Biasotti M, et al: Overlooked in the Undercounted: The Role of Mental Illness in Fatal Law Enforcement Encounters. Arlington, VA, Treatment Advocacy Center, 2015. Available at: https://www.treatmentadvocacycenter.org/wp-content/uploads/2023/11/Overlooked-in-the-Undercounted.pdf. Accessed June 1, 2023.

Hamilton L, Belenko S: Effects of pre-release services on access to behavioral health treatment after release from prison. Justice Q 33(6):1080–1102, 2016

Hampton DA: Re-entry: holistic approach to combat "the new civil death." Indiana Law Rev 54(3):597–634, 2021

Harper A, Ginapp C, Bardelli T, et al: Debt, incarceration, and re-entry: a scoping review. Am J Crim Justice 46(2):250–278, 2021 32837173

Hicks DL, Comartin EB, Kubiak S: Transition planning from jail: treatment engagement, continuity of care, and rearrest. Community Ment Health J 58(2):288–299, 2022 33835278

International Association of Chiefs of Police: Citation in Lieu of Arrest: Examining Law Enforcement's Use of Citation Across the United States. Alexandria, VA, 2016. Available at: https://www.theiacp.org/sites/default/files/all/ij/IACP%20Citation%20Final%20Report%202016.pdf. Accessed May 1, 2023.

Joudrey PJ, Nelson CR, Lawson K, et al: Law enforcement assisted diversion: qualitative evaluation of barriers and facilitators of program implementation. J Subst Abuse Treat 129:108476, 2021 34080562

Kentucky Department of Public Advocacy: Alternative Sentencing Worker Program. Frankfurt, KY, Kentucky Public Defenders Department of Public Advocacy, 2024. Available at: https://dpa.ky.gov/who-we-are/. Accessed September 16, 2024.

Kheibari A, Walker J, Clark J, et al: Forensic social work: why social work education should change. J Soc Work Educ 57(2):332–341, 2019

Kramer K, Flintoft J, Rushing Q, et al: Social Worker Defender Project: Program Manual. Lansing, Michigan, Indigent Defense Commission, 2020. Available at: https://michiganidc.gov/wp-content/uploads/2021/03/SWDP-Program-Manual.pdf. Accessed January 19, 2024.

Kubiak S, Roddy J, Comartin E, et al: Cost analysis of long-term outcomes of an urban mental health court. Eval Program Plann 52:96–106, 2015 25982871

Kubiak S, Comartin E, Milanovic E, et al: Countywide implementation of Crisis Intervention Teams: multiple methods, measures and sustained outcomes. Behav Sci Law 35(5–6):456–469, 2017 28983959

Lam C: Pretrial Services: An Effective Alternative to Monetary Bail. San Francisco, CA, Center on Juvenile and Criminal Justice, 2014. Available at: https://www.cjcj.org/media/import/documents/cjcj_pretrial_reform_july_2014.pdf. Accessed May 1, 2023.

Lange S, Rehm J, Popova S: The effectiveness of criminal justice diversion initiatives in North America: a systematic literature review. Int J Forensic Ment Health 10(3):200–214, 2011

LEAD Support Bureau. Case Management, LEAD Style. LEAD Support Bureau, n.d. Available at: https://leadbureau.org/key-methods/case-management/. Accessed May 21, 2024.

Michigan Courts: Wayne County Behavioral Health Pilot Project helping "familiar faces" in the justice system. Michigan Courts, July 13, 2022. Available at: https://www.courts.michigan.gov/news-releases/2022/july/wayne-county-behavioral-health-pilot-project-helping-familiar-faces-in-the-justice-system. Accessed June 1, 2023.

Munetz MR, Griffin PA: Use of the Sequential Intercept Model as an approach to decriminalization of people with serious mental illness. Psychiatr Serv 57(4):544–549, 2006 16603751

National Alliance on Mental Illness: State Legislation Report: Trends in State Mental Health Policy 2020–2021. Arlington, VA, National Alliance on Mental Illness, 2022. Available at: https://www.nami.org/NAMI/media/NAMI-Media/PDFs/NAMI_2020-21_State_Legislation_Report.pdf. Accessed March 3, 2023.

National Center for State Courts: State Courts Leading Change: Report and Recommendations. Arlington, VA, National Center for State Courts, October 2022. Available at: https://www.ncsc.org/__data/assets/pdf_file/0031/84469/MHTF_State_Courts_Leading_Change.pdf. Accessed January 9, 2024.

Neal M: Bail Fail: Why the U.S. Should End the Practice of Using Money for Bail. Washington, DC, Justice Policy Institute, 2012. Available at: http://www.justicepolicy.org/research/4364. Accessed March 3, 2023.

New York City Comptroller: NYC Bail Trends Since 2019. New York, NY, Office of the New York City Comptroller, March 22, 2022. Available at: https://comptroller.nyc.gov/reports/nyc-bail-trends-since-2019. Accessed June 1, 2023.

Pretrial Detention Reform Workgroup: Pretrial Detention Reform: Recommendations to the Chief Justice. Pretrial Detention Reform Workgroup, 2017. Available at: https://www.courthousenews.com/wp-content/uploads/2017/10/Calif-Bail-Reform-REPORT.pdf. Accessed September 10, 2024.

Pretrial Justice Institute: Rational and transparent bail decision making: moving from a cash-based to a risk-based process. Chicago, IL, MacArthur Foundation, 2012. Available at: https://www.safetyandjusticechallenge.org/wp-content/uploads/2015/05/Rational-and-Transparent-Bail-Decision-Making.pdf. Accessed March 1, 2023.

Rabuy B, Kopf D: Detaining the poor: how money bail perpetuates an endless cycle of poverty and jail time. Prison Policy Initiative, May 10, 2016. Available at: https://www.prisonpolicy.org/reports/incomejails.html. Accessed May 1, 2023.

Ray B, Kubiak SP, Comartin EB, et al: Mental health court outcomes by offense type at admission. Adm Policy Ment Health 42(3):323–331, 2015 24965770

Reaves B: Felony Defendants in Large Urban Counties, 2009: Statistical Tables (NCJ No 243777). Washington, DC, Bureau of Justice Statistics, December 2013. Available at: https://bjs.ojp.gov/library/publications/felony-defendants-large-urban-counties-2009-statistical-tables. Accessed May 1, 2023.

Ryan S, Brown CK, Watanabe-Galloway S: Toward successful postbooking diversion: what are the next steps? Psychiatr Serv 61(5):469–477, 2010 20439367

Sarteschi CM, Vaughn MG, Kim K: Assessing the effectiveness of mental health courts: a quantitative review. J Crim Justice 39(1):12–20, 2011

Scott DA, McGilloway S, Dempster M, et al: Effectiveness of criminal justice liaison and diversion services for offenders with mental disorders: a review. Psychiatr Serv 64(9):843–849, 2013 23728358

Seltzer T: Mental health courts: a misguided attempt to address the criminal justice system's unfair treatment of people with mental illnesses. Psychol Public Policy Law 11(4):570–586, 2005

Silva LR: Reaching for reentry: Indiana University Robert H. McKinney School of Law's contribution to the reentry movement. Indiana Law Rev 54(3):527–548, 2021

Sirotich F: The criminal justice outcomes of jail diversion programs for persons with mental illness: a review of the evidence. J Am Acad Psychiatry Law 37(4):461–472, 2009 20018995

Steinberg R, Keeney E: Shared roots and shared commitments: the centrality of social work to holistic defense. Hamishpat Law Review 22:211–242, 2016

Substance Abuse and Mental Health Services Administration: Guidelines for Successful Transition of People with Mental or Substance Use Disorders from Jail and Prison: Implementation Guide. (SMA) 16–4998. Rockville, MD, Substance Abuse and Mental Health Services Administration, January 2017. Available at: https://store.samhsa.gov/product/guidelines-successful-transition-people-mental-or-substance-use-disorders-jail-and-prison. Accessed June 1, 2023.

Substance Abuse and Mental Health Services Administration: National Guidelines for Behavioral Health Crisis Care: Best Practice Toolkit. Rockville, MD, Substance Abuse and Mental Health Services Administration, 2020. Available at: https://www.samhsa.gov/sites/default/files/national-guidelines-for-behavioral-health-crisis-care-02242020.pdf. Accessed June 1, 2023.

Vaske JC: North Carolina Judicial District 30B Pretrial Pilot Project Final Report. Part II: Evaluation Report. University of North Carolina Criminal Justice Innovation Lab, March 2020. Available at: https://cjil.sog.unc.edu/wp-content/uploads/sites/19452/2020/04/March-2020-Final-Report-30B-Project-Part-2.pdf. Accessed June 1, 2023.

Watson AC, Ottati VC, Morabito M, et al: Outcomes of police contacts with persons with mental illness: the impact of CIT. Adm Policy Ment Health 37(4):302–317, 2010 19705277

Watson AC, Compton MT, Draine JN: The Crisis Intervention Team (CIT) model: an evidence-based policing practice? Behav Sci Law 35(5–6):431–441, 2017 28856706

Reform in an Era of Mental Health and Crisis Services Innovation

Matthew L. Goldman, M.D., M.S.
Eric Rafla-Yuan, M.D.
Divya K. Chhabra, M.D.
Hosanna Fukuzawa, M.S.W.
Jessica Gaskin, M.S.W.
Kaitlyn Kok, B.S.
Leonard Swanson, M.S.W.

As communities across the United States increasingly recognize the limitations and potential dangers of a police-first response to people in need of urgent behavioral health services, a range of strategies have been used to instead provide behavioral health crisis responses led by specially trained clinicians and crisis workers. Increasing attention has been paid to interventions such as mental health promotion and crisis prevention; crisis call centers and suicide hotlines (including 988) operating in conjunction with 911; mobile crisis response teams; crisis stabilization facilities that accept police drop-offs as an alternative to jails or emergency departments; and postcrisis follow-up care. This chapter summarizes the range of crisis intervention approaches, as well as the significant momentum in policymaking at this critical moment of reckoning about the need to decriminalize mental illnesses.

Case Example: Ms. Johnston Continues Her Advocacy

On the heels of Ms. Johnston's successful involvement in her county's Stepping Up initiative (described at the beginning of Chapter 9), she could hardly believe what happened next: among the nine elected council members who oversaw local behavioral health funding, two of them had made mental health their top priority. The Mayor had held a recent press conference focused on mental health reform activities. What had changed? Why all of a sudden was mental health a political winner after years of advocacy with little response or engagement?

Through her involvement in the Stepping Up Initiative, Ms. Johnston learned that in the past few years, the community outcry about lack of access to the full array of mental health services had reached new heights. The murders of George Floyd, Daniel Prude, and so many others had rallied communities to seek alternatives to police response for people experiencing a mental health crisis. The pandemic had taken a toll on everyone's mental health, especially young people, who were having suicidal thoughts and attempts at historic levels. The opioid crisis was getting worse by the day, with overdose deaths reaching more than 100,000 people nationally; nearly everyone now knew someone who had died from opioid overdoses. And a federal initiative had created a new three-digit number—988—for people in mental health crisis to call and seek help, which was being implemented across the United States.

Local initiatives started to receive new funding. Ms. Johnston served as a key advisor to the development of a new public safety department, which was envisioned as a first-responder agency that was separate from the police and fire departments to oversee noncriminal community response. This department included a new mobile crisis program staffed by behavioral health specialists and people with lived experience of mental health or substance use conditions who could help engage with the people they responded to. She had seen 988 postings all over social media, and she recently learned of a new initiative aimed at embedding mental health clinicians in the local 911 call center so that calls could be handled by specialists rather than simply trigger police dispatch. There were even early discussions about creating a new behavioral health facility that she could take her patients to instead of the emergency department when a short period of evaluation and stabilization was needed, and even police would be able to drop off people there as a better option than jail. She was hopeful that it seemed like society had finally woken up, and the window of opportunity had opened to make real change for her patients and her community.

Law Enforcement Diversion Across the Crisis Service Continuum

For every instance that law enforcement interacts with a person in a behavioral health crisis, the opportunity exists to divert that person away from a criminal pathway and toward a health response. Localities are actively reconsidering how requests for emergency services are triaged, how first responders and transportation resources are being utilized, how crisis facilities are configured, and how transitions are facilitated in the aftermath of an acute event. These interventions span intercept 0 (community services) and intercept 1 (law enforcement) in the Sequential Intercept Model (see Chapter 9) and are promoted by the federal government through the "National Guidelines for Behavioral Health Crisis Care—Best Practice Toolkit" from the Substance Abuse and Mental Health Services Administration (SAMHSA) (2020b).

Crisis Calls

When someone is in crisis, they often pick up the phone to look for help. Until the recent launch of the 988 Suicide and Crisis Lifeline, there has never been an obvious single number to call or resource to reach out to, which has meant that calls for help would all too often result in a police encounter and potentially an unnecessary arrest. Some might search for a crisis line to seek out a listening ear and information about how to access local mental health services. Young people may feel more comfortable texting or chatting with a teen line that is staffed by people who specialize in engaging young people in crisis. Others, not knowing who else to call, may dial 911 because they feel unsafe with their thoughts or circumstances—or because they are a bystander observing someone else in public who appears to be in crisis—and 911 is the only number they know to call for help. And some, fearing the possibility that a phone call might lead to police banging down their front door, avoid reaching out to anyone at all. This complex and confusing landscape needs an overhaul, and initiatives across the United States have begun developing creative ways to connect people to the help they need without unnecessarily involving law enforcement.

988 SUICIDE AND CRISIS LIFELINE

The National Suicide Prevention Lifeline (NSPL) was established by SAMHSA in 2005. A network of independently operated and funded call centers largely staffed with volunteers was linked by a national toll-free number, (800) 273-TALK (Joiner et al. 2007). In July 2022, the 988 Suicide and Crisis Lifeline was launched as a way to increase access to the NSPL network of call centers by using an easier to remember three-digit number and expanding the scope beyond support for suicidal callers to, more broadly, support people in all types of crises related to mental health, substance use, and other psychosocial crises or needs (Hogan and Goldman 2021).

The evidence supporting crisis call lines has come primarily from the original version of the NSPL as well as the Veterans Crisis Line, which is reachable by dialing the same number. The NSPL has been shown to decrease suicidality during calls and connects one-third to one-half of callers to mental health referrals (Gould et al. 2007; Kalafat et al. 2007). Among callers who received outreach from a follow-up program within 48 hours of their having called the NSPL with suicidality, 80% reported that the follow-up call helped stop them from killing themselves and 90% reported that it kept them safe (Gould et al. 2018). Similarly, the Veterans Crisis Line, which fields calls in a population with substantially elevated suicide rates, led callers to experience reductions in distress and suicidal ideation during the call as well as increased contact and use of medical health care and behavioral health care (Britton et al. 2022, 2023; Hannemann et al. 2021). The chat platform of the NSPL was perceived as helpful among two-thirds of users, with approximately half of users reporting feeling less suicidal afterwards (Gould et al. 2021a). Of note, third-party callers, meaning people other than the person in crisis, showed higher rates of requesting transport to the emergency department (Gould et al. 2021b), which suggests that use of crisis lines by bystanders and other concerned parties may be more likely to involve first responders in call responses, including law enforcement.

Although this evidence base is robust for the role of lifelines in suicide prevention, little is known about the effectiveness of crisis call centers that serve a broader array of needs, which is increasingly common given the broader scope of the 988 Suicide and Crisis Lifeline. More research is needed to better understand outcomes among people who primarily call crisis lines for symptoms other than suicidal thoughts, such as anxiety, trauma-related symptoms, substance use relapse, or even psychosis and mania, particularly when the caller is a third-party bystander. Furthermore, although initial studies have examined 988 call rates by state (Kandula et al. 2023; Purtle et al. 2023), it is not yet known whether 988 is meeting one of its stated goals: diverting calls from 911 as a way to reduce the involvement of law enforcement in crisis response.

911 DIVERSION PROGRAMS

Of the 240 million calls to 911 each year, ~19% are related to behavioral health, according to an analysis of such calls in nine cities (Vera Institute of Justice 2022). Whereas 988 aims to draw calls away from the 911 system, for those calls that have already been placed to 911, the furthest upstream strategy to divert these calls from a default police response is to transfer them to a behavioral health specialist to handle the call before dispatch. By creating an opportunity for clinical triage, behavioral health personnel embedded in 911 settings are able to conduct de-escalation and interventions over the telephone, transfer appropriate calls to 988 and other crisis lines, dispatch civilian mobile crisis teams, and provide other alternatives that do not need to involve law enforcement unless there is significant concern for active violence, presence of weapons, or criminal activity.

Multiple 911 diversion initiatives have been implemented in cities across the United States over the past decade. In 2015, the Houston Police Department implemented a Crisis Call Diversion (CCD) program in partnership with local emergency and behavioral health departments. By routing behavioral health calls to mental health professionals rather than dispatching police officers or emergency medical services (EMS), they were able to divert more than 2,000 calls, resulting in more than $1.6 million in annual savings for first-responder agencies (Assey 2021). Similar programs in Pima and Maricopa Counties in Arizona have embedded behavioral health clinicians in 911 call centers with the goal of diverting calls before they would otherwise go to police (Assey 2021; Fix et al. 2023). The Crisis Intervention Team (CIT) International Best Practice Guide describes a case study of a 911 diversion program implemented in Broome County, New York, and includes an example of a 911 risk assessment tool that call takers can use to triage calls that are appropriate for behavioral health response in lieu of police dispatch (Usher et al. 2019).

The interplay between 911, 988, and other crisis lines and resource numbers (e.g., 211, 311, other local versions) is complex. Though many jurisdictions hope to someday realize the vision of having a single phone number for all mental health calls, the reality is that many members of the public will continue to call whatever phone number they think of first or seems most appropriate to them at the time. Therefore, 911 and crisis lines must work together to develop a shared understanding of what resources are most appropriate for which types of calls as a basis for implementing consistent triage protocols across programs. Ultimately, it should be the responsibility of crisis lines and other recipients of behavioral health crisis calls to achieve the goal of getting every call to the right place, preferably with as few transfers and delays as possible.

Mobile Crisis and Community Response

The murder of George Floyd in 2020 triggered widespread protests against police practices; as a result, many local jurisdictions set out to reform their crisis response systems. Clinical responses to crises that do not require the presence of law enforcement have spread rapidly since then (Balfour et al. 2022). Several models involve the presence of mental health professionals to attend to mental health crises in the community and make disposition decisions based on clinical risk assessment and treatment needs. Most models that include mental health professionals fall into one of three categories: 1) mobile crisis, 2) co-response, and 3) community response models. A fourth approach, CIT, involves a specialized law enforcement response without behavioral health staff and is detailed in Chapter 9.

In general, mobile crisis models tend to be based in behavioral health agencies, co-responder models are based in law enforcement agencies, and community response models are based in local emergency medical services, fire departments, or alternative first-responder agencies. Key differences between crisis models include where the call originates (e.g., 911, crisis lines), personnel and staffing, and primary call types they respond to. Figure 10–1 illustrates these differences and highlights the commonalities across the three groupings. Some model types and local examples are highlighted in the descriptions below. The response models are not mutually exclusive because communities can have multiple models attending to crises depending on severity. For example, a single community may have mobile crisis teams that respond to crisis line calls of known clients, whereas co-responder teams are used for calls with higher risk of danger (e.g., presence of weapons, active violence in progress). These interventions, which occur at prebooking intercepts, have been shown to decrease the proportion of people with mental illness entering jails (Swanson et al. 2023).

MOBILE CRISIS MODELS

Behavioral health specialists working as crisis responders are the core feature of mobile crisis teams. These programs were developed to de-

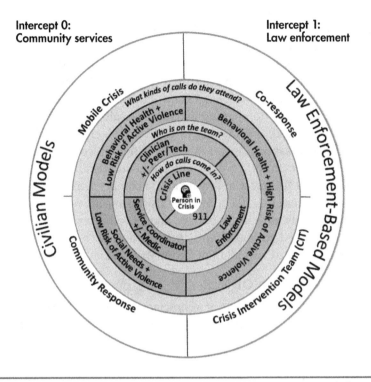

Figure 10–1. Conceptual diagram of crisis response models.

escalate crises and link individuals to ongoing care outside of a hospital or health care facility (Geller et al. 1995). A minimum expectation of mobile crisis teams is the inclusion of a clinician who can screen an individual for mental health or substance use concerns and triage them to an appropriate care plan based on a risk assessment. SAMHSA recommends inclusion of peer support workers (people with lived experience of mental health or substance use conditions who are trained to support other people experiencing similar challenges in a wide range of nonclinical activities) to build rapport and de-escalate (Substance Abuse and Mental Health Services Administration 2020b, 2022, 2023b). Mobile crisis team members are typically employed through a local community mental health agency or a contracted provider and primarily respond to calls that come in through community mental health call lines or similar crisis lines. Mobile crisis models predominantly respond to calls with a low risk of active violence, meaning that there are no weapons present and no active physical threats of harm to self or others. Some mobile crisis teams restrict eligibility criteria to known clients, public places, or daytime hours, although federal and state guidelines most often require them to serve all in need at any time (Centers for Medicare and Medicaid Services 2023; Substance Abuse and Mental Health Services Administration 2020b).

Although some regions have mobile crisis teams (Michigan Public Health Institute 2021), with a few existing for decades, not many studies have investigated their impact. Extant studies show mobile crisis teams have linked people to ongoing behavioral health services after a crisis (Currier et al. 2010; Kim and Kim 2017) and decreased risk of subsequent hospitalization (Guo et al. 2001). Although consumers and their families prefer these non-law-enforcement crisis response models (Pope et al. 2023), the variability in how to contact them can make access confusing (Odes et al. 2023). Mobile crisis teams are not expected to respond as rapidly as first responders, and law enforcement may not wait for a coordinated response with a mobile team to respond to 911 calls (Group for the Advancement of Psychiatry 2021).

CO-RESPONSE MODELS

A co-response team consists of a clinician and a law enforcement officer responding together to mental health crises. Co-response models seek to provide better ongoing connections to services for those experiencing a behavioral health crisis than traditional law enforcement can provide. Moreover, they seek to improve interdisciplinary communication and collaboration between the two agencies involved in the co-response team. The presence of a law enforcement officer allows co-response teams to attend calls with a higher risk of active violence, including calls where weapons are present.

Co-response models vary in structure. Sometimes, a clinician from a mental health agency is stationed at a law enforcement agency to attend to calls originating through 911, often via law enforcement referral. Mental health agency employees benefit from clinical supervision as well as access to electronic health records to verify and gain details about the client's history. In other cases, the law enforcement agency employs the clinician, and they attend to behavioral health crises and other social needs of people who interact with law enforcement. The clinician and officer may respond together, or the clinician may join as a secondary response when needed.

Several jurisdictions have found promising results from implementing co-response models compared with using traditional law enforcement responses to behavioral health crises. A systematic review of international co-response studies from 1999 through 2017, including models from Australia, the United Kingdom, Canada, and the United States, noted that co-response models showed lower rates of injury and arrest, increased voluntary transports to the hospital, decreased time spent at the hospital for a warm handoff, lessened time on scene, and improved information sharing and interagency collaboration. However, studies with a sufficient level of rigor were lacking (Puntis et al. 2018). Similar to those on mobile crisis teams, clinicians on a co-responder team can also initiate the screening process for inpatient hospitalization at the scene of an incident (Evangelista et al. 2016). A co-responder program in Indianapolis made fewer arrests than did typical police responders on similar calls (Bailey et al. 2022), and a Canadian co-responder program increased referrals to care while decreasing use of force and involuntary transport (Blais et al. 2022).

Although co-response teams are being implemented across and beyond the United States, the wide variation in services provided, operating procedures, and team composition make them difficult to evaluate as a group (Frederick et al. 2018; Puntis et al. 2018). Additionally, some have reported that law enforcement and co-response teams themselves are not always clear about which calls are appropriate for co-response. Clear communication, interagency collaboration, and detailed outlining of expectations are necessary to overcome implementation challenges (Bailey and Ray 2018; Bailey et al. 2018).

COMMUNITY RESPONSE MODELS

In contrast with behavioral health–based mobile crisis models and law enforcement–based co-responder models, some programs have attempted to divert 911 calls from law enforcement by routing social needs calls (nonemergency quality-of-life concerns such as those pertaining to disturbances, welfare, and basic needs) to community response models. These non–law enforcement first responders, such as paramedics who may or may not be paired with mental health clinicians, can respond to incidents with low risk of active violence, carrying out triage before deciding if law enforcement involvement is necessary (Irwin and Pearl 2020). Many community response calls may not be for active behavioral health crises, but there is a high prevalence of mental health and substance use needs among the population involved in such calls, particularly when calls are placed by third-party bystanders.

The Support Team Assisted Response (STAR; Denver, Colorado) and Crisis Assistance Helping Out On The Streets (CAHOOTS; Eugene, Oregon) models employ behavioral health clinicians and emergency medical technicians. San Francisco's Street Crisis Response Team (SCRT) model involved a behavioral health clinician, a peer support worker, and a community paramedic with specialized training in primary health care, health promotion, chronic disease management, and advanced clinical assessment (Shannon et al. 2023). These programs typically establish protocols with local first-response agencies (e.g., 911 dispatch, law enforcement) to field nonviolent 911 mental health crisis calls in lieu of law enforcement (Waters 2021). The two- or three-person teams can provide de-escalation, first aid, and basic needs services on scene, and can make referrals to other services. CAHOOTS has reported diverting as many as 8% of calls from law enforcement that otherwise would require an officer to be dispatched (Eugene Police Department Crime Analysis Unit 2020). STAR consists of a similar staffing model, and a peer-reviewed study of the STAR program noted a significant reduction in arrests within targeted precincts in Denver, Colorado (Dee and Pyne 2022).

Other community response teams, such as the Policing Alternatives and Diversion Initiative (PAD; Atlanta, Georgia) do not employ medical professionals and do not target mental health crises but instead bring social service specialists to nonemergency quality-of-life incidents. Albuquerque Community Safety is a recently formed public safety department in New Mexico that operates independently from and in collaboration with the Albuquerque Police and Fire departments and includes a civilian community responder program in addition to mobile crisis teams.

Despite the national recognition of the success realized with these programs, barriers remain to implementation across the United States. Many of these initiatives were supplemented by local funding, and not every community has the political will to invest in progressive community response models. Further, a tragic case highlighted that community response models often still rely on the discretion of dispatch and responding officers to call them. In Eugene, Oregon, the parents of a 33-year-old woman with schizophrenia met with law enforcement to inform them that their daughter had stopped taking medication, hoping to prevent a dangerous encounter. Unfortunately, certain patrol officers were not notified and pulled her over for a traffic infraction. The situation escalated to a physical struggle, and law enforcement shot and killed her in the spring of 2019. A subsequent report revealed the officers could have called CAHOOTS, had they recognized the symptoms of her mental illness. The tragedy demonstrates how crisis system issues can persist despite the existence of exemplar programs (Waters 2021).

Stabilization Facilities

Crisis stabilization units (CSUs)—also known as crisis receiving centers, crisis hubs, or crisis facilities—are specialized treatment centers designed to provide immediate to short-term care for individuals experiencing acute mental health or substance use crises. In addition to a primary focus on stabilization, prevention of symptom progression early in a crisis, and connection to ongoing care, these facilities preferentially serve as a rapid and accessible alternative for first responders, diverting individuals from emergency departments or jails, where the needs of an individual in crisis are often not adequately addressed (Love et al. 2023).

CSUs vary in their structure and services provided, but they typically offer a safe and therapeutic environment in which individuals can receive immediate assessment, psychiatric evaluation, supportive interventions, and referrals for ongoing care (McNeil 2020). Ideally, these facilities operate 24/7, ensuring around-the-clock availability for first responders such as mobile crisis teams, emergency medical services (EMS), or law enforcement to drop off individuals in crisis quickly and easily. By providing an alternative to incarceration or hospital admission, CSUs aim to effectively stabilize the underlying mental health or substance use disorders driving individuals' behavioral crises, while also minimizing overreliance on hospitals, emergency rooms, and the criminal legal system. As such, these units represent a shift toward decriminalizing mental illnesses by providing a dedicated setting for treatment and patient-centered community care rather than simply serving as a holding facility or extension of law enforcement.

Crisis stabilization units can be standalone, attached or adjacent to hospitals, or designated spaces within community mental health centers. Studies of these units have shown promise in terms of safe and effective crisis resolution (Zielinski et al. 2022), with improved engagement in follow-up care, reduced costs (Adams and El-Mallakh 2009), lower hospitalization and hospital readmission rates (Kim et al. 2020; Otterson et al. 2021), and increased satisfaction among individuals and their families (Ligon and Thyer 2000). By delivering immediate and targeted interventions, CSUs contribute to early intervention and support, while preventing escalation of crises and facilitating individuals' recovery and well-being.

Despite their potential benefits, a number of factors limit the implementation and effectiveness of CSUs. Key challenges include capacity, facility and program licensure with state and local agencies, and geographic availability of facilities. In some regions, particularly rural areas, the population density may not be enough to support a dedicated CSU. Low reimbursement rates and other constraints on funding, including the "institutions for mental disease" payment prohibition on federal reimbursements for mental health treatment facilities with more than 16 beds, may disincentivize state and local leaders from investing in new facilities. Facilities for youth face licensing challenges due to lack of guidelines for youth-specific settings, and facility-based care needs to be balanced with the benefits of instead stabilizing youth in their home and school environments. For all CSUs, adequate staffing, specialized training for staff members, and sufficient funding are crucial for ensuring effective operations. For CSUs to meet the growing demand for crisis services and provide comprehensive care to individuals in need, they must be adequately resourced and integrated as a part of a continuum of crisis care (Hirschtritt et al. 2023).

CSUs play a vital role in providing rapid and accessible care for individuals experiencing acute behavioral health crises. By offering an alternative to the very limited options individuals in crisis typically have available to them, such as emergency departments, these facilities aim to stabilize individuals, address their immediate needs, and connect them with appropriate follow-up care. Although CSUs have demonstrated positive outcomes in crisis resolution and diversion from more costly and less specialized settings, their limitations in terms of availability, accessibility, duration of care, and resource constraints highlight the need for continued investment and improvement in the full continuum of crisis services to ensure optimal support for individuals in crisis.

Postcrisis Follow-Up Care

Many crises require more than the brief period of support typically offered by a crisis intervention. Whether related to a stressful or traumatic experience, a diagnosable mental illness, a substance use disorder, or the combined impact of psychosocial adversities, the circumstances that lead a person to experience a crisis are typically complex and may require ongoing services and support. Not all people need specialty behavioral health care—increasing access to crisis services earlier in someone's experience makes it possible to avert a more serious crisis that could require intensive treatment. However, postcrisis follow-up services are important for all interventions across the crisis continuum.

The main evidence base for postcrisis follow-up has focused on suicidal patients seen in emergency departments. Follow-up contacts have been shown to decrease suicidal behavior (Luxton et al. 2013), and patient navigator programs can significantly decrease self-harm (Roberge et al. 2020). Follow-up telephone outreach is widely viewed as a low-cost and important practice to prevent repeated suicide attempts, including when paired with development of a suicide prevention safety plan (Catanach et al. 2019; McKeon 2019; Stanley et al. 2015).

Although the benefits of follow-up services are not well studied specifically in mobile crisis or crisis stabilization settings or for presenting issues other than suicidality, there is broad consensus that follow-up is essential to avoid creating crisis services that become a "bridge to nowhere." There is real risk that underresourced crisis services could become a series of revolving doors that cycle people through traumatic experiences even at the hands of behavioral health specialists. A major need for investment in both postcrisis follow-up clinical services and research funding to better clarify best practices in this area is clear.

Role of Prevention in Crisis Response Services

Crisis response systems are a necessary element in managing acute situations as they arise in the context of mental illnesses or substance use disorders. However, preventing these situations from arising in the first place is essential to ultimately reduce the impact of behavioral health disorders on communities. Examples of pertinent prevention strategies include the expansion of access to mental health services; policies and training that can prevent diagnostic overshadowing (i.e., citing a more severe diagnosis such as schizophrenia when a more moderate or transient diagnosis may be more accurate) and polypharmacy (i.e., when multiple medications are prescribed for a condition that may be better treated with a single option having fewer potential side effects and interactions); incorporation of mental health services in community, primary care, and criminal legal system settings; and attention to psychosocial adversities and social determinants of health in mental health and crisis services (e.g., poverty, housing instability, exposure to trauma or violence, job insecurity).

From 2008 to 2019, the number of U.S. adults with mental illnesses increased by 30%, from 39.8 million to 51.5 million, and the pandemic further exacerbated this trend (Auerbach and Miller 2020; Substance Abuse and Mental Health Services Administration 2020a). Barriers include a shortage of mental health professionals, lack of access to insurance including Medicaid, and gaps in insurance coverage for mental illnesses. As a result, many individuals—adults and youth alike—do not receive mental health services until a crisis occurs and they are sent to an emergency department.

Increasing access to services can be achieved by integrating mental health services into primary care through the collaborative care model (Raney 2015), which involves a primary care provider as the team leader, behavioral health care managers, psychiatrists, and other health professionals working at the "top of their license" in a primary care setting in an efficient way, focusing on patients with more severe issues first. Research findings show that this model improves access to mental health care and clinical outcomes in a variety of settings and populations, including underrepresented minorities (Hu et al. 2020).

Meeting people where they are, whether it is in community centers, the home, schools, or the criminal legal system, can prevent acute crises from emerging. Specifically in the criminal legal system, access to mental health services could be provided at various points across the system such as diversion programs, mental health courts, specialized probation teams, forensic assertive community treatment teams, and reentry programs (Bonfine and Nadler 2019). In addition, some studies show that the inclusion of adequate mental health services in jails and prisons can improve mental health outcomes and decrease recidivism (Wallace and Wang, 2020). These programs are detailed further in Chapter 9.

For many individuals with mental health concerns, entry into the criminal legal system can occur at a young age. Young people in the criminal legal or foster care systems—or both, which is common given the disproportionate rate of entry from foster care into the criminal legal system—are more likely to be misdiagnosed with conduct disorder and psychotic disorders (Zito et al. 2008). This clinical history can translate to schizophrenia diagnoses being perpetuated into adulthood, with trauma symptoms often getting missed in the process of the client receiving the wrong diagnosis. Even if clients are diagnosed with and meet criteria for conduct disorder, the effects of trauma and the diagnoses of anxiety disorders, depressive disorders, and PTSD are often missed. These trends are disproportionately observed among Black and Latinx youth, specifically boys (Muroff et al. 2008).

One major consequence of misdiagnosis is exposure to inappropriate psychotropic medications. In one study, youth involved in the foster care system were three times more likely to receive psychotropic medications and incomplete medication trials than other children on Medicaid. They were also more likely to receive multiple psychiatric medications at once, often without a full trial of each medication before adding another. Misdiagnoses and polypharmacy often carry over into adulthood, meaning that many do not receive proper treatment for the entirety of their mental illness trajectory. This pattern calls for focused training on the risks of misdiagnosis for providers who may not be well versed in these disparities and alternative solutions to behaviors likely caused by trauma. Additionally, research on intentional deprescribing (systematically removing and refining a patient's psychopharmacological treatments) is lacking, which often leads providers to continue multiple medications.

In addition to a lack of research on how the process of deprescribing can be executed systematically, effectively, and reliably, many professionals are not trained on what we do know thus far about deprescribing. Regulations and policy changes around polypharmacy could serve as a safeguard to this issue, particularly with both children and adults who lack consistent care; Black, Indigenous, and people of color (BIPOC) communities; and those who are involved in the criminal legal and foster care systems (Tamburello et al. 2023). For instance, California began tightening its control over psychotropic prescribing for children receiving Medi-Cal and even more safeguards around prescribing for foster care youth, leading to declining rates of antipsychotic prescriptions for foster care youth ages 0–17 and a 52% reduction for Black youth in foster care (Nunes et al. 2022).

Social determinants of mental health such as poor education, exposure to adverse childhood experiences, poverty, food insecurity, housing instability, and job insecurity put individuals at an increased risk of both physical and mental illness. These factors have a key influence on mental illnesses, substance use disorders, and ultimately, acute crises. Considering social determinants of mental health in clinical services and other settings (e.g., schools) can play an important role in the prevention of crises and must also be considered at the local, state, and federal levels in imagining how policy change and legislation can influence these factors, such as increasing access to affordable housing and minimum wage legislation (Compton and Shim 2015).

National Legislation and Policy Promoting Crisis Services

Beginning in 2020, significant national legislative and policy advances have promoted crisis services and have the potential to reshape the landscape of care for mental health and substance use disorders. These advances build on decades of advocacy and policy work that has paved the way for ongoing reform efforts. Contextualizing this stepwise progress helps to understand the current focus on reforming crisis response systems today.

Setting the Stage for Crisis Response Services

The late 1960s and early 1970s witnessed the deinstitutionalization movement, which aimed to shift people with mental health conditions out of large state psychiatric institutions and into community-based care settings when appropriate and feasible. This transformation underscored the importance of services capable of responding in the community as a necessary component of a comprehensive mental health care system, although many of those goals were never realized owing to lack of investment. The era also saw important advances in emergency response. The first 911 phone call was made in 1968, and much of the foundation of the 911 and emergency medical system (EMS) is based in the Emergency Medical Systems Services Act of 1973, which set requirements for a coordinated EMS system and provided states and localities with guidance and funding (Figure 10–2). Notably, these advances in EMS response did not translate into changes for response to behavioral health emergencies.

The emergence of co-response teams and the CIT model in the 1980s through recent years marked a development along this path, recognizing that standard police training or engaging police officers alone were insufficient when responding to emergencies related to mental health and substance use. Co-response teams, piloted in cities such as Seattle, Los Angeles, and New York, pair teams of police officers with mental health professionals. CIT provides additional training to law enforcement personnel and emphasizes the importance of partnerships between law enforcement, behavioral health professionals, and people living with behavioral health conditions to improve community responses to mental health crises (Usher et al. 2019) (see Chapter 9). Notably, both models rely on armed law enforcement officers as a primary means of aiding individuals experiencing a mental health or substance use crisis.

Building Momentum for Crisis Care Through Mental Health Legislative Reform

In the 1990s, the passage of the Mental Health Parity Act of 1996 (MHPA) required large employer-sponsored group insurance plans to apply the same lifetime and annual dollar limits for mental health benefits as those for medical and surgical benefits. Although riddled with loopholes, it was the first congressional action toward mental health parity, the concept that mental illness and substance use disorder treatment should receive equal coverage as treatment for other health issues (Goodell 2014). Parity was further reinforced by passage of the Mental Health Parity and Addiction Equity Act of 2008 (introduced by the same members of Congress as the original MHPA) and by inclusion of mental health as an Essential Health Benefit under the Affordable Care Act in 2010. Financial support, typically by insurer coverage, is a continuing important requirement for the development of sustainable crisis services.

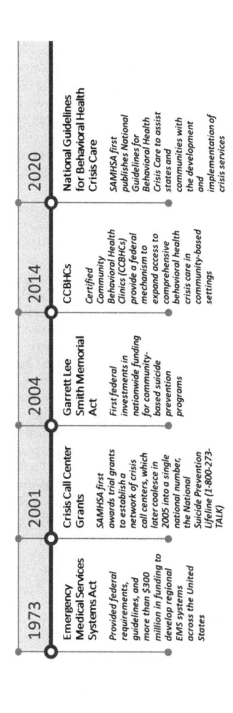

Figure 10-2. Timeline of landmark initiatives for 988 and crisis response (1973–2020).

Note. SAMHSA=Substance Abuse and Mental Health Services Administration.

The implementation of the Garrett Lee Smith Memorial Act in the early 2000s marked the first funding for community-based, comprehensive suicide prevention programs on a nationwide basis (Goldston and Walrath 2023). At times, these included crisis response programming, crisis centers, and crisis hotlines. Compared with communities matched on other metrics, communities implementing Garrett Lee Smith suicide prevention activities demonstrated lower population rates of suicide attempts and lower mortality among young people (Goldston and Walrath 2023). Although the program is focused on suicide prevention, the success of the Garrett Lee Smith program and its consistent congressional reauthorization has illustrated the effect of sustained federal leadership and support for these services.

In 2014, Congress passed legislation to designate and fund a demonstration program for Certified Community Behavioral Health Clinics (CCBHCs) to expand access to mental health and substance use disorder treatment services, including, among other services, comprehensive behavioral health crisis care in community-based settings (Substance Abuse and Mental Health Services Administration 2023a). In addition to providing comprehensive treatment for mental illnesses and substance use disorders, CCBHCs must adhere to specific standards for implementing 24/7 crisis care, providing mobile crisis services, building partnerships with local law enforcement agencies and hospitals, and providing ongoing connections to treatment. Furthermore, as a requirement for certification, CCBHCs must provide services to anyone seeking help for a mental health or substance use condition, regardless of their diagnosis, place of residence, or ability to pay. This greatly improves the ability of CCBHCs to provide crisis services to anyone, anywhere, anytime. CCBHCs have shown substantial improvement in expanding community access to crisis care, forged new pathways for connections to treatment, and supported a significant decrease in hospitalizations, emergency department visits, and incarceration. Although CCBHCs are promising, widespread implementation was hampered by the initial demonstration program that was limited to only eight states, and the CCBHC model's impact on increasing access to crisis services has not yet been examined in detail (Congressional Research Service 2023).

Congress Takes Up 988 and Crisis Services

As shown in Figure 10–3, in the years 2019–2022 an exponentially increased number of federal developments for crisis response debuted, including the passage and implementation of 988, the new three-digit

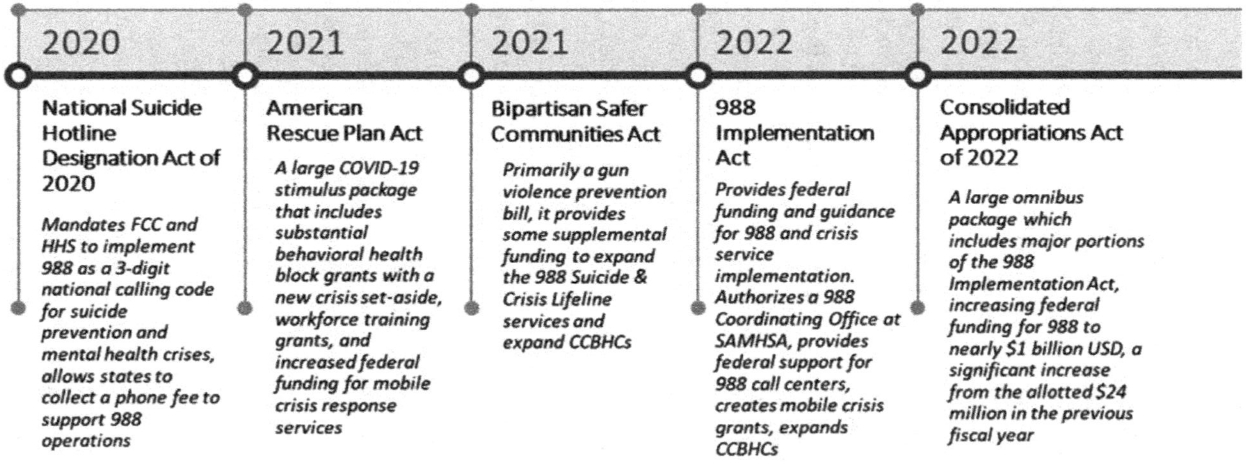

Figure 10–3. Timeline of landmark initiatives for 988 and crisis response (2020–2022).

Note. CCBHC=Certified Community Behavioral Health Clinic; FCC=Federal Communications Commission; HHS=U.S. Department of Health and Human Services.

hotline number; increased funding for crisis response services through a variety of mechanisms; and expansion of CCBHCs.

The 988 Suicide and Crisis Lifeline was set in motion by the passage of the National Suicide Hotline Designation Act of 2020, after reports from the Federal Communications Commission (FCC), SAMHSA, and the Veterans Administration identified gaps in the effectiveness of the existing National Suicide Prevention Lifeline and the potential value of converting to a three-digit number (Substance Abuse and Mental Health Services Administration 2023d; Hogan and Goldman 2021). These reports were themselves required by the National Suicide Hotline Improvement Act of 2018. In addition to requiring 988 to be accessible as the new three-digit number by July 16, 2022, the National Suicide Hotline Designation Act of 2020 also allowed states to enact a telecommunication fee to help support 988 operations, including crisis response and stabilization (National Suicide Hotline Designation Act 2020); only nine states have so implemented the fee at the time of this writing (National Alliance on Mental Illness 2023). Importantly, the Act also required the federal government to "develop strategies for providing access to competent, specialized services to lesbian, gay, bisexual, transgender, and queer (LGBTQIA+) youth; other minority groups; and rural individuals and other high-risk groups," marking congressional recognition of the importance of equitable and accessible crisis services (National Suicide Hotline Designation Act 2020).

Paired with congressional activity were initiatives by SAMHSA, mental health professionals, and advocates to develop a crisis continuum of care. With a tagline of "someone to contact, someone to respond, and a safe place to go," the crisis continuum of care was billed as a parallel to services provided for other types of medical emergencies. In 2020, SAMHSA released its best practice toolkit entitled, "National Guidelines for Behavioral Health Crisis Care—Best Practice Toolkit," in which such a continuum was described (Substance Abuse and Mental Health Services Administration 2020b). Other important conceptual shifts included expanding the purpose of 988 from a sole focus on suicide prevention to being an initial access point for crisis care with a purpose of assisting callers in crisis as well as triage and connection to higher levels of crisis care when appropriate. Today, SAMHSA describes 988 as being responsive to "suicidal, substance use, or mental health crisis, or any other kind of emotional distress" (Substance Abuse and Mental Health Services Administration 2023c).

Despite these significant policy advances, none of the previously discussed initiatives authorized or appropriated federal funding for the implementation or administration of the new 988 program or related services. Through the dedicated work of advocates and policy-makers, these came in 2021 and 2022 through vehicles such as the American Rescue Plan Act, the Bipartisan Safer Communities Act, and the Consolidated Appropriations Acts of 2021 and 2022. These pieces of legislation contained measures such as the significantly increased mental health block grant funding to states with a new set-aside for crisis services, the first dedicated funding for 988 call centers, specific support for language accessibility, funding for specialized services for high-risk populations, grants and increased Medicaid reimbursements for mobile crisis teams, the creation of a 988 and Behavioral Health Crisis Coordinating Office at SAMHSA, and the expansion of CCBHC planning grant eligibility to all 50 states. Notably, all of these measures were drawn from or solidified by the 988 Implementation Act of 2022, a bipartisan effort to support comprehensive implementation of 988 and non-law-enforcement-based crisis services across the country. Provisions requiring all public and private health insurance companies to provide coverage for crisis services did not garner enough support to pass, but in sum, by early 2023, federal funding for 988 and crisis services had risen exponentially to an amount of more than $1 billion, marking a substantial shift in the development of national policy advances and investments in crisis services.

Medicaid and Crisis Services

Medicaid, the federal- and state-funded program designed to provide health coverage for low-income individuals and families, plays a critical role in mental health funding within the U.S. health care system (Medicaid and CHIP Payment and Access Commission 2015). Unfortunately, the nation's failure to broadly support mental health systems through adequate insurance reimbursements as well as general programmatic funding has resulted in an overreliance on Medicaid funding to develop mental health system infrastructure. This is also true for mental health crisis services, which aim to serve any individual in need, regardless of their insurance status. Unlike police and fire departments that generally receive most of their operational funding through municipal budgetary allocations, mental health services are typically reimbursed per encounter from a health insurance plan.

Insurance reimbursements for crisis services are in a state of transition. Crisis programs often receive reimbursement from Medicaid, but commercial insurance seldom reimburses for crisis services despite laws requiring them to cover mental health services in parity with medical services (Goodell 2014). In contrast, EMS providers receive higher-paying commercial insurance reimbursements and use the funds to off-set lower Medicaid reimbursement rates. As a result, crisis programs have struggled to scale up on Medicaid alone.

Being underinsured or uninsured can impede access to lifesaving services. For example, people who are uninsured or whose insurance plans have high deductibles may be reluctant to call an ambulance to avoid the high cost of emergency care (Chou et al. 2021). Although out-of-pocket costs have yet to be described as a common deterrent for people seeking crisis care, this phenomenon will need to be monitored as insurance coverage for crisis services increases.

Despite these challenges, Medicaid remains a primary source of crisis service funding nationwide. To supplement the limitations of Medicaid reimbursements for crisis services, Congress passed a Medicaid-enhanced Federal Medical Assistance Percentage (FMAP) match in the American Rescue Plan Act for mobile crisis services provided to Medicaid beneficiaries (Randi 2021). This enhanced federal share of Medicaid funding provides incentives to states to reimburse for mobile crisis services and offers flexibility for states to define staffing requirements for the team, as long as the team includes at least one qualified mental health professional to conduct a behavioral health assessment. However, to qualify for enhanced funding, mobile crisis teams must be available 24/7, which many jurisdictions have not yet achieved. Furthermore, the American Rescue Plan Act legislation did not solve the reimbursement limitations of crisis service infrastructure depending on Medicaid insurance status or challenges around the required presence of a diagnosed behavioral health disorder.

Another Medicaid restriction arises for individuals who are incarcerated. Although the right to health care for people who are incarcerated or in custody was established by the Supreme Court in 1976 in *Estelle v. Gamble*, in practice, many states and localities provide limited mental health services to incarcerated individuals, as evidenced by numerous state and federal lawsuits. Additionally, Medicaid, the predominant insurance provider of individuals with serious mental illness (SMI), has an "inmate exclusionary policy" precluding reimbursement for services while an individual is detained (Alsan et al. 2023). This means that incarcerated people have no realistic avenue to obtain care from community mental health providers, sharply limiting access to discharge planning services, and importantly, often are unable to transition to community-based care on release. These disruptions in care cause undue delay and lower the chance for stabilization in the community after release, ultimately increasing the risk of recidivism (Simes and Jahn 2022). Responding to these challenges, the Centers for Medicare and Medicaid Services announced a state option for a Section 1115 Medicaid demonstration waiver, which would allow for health care coverage of incarcerated, Medicaid-eligible individuals 30 to 90 days before release. California was the first state receiving approval, in 2023, for client coverage 90 days before release from incarceration (Centers for Medicare and Medicaid Services 2023).

Crisis Services and Equity

Inequity and discrimination in mental health care cast a shadow over numerous segments of society, including BIPOC communities and people identifying as LGBTQIA+, living with disabilities, experiencing homelessness, living in rural communities, and others. Within the landscape of crisis services, acknowledging and confronting these disparities is paramount, particularly given the heightened vulnerability of these groups to receiving a law enforcement response during a psychiatric emergency and their subsequent risk of poorer outcomes (Rafla-Yuan et al. 2021).

Marginalized communities, in particular, face systemic challenges in accessing mental health care. Simultaneously, they often experience overexposure to law enforcement and the resulting public health harms, including adverse mental health, increased risk behaviors, and decreased overall safety, in addition to a higher likelihood of ensnarement in the criminal legal system (Esposito et al. 2021). Compounding these challenges is the distressing reality that individuals with SMI are at a significantly elevated risk of experiencing police force and injury in police encounters compared with the general public (Laniyonu and Goff 2021).

By transitioning from law enforcement to mental health teams with specialized training and establishing services and facilities that are specifically designed to support individuals experiencing psychiatric crises, several detrimental consequences associated with law enforcement response can be avoided (Rafla-Yuan et al. 2021). Mobile crisis response teams with specialized training can offer compassionate and informed interventions that prioritize de-escalation, engagement, and linkage to ongoing care. Purposefully built crisis stabilization facilities can better provide a therapeutic environment in which individuals in crisis are not subjected to the distressing atmosphere of a police encounter or an emergency department, thereby potentially averting worsened anxiety or trauma.

A number of strategies can additionally bolster equitable access to quality crisis services (Goldman and Vinson 2022). Incorporating peer support workers within crisis response teams can offer a unique perspective and foster a sense of understanding and empathy for individuals in crisis. Collaborating closely with established local community partners and organizations, particularly those trusted within marginalized communities, can help enhance trust, community awareness, and engagement. Transparency in sharing protocols and ensuring patient privacy increases the likelihood that individuals who use crisis services feel the same level of confidence as they would accessing any other kind of medical care. Technological solutions may improve accessibility for those who are deaf, hard of hearing, or have difficulty communicating by standard voice phone call. Additionally, engaging in outreach initiatives to educate underserved populations about available crisis services can play a pivotal role in ensuring equity in access.

Ultimately, shifting the paradigm away from armed law enforcement as the default response to psychiatric emergencies and investing in clinical and community-based solutions presents an opportunity to rectify historic inequities and improve outcomes, particularly for historically marginalized communities that have borne the brunt of overpolicing and inadequate crisis interventions. Additionally, sustainable funding must be incorporated to ensure that crisis services provide equitable and quality care to all.

Crisis Services as a Civil Right

In addition to health-related legislation and policy activities, recent advances in the activity of the U.S. Department of Justice addressing mental health issues through a disability-rights lens have been important for crisis services. Recognizing that "people with disabilities should have full lives with equal opportunities, respect, and dignity," the Civil Rights Division of the Department of Justice has increased attempts to hold jurisdictions accountable for responding to individuals with mental illnesses, including those experiencing mental health crises, as a disability rather than a crime (U.S. Department of Justice 2022). Additionally, through the integration mandate of the Americans with Disabilities Act, the Department of Justice maintains that needless incarceration and avoidable encounters with law enforcement of individuals with mental illnesses violate federal law. A number of states and localities have already been investigated for violation of the integration mandate. These regulatory actions provide powerful incentives for state and local policymakers to ensure that sufficient community mental health services are in place, including crisis response services.

Conclusion

The clinical, social, and policy advances described in this chapter have significantly promoted crisis services and reshaped the landscape of behavioral health care in the United States. These changes have built on decades of advocacy and policy work, laying the foundation for ongoing reform efforts. The shift to community-based care, the importance of mental health parity and sustained funding, and the designation and equitable implementation of the 988 hotline and a larger crisis continuum of care all have played crucial roles in improving crisis response systems nationwide. These structural changes to crisis response have offered solutions to disentangling people with mental illness from criminal legal systems. Although this progress is promising, more work is needed to establish causal linkages between increases in these upstream interventions and decreases in downstream criminal legal involvement. Further work is needed to ensure consistent and equitable clinical quality, insurance coverage, and access to crisis services that respond effectively and uphold the dignity of those they aim to serve.

KEY POINTS

- For every instance that law enforcement interacts with a person in a behavioral health crisis, there is an opportunity to divert that person away from a criminal pathway and toward a specialized health response.

- Diversion is possible through a range of program models across the crisis continuum, including crisis call centers, mobile crisis and community response, stabilization facilities, and postcrisis follow-up care.

- Prevention of crises can reduce the burden of mental health and substance use conditions through expanding access to services, reducing problematic practices (e.g., overdiagnosis, misdiagnosis, overprescribing of psychiatric medications), and addressing social determinants of health in mental health and crisis service settings.

- Decades of mental health policy advocacy and reforms have set the stage for the significant increase in crisis system legislative activity and financial investments in recent years, which has brought about structural solutions with the potential to disentangle people with mental illness from criminal legal systems.

- Further work is needed to ensure consistent and equitable clinical quality, insurance coverage, and access to crisis services that respond effectively and uphold the dignity of those they aim to serve.

References

Adams CL, El-Mallakh RS: Patient outcome after treatment in a community-based crisis stabilization unit. J Behav Health Serv Res 36(3):396–399, 2009 18766444

Alsan M, Yang CS, Jolin JR, et al: Health care in U.S. correctional facilities: a limited and threatened constitutional right. N Engl J Med 388(9):847–852, 2023 36856624

Assey D: Tips for Successfully Implementing a 911 Dispatch Diversion Program. New York, The Council of State Governments Justice Center, 2021. Available at: https://csgjusticecenter.org/publications/tips-for-successfully implementing-a-911-dispatch-diversion-program/. Accessed December 26, 2023.

Auerbach J, Miller BF: COVID-19 exposes the cracks in our already fragile mental health system. Am J Public Health 110(7):e1–e2, 2020 32271609

Bailey K, Ray B: Evaluation of the Indianapolis Mobile Crisis Assistance Team: Report to the Indianapolis Office of Public Health and Safety. Indianapolis, Indiana University Public Policy Institute, 2018. Available at: https://www.us-amsa.org/wp-content/uploads/2021/09/EVALUATION-OF-THE-INDIANAPOLIS-MOBILE-CRISIS-ASSISTANCE-TEAM-2018.pdf. Accessed December 26, 2023.

Bailey K, Paquet SR, Ray BR, et al: Barriers and facilitators to implementing an urban co-responding police-mental health team. Health Justice 6(1):21, 2018 30467739

Bailey K, Lowder EM, Grommon E, et al: Evaluation of a police-mental health co-response team relative to traditional police response in Indianapolis. Psychiatr Serv 73(4):366–373, 2022 34433289

Balfour ME, Hahn Stephenson A, Delany-Brumsey A, et al: Cops, clinicians, or both? Collaborative approaches to responding to behavioral health emergencies. Psychiatr Serv 73(6):658–669, 2022 34666512

Blais E, Landry M, Elazhary N, et al: Assessing the capability of a co-responding police-mental health program to connect emotionally disturbed people with community resources and decrease police use-of-force. J Exp Criminol 18(1):41–65, 2022

Bonfine N, Nadler N: The perceived impact of sequential intercept mapping on communities collaborating to address adults with mental illness in the criminal justice system. Adm Policy Ment Health 46(5):569–579, 2019 30969391

Britton PC, Karras E, Stecker T, et al: Veterans crisis line call outcomes: distress, suicidal ideation, and suicidal urgency. Am J Prev Med 62(5):745–751, 2022 35063305

Britton PC, Karras E, Stecker T, et al: Veterans crisis line call outcomes: treatment contact and utilization. Am J Prev Med 64(5):658–665, 2023 36805255

Catanach B, Betz ME, Tvrdy C, et al: Implementing an emergency department telephone follow-up program for suicidal patients: successes and challenges. Jt Comm J Qual Patient Saf 45(11):725–732, 2019 31575455

Centers for Medicare and Medicaid Services: HHS approves California's Medicaid and Children's Health Insurance Plan (CHIP) demonstration authority to support care for justice-involved people. CMS.gov Newsroom, January 26, 2023. Available at: https://www.cms.gov/newsroom/press-releases/hhs-approves-californias-medicaid-and-childrens-health-insurance-plan-chip-demonstration-authority. Accessed December 26, 2023.

Chou SC, Hong AS, Weiner SG, et al: Impact of high-deductible health plans on emergency department patients with nonspecific chest pain and their subsequent care. Circulation 144(5):336–349, 2021 34176279

Compton MT, Shim RS: The Social Determinants of Mental Health. Washington, DC, American Psychiatric Publishing, 2015

Congressional Research Service: Certified Community Behavioral Health Clinics (CCBHCs). In Focus, September 15, 2023. Available at: https://sgp.fas.org/crs/misc/IF12494.pdf. Accessed December 26, 2023.

Currier GW, Fisher SG, Caine ED: Mobile crisis team intervention to enhance linkage of discharged suicidal emergency department patients to outpatient psychiatric services: a randomized controlled trial. Acad Emerg Med 17(1):36–43, 2010 20015106

Dee TS, Pyne J: A community response approach to mental health and substance abuse crises reduced crime. Sci Adv 8(23):eabm2106, 2022 35675395

Esposito M, Larimore S, Lee H: Health policy brief: aggressive policing, health, and health equity. Health Affairs, April 30, 2021. Available at: https://www.healthaffairs.org/do/10.1377/hpb20210412.997570/full. Accessed December 26, 2023.

Estelle v. Gamble, 429 U.S. 97 (1976)

Eugene Police Department Crime Analysis Unit: CAHOOTS Program Analysis. Eugene, OR, Eugene Police Department Crime Analysis Unit, 2020. Available at: https://www.eugene-or.gov/DocumentCenter/View/56717/CAHOOTS-Program-Analysis. Accessed December 26, 2023.

Evangelista E, Lee S, Gallagher A, et al: Crisis averted: how consumers experienced a police and clinical early response (PACER) unit responding to a mental health crisis. Int J Ment Health Nurs 25(4):367–376, 2016 26931611

Fix RL, Bandara S, Fallin MD, Barry CL: Creating comprehensive crisis response systems: an opportunity to build on the promise of 988. Community Ment Health J 59(2):205–208, 2023 35997872

Frederick T, O'Connor C, Koziarski J: Police interactions with people perceived to have a mental health problem: a critical review of frames, terminology, and definitions. Victims and Offenders 12(8):1037–1054, 2018

Geller JL, Fisher WH, McDermeit M: A national survey of mobile crisis services and their evaluation. Psychiatr Serv 46(9):893–897, 1995 7583498

Goldman ML, Vinson SY: Centering equity in mental health crisis services. World Psychiatry 21(2):243–244, 2022 35524591

Goldston DB, Walrath C: The Garrett Lee Smith Memorial Act: a description and review of the suicide prevention initiative. Annu Rev Clin Psychol 19(1):261–275, 2023 36716748

Goodell S: Health policy brief: mental health parity. Health Affairs, April 3, 2014. Available at: https://www.healthaffairs.org/do/10.1377/hpb20140403.871424/full. Accessed December 26, 2023.

Gould MS, Kalafat J, Harrismunfakh JL, et al: An evaluation of crisis hotline outcomes. Part 2: suicidal callers. Suicide Life Threat Behav 37(3):338–352, 2007 17579545

Gould MS, Lake AM, Galfalvy H, et al: Follow-up with callers to the National Suicide Prevention Lifeline: evaluation of callers' perceptions of care. Suicide Life Threat Behav 48(1):75–86, 2018 28261860

Gould MS, Chowdhury S, Lake AM, et al: National Suicide Prevention Lifeline crisis chat interventions: evaluation of chatters' perceptions of effectiveness. Suicide Life Threat Behav 51(6):1126–1137, 2021a 34331471

Gould MS, Lake AM, Kleinman M, et al: Third-party callers to the national suicide prevention lifeline: seeking assistance on behalf of people at imminent risk of suicide. Suicide Life Threat Behav 52(1):37–48, 2021b 34032311

Group for the Advancement of Psychiatry: Roadmap to the Ideal Crisis System: Essential Elements, Measurable Standards and Best Practices for Behavioral Health Crisis Response. Washington, DC, National Council for Mental Wellbeing, 2021. Available at: https://www.thenationalcouncil.org/resources/roadmap-to-the-ideal-crisis-system. Accessed December 26, 2023.

Guo S, Biegel DE, Johnsen JA, et al: Assessing the impact of community-based mobile crisis services on preventing hospitalization. Psychiatr Serv 52(2):223–228, 2001 11157123

Hannemann CM, Katz IR, McCarthy ME, et al: Suicide mortality and related behavior following calls to the Veterans Crisis Line by Veterans Health Administration patients. Suicide Life Threat Behav 51(3):596–605, 2021 33373061

Hirschtritt ME, Howard CA, Simon GE: Fulfilling the goals of 988 through crisis stabilization care. Psychiatr Serv 74(8):889–891, 2023 36718601

Hogan MF, Goldman ML: New opportunities to improve mental health crisis systems. Psychiatr Serv 72(2):169–173, 2021 32988327

Hu J, Wu T, Damodaran S, et al: The effectiveness of collaborative care on depression outcomes for racial/ethnic minority populations in primary care: a systematic review. Psychosomatics 61(6):632–644, 2020 32381258

Irwin A, Pearl B: The Community Responder Model. Washington, DC, Center for American Progress, 2020. Available at: https://www.americanprogress.org/article/community-responder-model. Accessed December 26, 2023.

Joiner T, Kalafat J, Draper J, et al: Establishing standards for the assessment of suicide risk among callers to the national suicide prevention lifeline. Suicide Life Threat Behav 37(3):353–365, 2007 17579546

Kalafat J, Gould MS, Munfakh JL, et al: An evaluation of crisis hotline outcomes. Part 1: nonsuicidal crisis callers. Suicide Life Threat Behav 37(3):322–337, 2007 17579544

Kandula S, Higgins J, Goldstein A, et al: Trends in crisis hotline call rates and suicide mortality in the United States. Psychiatr Serv 74(9):978–981, 2023 36872897

Kim AK, Vakkalanka J, Tate J, et al: 405 Crisis stabilization unit reduces admission rates for suicidal patients in a Midwest emergency department. Ann Emerg Med 76(4):S155, 2020

Kim S, Kim H: Determinants of the use of community-based mental health services after mobile crisis team services: an empirical approach using the Cox proportional hazard model. J Community Psychol 45(7):877–887, 2017

Laniyonu A, Goff PA: Measuring disparities in police use of force and injury among persons with serious mental illness. BMC Psychiatry 21(1):500, 2021 34641794

Ligon J, Thyer BA: Client and family satisfaction with brief community mental health, substance abuse, and mobile crisis services in an urban setting. Crisis Intervention and Time-Limited Treatment 6(2):93–99, 2000

Love K, Bolton JM, Hunzinger E, et al: Needs assessment of clients accessing a community mental health crisis stabilization unit. Community Ment Health J 59(2):400–408, 2023 36040635

Luxton DD, June JD, Comtois KA: Can postdischarge follow-up contacts prevent suicide and suicidal behavior? A review of the evidence. Crisis 34(1):32–41, 2013 22846445

McKeon R: Telephonic follow up for suicidal patients discharged from the emergency department: why it is crucial. Jt Comm J Qual Patient Saf 45(11):722–724, 2019 31668329

McNeil SE: Crisis Stabilization Services, in Models of Emergency Psychiatric Services That Work. Edited by Fitz-Gerald MJ, Takeshita J. Springer International, 2020, pp 51–59

Medicaid and CHIP Payment and Access Commission: Behavioral Health in the Medicaid Program—People, Use, and Expenditures. Washington, DC, MACPAC, 2015. Available at: https://www.macpac.gov/publication/behavioral-health-in-the-medicaid-program%e2%80%95people-use-and-expenditures. Accessed December 26, 2023.

Michigan Public Health Institute: Michigan Behavioral Health Crisis Services: CMHSP 2020 Survey Results. Okemos, MI, Michigan Public Health Institute, 2021. Available at: https://cmham.org/wp-content/uploads/2021/06/CMHSP-Crisis-Survey-Report-Full-Final.pdf. Accessed December 26, 2023.

Muroff J, Edelsohn GA, Joe S, et al: The role of race in diagnostic and disposition decision making in a pediatric psychiatric emergency service. Gen Hosp Psychiatry 30(3):269–276, 2008 18433660

National Alliance on Mental Illness: 988 Crisis Response State Legislation Map. Arlington, VA, National Alliance on Mental Illness, 2023. Available at: https://reimaginecrisis.org/map/. Accessed December 26, 2023.

National Suicide Hotline Designation Act of 2020, Pub. L. No. 116–172, § 4, 134 Stat. 832, 833 (2020)

Nunes JC, Naccarato T, Stafford RS: Antipsychotics in the California foster care system: a 10-year analysis. J Child Adolesc Psychopharmacol 32(7):400–407, 2022 35834606

Odes R, Manjanatha D, Looper P, et al: How to reach a mobile crisis team: results from a national survey. Psychiatr Serv 74(10):1084–1085, 2023 36935621

Otterson SE, Fristad MA, McBee-Strayer S, et al: Length of stay and readmission data for adolescents psychiatrically treated on a youth crisis stabilization unit versus a traditional inpatient unit. Evid Based Pract Child Adolesc Ment Health 6(4):484–489, 2021

Pope LG, Patel A, Fu E, et al: Crisis response model preferences of mental health care clients with prior misdemeanor arrests and of their family and friends. Psychiatr Serv 74(11):1163–1170, 2023 37070262

Puntis S, Perfect D, Kirubarajan A, et al: A systematic review of co-responder models of police mental health 'street' triage. BMC Psychiatry 18(1):256, 2018 30111302

Purtle J, Lindsey MA, Raghavan R, et al: National Suicide Prevention Lifeline 2020 in-state answer rates, stratified by call volume rates and geographic region. Psychiatr Serv 74(2):204–205, 2023 35833253

Rafla-Yuan E, Chhabra DK, Mensah MO: Decoupling crisis response from policing: a step toward equitable psychiatric emergency services. N Engl J Med 384(18):1769–1773, 2021 33951369

Randi O: American Rescue Plan Act allows states to expand mobile crisis intervention services for children and youth through Medicaid. National Academy for State Health Policy, August 2, 2021. Available at: https://nashp.org/american-rescue-plan-act-allows-states-to-expand-mobile-crisis-intervention-services-for-children-and-youth-through-medicaid. Accessed December 26, 2023.

Raney LE: Integrating primary care and behavioral health: the role of the psychiatrist in the Collaborative Care Model. Am J Psychiatry 172(8):721–728, 2015 26234599

Roberge J, McWilliams A, Zhao J, et al: Effect of a virtual patient navigation program on behavioral health admissions in the emergency department: a randomized clinical trial. JAMA Netw Open 3(1):e1919954, 2020 31995214

Shannon B, Baldry S, O'Meara P, et al: The definition of a community paramedic: an international consensus. Paramedicine 20(1):4–22, 2023

Simes JT, Jahn JL: The consequences of Medicaid expansion under the Affordable Care Act for police arrests. PLoS One 17(1):e0261512, 2022 35020737

Stanley B, Brown GK, Currier GW, et al: Brief intervention and follow-up for suicidal patients with repeat emergency department visits enhances treatment engagement. Am J Public Health 105(8):1570–1572, 2015 26066951

Substance Abuse and Mental Health Services Administration: Key substance use and mental health indicators in the United States: Results from the 2019 National Survey on Drug Use and Health (HHS Publ No PEP20-07-01-001, NSDUH Series H-55). Rockville, MD, Substance Abuse and Mental Health Services Administration, 2020a. Available at: https://store.samhsa.gov/product/results-2019-national-survey-drug-use-and-health-nsduh-key-substance-use-and-mental-health. Accessed December 26, 2023.

Substance Abuse and Mental Health Services Administration: National Guidelines for Behavioral Health Crisis Care—Best Practice Toolkit. Rockville, MD, Substance Abuse and Mental Health Services Administration, 2020b. Available at: https://www.samhsa.gov/sites/default/files/national-guidelines-for-behavioral-health-crisis-care-02242020.pdf. Accessed December 26, 2023.

Substance Abuse and Mental Health Services Administration: Peer Support Services in Crisis Care (HHS Publ No PEP22–06–04–001). Rockville, MD, Substance Abuse and Mental Health Services Administration, 2022. Available at: https://store.samhsa.gov/sites/default/files/pep22–06–04–001.pdf. Accessed December 26, 2023.

Substance Abuse and Mental Health Services Administration: Certified Community Behavioral Health Center (CCBHC) Certification Criteria. Rockville, MD, Substance Abuse and Mental Health Services Administration, 2023a. Available at: https://www.samhsa.gov/sites/default/files/ccbhc-criteria-2023.pdf. Accessed December 26, 2023.

Substance Abuse and Mental Health Services Administration: National Model Standards for Peer Support Certification (HHS Publ No PEP23–10–01–001). Rockville, MD, Substance Abuse and Mental Health Services Administration, 2023b. Available at: https://www.samhsa.gov/about-us/who-we-are/offices-centers/or/model-standards. Accessed December 26, 2023.

Substance Abuse and Mental Health Services Administration: 988 Frequently Asked Questions. Rockville, MD, Substance Abuse and Mental Health Services Administration, 2023c. Available at: https://www.samhsa.gov/find-help/988/faqs. Accessed December 26, 2023.

Substance Abuse and Mental Health Services Administration: 988 Suicide and Crisis Lifeline. Rockville, MD, Substance Abuse and Mental Health Services Administration, 2023d. Available at: https://www.samhsa.gov/find-help/988. Accessed December 26, 2023.

Swanson L, Nelson V, Comartin EB, et al: Assessing county-level behavioral health and justice systems with the sequential intercept model practices, leadership, and expertise scorecard. Community Ment Health J 59(3):578–594, 2023 36322279

Tamburello A, Penn J, Negron-Muñoz R, Kaliebe K: Prescribing psychotropic medications for justice-involved juveniles. J Correct Health Care 29(2):94–108, 2023 36637811

U.S. Department of Justice: Assistant Attorney General Kristen Clarke delivers remarks at the 3rd Annual Sozosei Summit to decriminalize mental illness. Office of Public Affairs, December 7, 2022. Available at: https://www.justice.gov/opa/speech/assistant-attorney-general-kristen-clarke-delivers-remarks-3rd-annual-sozosei-summit. Accessed December 26, 2023.

Usher L, Watson AC, Bruno R, et al: Crisis Intervention Team (CIT) Programs: A Best Practice Guide for Transforming Community Responses to Mental Health Crises. Memphis, TN, CIT International, 2019. Available at: https://www.citinternational.org/resources/Best%20Practice%20Guide/CIT%20guide%20desktop%20printing%202019_08_16%20(1).pdf. Accessed December 26, 2023.

Vera Institute of Justice: 911 Analysis: Call Data Shows We Can Rely Less on Police. Washington, DC, Vera Institute of Justice, 2022. Available at: https://www.vera.org/downloads/publications/911-analysis-we-can-rely-less-on-police.pdf. Accessed December 26, 2023.

Wallace D, Wang X: Does in-prison physical and mental health impact recidivism? SSM Popul Health 11:100569, 2020 32258357

Waters R: Enlisting mental health workers, not cops, in mobile crisis response. Health Aff (Millwood) 40(6):864–869, 2021 34097522

Zielinski MJ, Praseuth A, Gai MJ, et al: Crisis stabilization units for jail diversion: a preliminary assessment of patient characteristics and outcomes. Psychol Serv 19(4):630–636, 2022 35099227

Zito JM, Safer DJ, Sai D, et al: Psychotropic medication patterns among youth in foster care. Pediatrics 121(1):e157–e163, 2008 18166534

Equity in Mental Health and Criminal Legal System Reform

Samuel W. Jackson, M.D.
Matthew L. Edwards, M.D.

This book describes the contexts that often lead to arrest and entanglement with the misdemeanor criminal legal system—events that result in criminalizing individuals with serious mental illness (SMI). Most chapters draw largely on data from a mixed methods multisite study of the use and processing of misdemeanor charges in Atlanta, Chicago, Manhattan, and Philadelphia, as well as qualitative interviews in Georgia with people with mental illnesses and their family members about their experiences with misdemeanor arrests.

Chapter 9 ("The Current Era of Multifaceted Criminal Legal System Reform") and Chapter 10 ("Reform in an Era of Mental Health and Crisis Services Innovation") review reform efforts in the criminal legal, mental health, and crisis service systems. In this chapter, we focus on reforms within these three systems that consider the problem of racial inequities. We argue that meaningful attempts to reform these systems must consider the disparate outcomes that racialized people with mental illnesses and criminal legal system involvement experience. By framing race, racialization, and racism in this context, we demonstrate that racial equity must be an explicit focus and that each system must engage in reform to achieve equity.

Framing Concepts in Racial Equity

An explicit goal of this chapter is to frame concepts in racial equity and highlight how race shapes the lived experiences of individuals with mental illnesses as they encounter the mental health and criminal legal systems. Addressing racial equity in these systems requires an understanding of how SMI, race, and criminal legal involvement interact.

In Pursuit of Equity

Although equity, equality, and justice are often used interchangeably, these concepts are distinct. Addressing health inequities and disparities through an equity lens is fundamentally different than through an equality lens, requires different approaches, and may lead to different health and social outcomes. Whereas equality implies treating all individuals the same, equity goes further to ensure that individuals have what they need to achieve equal outcomes. Moreover, race-neutral interventions—policies, practices, and opportunities that treat everyone equally—may maintain or worsen existing inequities. This approach also selectively focuses on the *what* of the problem (e.g., rates of misdemeanor charges in Black men with SMI compared with White men with SMI) rather than the *how*. In contrast, reforms pursuing equity recognize the need to address the limiting conditions for individuals to achieve equal outcomes. Only by addressing *how* public policies and social norms lead to unequal and unjust distribution of opportunities and the social determinants of ill health can we ensure equal outcomes (Shadravan and Barceló 2021; Shim et al. 2015).

Intersectionality

Recognizing that our diverse identities, experiences, and exposures differentially affect our lives and outcomes lies at the center of a focus on equity. Individuals from racially and ethnically oppressed backgrounds who experience SMI are ensnared in the criminal legal system at every level. *Intersectionality,* a term originally coined by legal scholar Kimberlé Crenshaw (1989), explains how occupying multiple devalued social categories can "multiply burden" and lead to oppression. This type of synergism means that the collective toll on an individual from a marginalized or multiply marginalized background with an SMI and multiple misdemeanors is greater than the sum of their separate effects (Crenshaw 1989). We know that intersectionality shapes and structures the experiences of individuals who live at the cross-sectional margins of society, despite their absence in research, decision-making, and policy interventions. Research, policy, and programming often do not consider intersectionality, which prevents identifying and addressing how inequities mutually reinforce one another. Intersectional data, like intersectional lives, tend to be invisible to the public eye (Shadravan et al. 2021). Yet, collecting these data and addressing inequities is especially important for people who live at intersecting axes of oppression (Crenshaw 1989; Shadravan et al. 2021).

Race, Racialization, and Racism

How race is defined, how racial categories structure health and social outcomes, and who defines race serve as a backdrop to any discussion of structural racism and racial inequity. Race, often used subjectively to refer to physical features such as skin color, ancestry, or shared culture, is a malleable social concept based on social, historical, and political forces and self-identification (Omi and Winant 2014). Race is a social rather than a biological construct. It is a salient social classification that stratifies societal roles and positions, structuring inequality in the process (Bailey et al. 2017; Hoffman et al. 2016; Omi and Winant 2014). *Racialization* refers to the process of assigning racial meaning to individuals, objects, or concepts, or defining individuals by racial categories, often as a basis for social exclusion (Murji and Solomos 2005; Wright 2015).

Structural racism refers to the process in which mutually reinforcing systems, including housing, education, employment, media, health care, and the carceral systems, limit the opportunities, resources, rights, power, and well-being of individuals and populations based on their physical characteristics (Bailey et al. 2017). Structural racism reifies racially discriminatory beliefs, values, and outcomes (Hoffman et al. 2016; Pérez-Stable 2021). The tacit justification for racism is *racial essentialism,* the belief that social identities have distinct and unchanging characteristics (Haslam et al. 2000; Shim and Vinson 2021). Structural and interpersonal racism shapes people's experiences and outcomes in mental health care and criminal legal systems. Such racism must be accounted for and corrected during any meaningful reform efforts.

This chapter focuses on racialization because race plays a strong and persistent role in structuring societal inequity in the United States. Consistent with the focus of the social science literature, the studies of misdemeanor criminal legal system involvement focus heavily on the Black race. Nevertheless, we recognize that other people of color as well as people of different nationalities and diverse sexual, gender, and religious backgrounds, within and outside the United States, are also affected by structural discrimination, requiring similar pursuits of equity.

Racial Inequity

Racist processes have produced profound inequities across nearly every socioeconomic category in the United States (see Table 11–1). These include inequities in health, income, wealth, education, and employment. Black Americans have the highest infant mortality rate of any racial or ethnic group (Ely and Driscoll 2021). Black households possess only 7% of the wealth of White households (Bennett et al. 2022). The academic achievement gap between Black and White children is estimated to be around 2 years of schooling, with the COVID-19 pandemic widening this difference (Goldhaber et al. 2022), and Black Americans have the highest unemployment rate among any racial or ethnic group (Bureau of Labor Statistics 2023). Explicitly racist federal policies and interpersonal discrimination by the housing system have created extreme neighborhood segregation and home ownership disparities, which in turn contribute to the massive education and wealth gaps, both of which are fundamental causes of racial differences in health (Jones et al. 2020; Massey and Denton 1998; Williams and Collins 2001).

Racial inequities also permeate educational attainment, produced partly by the interplay of racist processes within the education, mental health, and juvenile legal systems. Racialized minorities are more likely to be dismissed or expelled from school for disruptive behavior, and disruptive behavior is more often pathologized or misdiagnosed as oppositional defiant disorder and conduct disorder (compared with ADHD) in Black children relative to White children (Coker et al. 2016; Fadus et al. 2020; Morgan et al. 2013; Skiba et al. 2014). Systemic and interpersonal biases contribute to the underdiagnosis of ADHD and overdiagnosis of disruptive behavior disorders. Clinicians more often view the behavior of racially and ethnically oppressed people as dan-

Table 11–1. Examples of racial and ethnic inequities in the United States

	Total	Black non-Hispanic	White non-Hispanic	Hispanic (any race)	Asian non-Hispanic	Non-Hispanic Native American or Alaska Native	Non-Hispanic Pacific Islander	Two or more non-White ethnicities
Infant mortality per 1,000 live births, 2019	5.4	10.6	4.5	5	3.4	7.9	8.2	—
Life expectancy at birth (years), 2021	76.1	70.8	76.4	77.7	83.5	65.2	—	—
High school dropout rate of 16- to 24-year-olds, 2021	5.2	5.6	4.1	7.8	1.8	10.2	7.6	5.1
Jail incarceration rates per 100,000, 2021	192	528	157	145	19	316	110	25
Unemployment rate, 2021	5.3	8.6	4.7	6.8	5.0	8.2	6.9	8.2
Supplemental poverty measure rates, 2021	7.8	11.3	5.7	11.2	9.5	12.4	12.4	7.3
Median household wealth ($), 2019	—	14,100	187,300	31,700	206,400	—	—	—
Percentage uninsured, 2021	8.6	9.6	5.7	17.7	5.8	18.8	10.1	7.5

Table 11-1. Examples of racial and ethnic inequities in the United States *(continued)*

	Total	Black non-Hispanic	White non-Hispanic	Hispanic (any race)	Asian non-Hispanic	Non-Hispanic Native American or Alaska Native	Non-Hispanic Pacific Islander	Two or more non-White ethnicities
Adults reporting fair or poor health status (%), 2021	16.3	20.7	14.5	22.6	8.6[a]	25.8	8.6[a]	—
Adults with any mental illness who received treatment (%), 2021	47.2	39.4	52.4	36.1	25.4	—	—	52.2
Diabetes deaths per 100,000, 2021[b]	25.4	46.3	22.4	29.4	18.1	51.0	54.4	14.9
Heart disease deaths per 100,000, 2021[c]	174	226	180	119	86	155	182	75

—= Comparable data points were not readily available.

[a]Non-Hispanic Asian and Pacific Islander groups were combined in this data set.

[b]Based on standard U.S. population.

[c]Based on standard U.S. population.

Source. Ely and Driscoll 2021 (infant mortality); Arias et al. 2022 (life expectancy); National Center for Education Statistics 2023 (high school); Bureau of Justice Statistics 2021a (jail); Bureau of Labor Statistics 2023 (unemployment); Creamer et al. 2022 (poverty); Bennett et al. 2022 (household wealth); Branch and Conway 2022 (health insurance); KFF 2021a (poor health); Substance Abuse and Mental Health Services Administration 2023 (mental illness); KFF 2021b (diabetes deaths); KFF 2021c (heart disease).

gerous and insubordinate, resulting in conduct disorder and oppositional defiant disorder diagnoses compared to non-Hispanic White
children with similar behavior who tend to receive mood, anxiety, development, or adjustment disorder diagnoses (Clark 2007; Fadus et al.
2020; Feisthamel and Schwartz 2009). Moreover, Black and Latinx children are less likely to be referred to mental health services by a school
professional, and if they are referred, they are less likely to be able to
pay (Fadus et al. 2020). When a child is misdiagnosed with a disruptive
behavior disorder in place of ADHD, the child loses important supportive services and experiences more exclusionary disciplinary practices
(Fadus et al. 2020). These intermediate outcomes are even stronger predictors of future harmful consequences such as dropout from school
and penetration into the juvenile legal system (Fadus et al. 2020).

   While an exhaustive list of racial inequities and their contexts is beyond the scope of this chapter, these few examples serve as a framework to identify and address disparities within the mental health and
criminal legal systems.

Racism in the Criminal Legal System

Racialized outcomes in criminal legal system involvement exist at every
level. Racist policies and processes increase points of contact between
Black youth and the criminal legal system starting at a young age. Zero
tolerance policies in schools, which mandate predetermined, punitive
consequences regardless of the situational context of behavior, result in
significant increases in suspensions, expulsions, and law enforcement
referrals, disproportionately impacting Black youth. In what has been
called a "school-to-prison pipeline," Black youth are more likely to attend inadequately resourced and staffed schools, have limited access to
behavioral health interventions, and are about 2.5 times more likely to
be suspended than their White peers, with suspension, expulsion, or
being held back being among the largest predictors of future arrest
(Barnes and Motz 2018).

   Racial disparities in the juvenile legal system mirror racial disparities in schools. Police tend to perceive Black male youth as less childlike,
overestimating their age by 4 years, and in doing so, perceive Black
boys as less innocent than White boys (Goff et al. 2014). Unsurprisingly,
Black youth who are not engaged in criminalized behavior are more
likely to be stopped by police than White youth (Harris et al. 2020), 2.4
times more likely to be arrested, more likely to be referred to court, and
more likely to be placed in an out-of-home facility after being adjudi-

cated (Bishop et al. 2010; Development Services Group 2022). Additionally, Black children are more likely to receive incarceration, probation, or parole rather than treatment, and when they are referred to treatment, the facilities are more likely to be of poor quality (Raz 2018).

As in childhood, Black adults are disproportionately policed, and their behavior is criminalized compared to their non-Hispanic White counterparts. Black Americans are more likely to be subjected to traffic stops (Baumgartner et al. 2017; Voigt et al. 2017) and spoken to disrespectfully, regardless of the severity of the infraction or outcome of the stop (Baumgartner et al. 2017). In one study of Oakland, California, traffic stops, even after analyses controlled for dozens of factors related to police decision-making, including crime rates and individual demographic variables, being Black was still associated with an increased likelihood of being stopped, handcuffed, searched, and arrested, despite the officer being no more likely to find contraband on African Americans compared with other races (Hetey et al. 2016). Similar data exist across the country (Baumgartner et al. 2017).

Despite no significant differences in illicit drug use, similar self-reports of criminal offending, and (in some studies) lower rates of drug trafficking than White Americans, Black Americans are more likely to be arrested when caught doing something illegal (Blankenship et al. 2018), to be detained while awaiting trial, to receive a felony conviction, to be sentenced to jail or prison, and to be placed on probation than their White counterparts (Pettit and Gutierrez 2018). In fact, on average, Black males receive 20% longer sentences than White men for the same crime (Pryar et al. 2017). High incarceration rates in certain communities have been shown to increase policing and surveillance tactics, creating a reinforcing loop (Pettit and Gutierrez 2018; Pryar et al. 2017). Paradoxically, post-arrest diversion programs meant to break this cycle have also been less accessible to Black men and women ensnared in the criminal legal system (Pettit and Gutierrez 2018; Pryar et al. 2017).

Taken as a whole, these racialized disparities in criminal legal system outcomes mean Black Americans are 5.1 times more likely than White Americans to be incarcerated in state prisons (Vinson et al. 2020). And while Black Americans make up only 13.6% of the U.S. population (U.S. Census Bureau 2023), they make up 35% of the total jail population (Bureau of Justice Statistics 2021a) and are the single largest racial demographic group in prison (Bureau of Justice Statistics 2021b). The risk of lifetime imprisonment for Black men rose from one in five in the mid-1980s to nearly *one in two* in 2004 before falling to roughly one in six in 2016. This rate remains higher than ever recorded for White males (Massoglia and Pridemore 2015; Roehrkasse and Wildeman 2022).

Being convicted of a crime also has significant socioeconomic and health impacts, particularly for Black Americans (Pager 2007). In a field study examining the effect of having a criminal record in the job market in Milwaukee, ex-offenders received less than half the callbacks of equally qualified applicants without criminal backgrounds (Western and Wildeman 2009). Strikingly, young Black men without criminal records received a similar number of callbacks for jobs as White men just out of prison (Western and Wildeman 2009). The results were similar for felony convictions, even without spending time in prison or jail (Western and Wildeman 2009). Moreover, incarceration is strongly associated with extended periods of unemployment, underemployment, lower wages, and slower wage growth (Pryar et al. 2017).

The economic and health consequences extend beyond the individuals in the criminal legal system, reverberating throughout their families and communities. Families with incarcerated family members have increased financial debt and economic insecurity, leading to increased rates of housing instability (Gatewood et al. 2023). Children of recently incarcerated fathers are three times more likely to experience homelessness than children without incarcerated fathers, and more than 10% of Black children have at least one parent incarcerated (Wakefield and Wildeman 2013). Paternal incarceration increases the odds of infant death in the first year of life by 49%, slightly higher than the effect of maternal smoking, which increases the odds of infant mortality by 46% (Wildeman and Muller 2012). Children with parents in the criminal legal system also endure worse mental health and behavioral issues (Pettit and Gutierrez 2018), and parental incarceration is a significant driver of adverse childhood experiences (ACEs) that contribute to poor health and social outcomes across the life course (Pettit and Gutierrez 2018; Wildeman and Muller 2012). As such, parental incarceration is an important contributor to racial disparities in childhood health and well-being (Asad and Clair 2018; Western and Wildeman 2009; Wildeman and Wang 2017).

Such profound racial disparities, perpetuated through criminal legal system involvement, are perhaps best understood through the concept of racialized legal status as a social determinant of health. Racialized legal status is a social status created by ostensibly race-neutral legal classification that gets "colored" over time through its disparate impact on racial or ethnic minorities. This concept can be applied more broadly to understand how the law uses various legal statuses (e.g., immigration status, criminal status) to produce racial and ethnic health disparities. As a social determinant of health, an individual's racialized legal status excludes them from material and societal benefits, resulting in further inequities. However, an individual's racialized legal status has larger effects on their community (e.g., increased stress to family members and other racial/ethnic in-group members) regardless of legal status (Stacy and Cohen 2017).

Consider "Ban the Box" initiatives, which refer to ostensibly well-intentioned efforts to improve outcomes for individuals ensnared in the criminal legal system by removing discriminating questions about an applicant's criminal record from job applications and, thus, hiring decisions. Paradoxically, these initiatives to remove discrimination in hiring at the local and national level can increase racial disparities in employment. In one study, White applicants received 7% more callbacks than Black applicants before the Ban the Box reform but 45% more callbacks than Black applicants after removing the criminality box (Asad and Clair 2018). Although Ban the Box initiatives aimed to reduce the racial gap between Black and White individuals who received job offers, they led to an unexpected increase in racial disparities in hiring. Thus, without Black applicants being able to prove their lack of a criminal record, employers likely used Black race and male gender as a proxy for criminal status (Asad and Clair 2018; Stacy and Cohen 2017). As such, Ban the Box provides yet another example of how racialized legal statuses shape outcomes for racially and ethnically oppressed people.

Racism in the Mental Health System

Studies show that racialized minorities experience inequitable access and disparate outcomes and are more likely to enter and experience mental health treatment through coercive means (Yeh et al. 2002). Black Americans are less likely to receive mental health care (Substance Abuse and Mental Health Services Administration 2023), and when they do receive care, it is more likely to be of poorer quality. This decreased access occurs despite an equal or even greater willingness to receive treatment for a mental illness (Shim et al. 2009). A recent large, cross-sectional study of older adults with depression found that Black participants had 10% higher 8-item Patient Health Questionnaire scores (a measure of depression) and were more likely to report sadness, anhedonia, and psychomotor symptoms. However, they were 61% less likely to report any treatment (i.e., medication or therapy) than non-Hispanic White participants, even after controlling for potentially confounding variables (Vyas et al. 2020). Further, when Black Americans do receive mental health care, it is more likely to be from a primary care physician and less likely from a mental health specialist such as a psychiatrist or therapist (Alegría et al. 2008; Cook et al. 2014; Wielen et al.

2015). Largely because of this inequitable access to quality care, Black Americans have greater mental illness persistence and severity (Vyas et al. 2020).

A study by Kugelmass (2016) showed a significant difference in accessibility for Black participants seeking psychotherapy, differences that were based on perceived race and social class backgrounds. In his phone-based audit experiment, a Black working class man with health insurance who called 80 therapists in his insurance network requesting a weekday evening appointment found only one offer. In contrast, 16 of 80 calls (20%) made by a White working class woman—with identical insurance coverage—produced an offer. Even comparing matched middle class groups, Black middle class participants seeking a psychotherapist were significantly less likely than their White counterparts to be offered an appointment. These results shed light on conscious and unconscious discriminatory biases, even among highly trained clinicians, and the lack of mental health care system access (Kugelmass 2016).

When racialized minorities receive specialized mental health treatment, they are also more likely to enter treatment through "coercive" channels (Yeh et al. 2002, p. 58), such as through the juvenile legal system, child protective services, involuntary inpatient treatment, outpatient civil commitment, and crisis services (Fadus et al. 2020; Raz et al. 2021; Shea et al. 2022; Swanson et al. 2009; Yeh et al. 2002). Although this is not an example of a carceral disparity, in many ways, it resembles one. A prospective cohort study in Boston found that Black patients on an inpatient psychiatric unit were more likely than White patients to be admitted involuntarily, even after adjusting for confounding variables (Shea et al. 2022). An analysis of New York State's outpatient commitment program found that Black adults were about five times more likely to receive court-ordered outpatient treatment than White adults (Swanson et al. 2009). The study found that the disproportionate application of outpatient civil commitment was better explained by overlapping "upstream" social disparities, such as the increased prevalence of SMI and a greater reliance on public services in Black communities (Swanson et al. 2009).

Similarly, racially and ethnically oppressed people are more likely to have traumatic experiences while receiving treatment. When admitted to an inpatient unit, pediatric and adult Black patients are more likely to be physically and chemically restrained and placed in seclusion (Daniels et al. 2023; Pedersen et al. 2023). These racist practices result in racial and ethnic minority groups being more likely to suffer physical and psychological harm and even die while receiving psychiatric care (Dotson et al. 2022). Although race itself has been associated with increased rates of restrictive practices, a review of this literature highlights again how the intersectionality of other social determinants of poor health, such as immigration status, with race creates multiple sources of disadvantage for certain minority groups within the mental health system.

The Narrative of the Numbers

Facts alone are not enough. Explaining disparities such as these by documenting disparate behavior and risk, highlighting only those facts and figures without dispute, is tempting. Yet, there is some evidence that simply collating gross inequities may make some individuals less—not more—likely to support racial equity initiatives (Hetey and Eberhardt 2018).

Presenting evidence of disparities in the criminal legal system, stratified by race or mental health status, may unintentionally reinforce stereotypical associations that Black Americans and those with mental illness are criminals, and that criminals are Black and have mental illness. When these associations occur, the disparities maintain the status quo, reify false race-based beliefs, and lead to disparate outcomes such as the overrepresentation of Black people with mental illness in jails and prisons (Hetey and Eberhardt 2018).

What strategies should policy reforms take if presenting evidence of these disparities is insufficient and may have a paradoxical effect? And what can be done to remedy these incorrect beliefs and assumptions, change unequal practices, and mitigate or reverse disparate outcomes? Understanding the historical context is vital in informing our understanding, approaches, and policies. Ramos's (2019) historical analysis of these precedents in the context of the biology of race and violence in Los Angeles illustrates how policy reforms can have unintended effects.

Although community policing was initially conceived to be a desirable, local, and commonsense solution to the challenges and inequities in our most vulnerable communities, the overpolicing of some communities, driven largely by "tough-on-crime" policies and the "broken windows" approach (Ramos 2019) has led to disproportionately more people of color being arrested for minor offenses. Worsening unemployment and poverty of the 1970s, as structural products of the transition of a labor economy to a lower-paying service economy (Dunlap and Johnson 1992), and the uneven development between neighborhoods of color and White neighborhoods, are thought to have been the largest drivers for engaging in informal economies that lead to arrest and incarceration (Ramos 2019; Raz 2013). Instead of addressing poverty and unemployment, politicians and voters interpreted rioting, crime, drug use, and family dysfunction as problems related to race rather than socioeconomic problems, requiring tougher policing strategies (Ramos 2019). The response was a "broken windows" approach during the 1980s and 1990s that directed police to have zero tolerance when addressing low-level street activity to prevent more dangerous forms of crime (Ramos 2019). The logic of these popular policies was that disorder and crime were inseparably linked, whereby disorder predicts the development of crime (Ramos 2019). When coupled with the larger criminalization of drug use during the 1970s through the 1990s—especially in the absence of adequate addiction treatment—individuals from these marginalized groups were more likely to come into contact with the criminal legal system.

At the same time, ostensibly progressive ideas of racial sameness in psychiatry sought to explain racial differences in violent behavior during the 1960s and 1970s. For example, Louis J. West, former chairman of psychiatry at the University of California, Los Angeles, School of Medicine and director of the Neuropsychiatric Institute, viewed violent behavior in Black communities as a consequence of marginalized individuals' increased exposure to trauma and other early adverse childhood experiences (Ramos 2019). Moreover, West believed that these exposures led to neurobiological changes that underpinned later violent or deviant behavior (Ramos 2019). He hoped to demonstrate how these racial differences—that were explained by biology—were not intrinsic to racially and ethnically oppressed people.

West, along with J. Alfred Cannon, then chair of psychiatry at the Martin Luther King Jr. Health Center and Drew Postgraduate Medical School (King/Drew), with support from then-Governor Ronald W. Reagan, helped redirect NIMH funding away from community treatment services toward biologically based research that contributed to the "medicalized criminalization of poor people of color" (Ramos 2019). Because West sought to explain violence through "neutral" biological terms, he believed that biological explanations would supplant race and racism as explanations of violence. Cannon understood violence and deviance as a consequence of communities' social and economic marginalization and history of racial oppression. While these two thought leaders understood behavior differently, both were examples of efforts to adopt race neutrality and colorblindness as a means to remove the influence of race and racism from social structures. By framing these explanations in medicalized terms of biological and psychological development, however, West, Cannon, and their contemporaries "inadvertently pathologized poverty and blamed racially oppressed families for their shortcomings rather than addressed the underlying issues and social structures that explained these inequities" (Edwards et al. 2021, p. 57). The net effect was to expand the population of mentally ill people by designating behavior associated with urban crime and disruptive activity as pathological. Further pathologizing of behaviors, such as through the War on Drugs (announced in 1971 and continued through the 1980s and 1990s), became a key part of the burgeoning carceral society, further bolstering police targets for broken-windows approaches during the 1980s (Ramos 2019).

The increase in police contact with poor, minoritized, and mostly urban racial groups occurred during an era of minimum sentencing guidelines and harsh penalties for minor and especially repeated offenses, leading to widespread racial, gender, and socioeconomic inequities (Dunlap and Johnson 1992; O'Hear 2009). Specifically, the War on Drugs produced massive and racially disproportionate increases in the number of incarcerated Black men (O'Hear 2009). With a particular focus on crack cocaine, the Anti-Drug Abuse acts of 1986 and 1988 gave rise to the most recognized mandatory minimum sentencing law, the 100:1 crack:powder cocaine ratio. This law made it such that a given quantity of crack cocaine (disproportionately used by Black Americans) resulted in the same sentence that would be imposed for 100 times that quantity of powder cocaine (overwhelmingly used by White Americans) (O'Hear 2009). These sentencing guidelines created racial sentencing disparities in which the average federal sentence for crack cocaine was 119 months (O'Hear 2009). In comparison, the average sentence for the powder form of the same drug was 78 months—a difference of nearly 3.5 years of life behind bars (O'Hear 2009). These minimum sentencing laws governed drug-related offenses for decades, ending with the Fair Sentencing Act of 2010, which changed the ratio from 100:1 to 18:1 and eliminated the 5-year mandatory minimum sentence for cocaine possession.

The "tough-on-crime" policing and increasingly aggressive sentencing policies from the 1970s through the 1990s, which followed most of the deinstitutionalization of people with SMI out of state mental hospitals, substantially expanded the number of incarcerated people with SMI. Although no evidence exists of transinstitutionalization from state mental hospitals to prisons from 1950 to 1980 before harsh sentencing was enacted, one analysis does show significant transinstitutionalization from 1980 to 2000, particularly for White men (Raphael and Stoll 2013). The authors of that study concluded that primarily due to increased sentencing policies in most states, for the year 2000, "there are 40,000–72,000 incarcerated individuals who in years past would likely have been mental hospital inpatients. … this increase constitutes 14% to 26% of the mentally ill incarcerated population" (Raphael and Stoll 2013, p. 219). Transinstitutionalization, however, continues to be debated, with critiques stating that while the proportion of people with SMI in jails and prisons indeed rose between 1990 and 2000, there were low levels of arrest following discharge from state hospitals and major demographic differences among state psychiatric hospital patients compared with incarcerated individuals (Prins 2011). Regardless, the massive increase in the number of incarcerated individuals with SMI following harsh sentencing policy decisions has led to jails and prisons becoming the largest mental health institutions in the country (Al-Rousan et al. 2017; Ramos 2019). These trends suggest that the safeguarding and treatment function of state hospitals was partly transferred to the carceral system in the wake of deinstitutionalization (Ramos 2019). These obscured distinctions between the roles of prisons and psychiatric institutions highlight how the United States approaches individual safety and well-being (especially as it pertains to race) through an intertwined criminal legal and psychiatric authority (Ramos 2019).

Systems work exactly how they are designed to work and for the people who created them. Mental health and criminal legal system design has historically discounted the lived experiences of minoritized voices, referred to as *epistemic injustice* (i.e., discrediting people based on their social status) (Del Pozo and Rich 2021). Understanding how this deprives systems of knowledge and devalues the experiences of those disadvantaged by these pervasive inequities is a vital first step in approaching equitable reform (Del Pozo and Rich 2021).

Racial Equity in Criminal Legal Reform for People With Serious Mental Illness

In one of the studies of people with SMI and misdemeanors that provide the foundation for this book, Black race was significantly associated with the number of arrests, second only to lower educational attainment (Compton et al. 2022). These two unsurprising findings reaffirm the importance of including racial equity in multisystem reform (e.g., criminal legal system, education, mental health). Moreover, we contend that any system or systems that do not include racial equity as a focus will not lead to racial equity as an outcome.

Race is one of the most important factors associated with the entanglement of people with SMI in the criminal legal system. As such, race should be considered in reforming the criminal legal and mental health systems. Because the burden of entanglement among people with SMI is disproportionately felt in marginalized communities, reforms should be most accessible to populations with the greatest need (e.g., Black people, those with the lowest educational attainment). Structuring reform to prioritize accessibility by the highest-needs groups at the onset improves the likelihood that those groups would benefit (Shadravan et al. 2021).

Ensuring broader access to race-neutral programs is not enough. Using the attorney-client relationship as an example, legal scholar and sociologist Matthew Clair (2020) demonstrated that when defendants from marginalized backgrounds (i.e., poor and racially and ethnically oppressed people) know their legal rights and more actively engage in trying to fight their cases, they often experience poorer legal outcomes. Privileged defendants, by contrast (e.g., middle-class, White working class individuals), are more likely to entrust their defense to their lawyers, accede to judges' authority, and consequently receive opportunities for rehabilitation and treatment. In this instance, attempts to advocate for themselves in the criminal legal system often have the opposite effect on people from marginalized backgrounds. Thus, even constitutionally granted access to legal representation does not ensure equity in the criminal legal system (Clair 2020).

Race-conscious interventions, such as affirmative action policies that prioritize racial groups, have suffered from legal challenges and low public support. By contrast, race-neutral programming that addresses racial disparities without directly targeting benefits exclusively to racial minority groups tends to garner more public and political support (Sniderman et al. 1996). Yet race-neutral approaches often fail to do what they set out to do and sometimes worsen racial inequities. For example, race-neutral solutions such as general economic growth theory and antidiscrimination enforcement of loan denials focus on people of all races and attempt to ensure no adverse impact on the majority groups. Without addressing the underlying cause of racial income inequity, for example, there is no consistent pattern of narrowing racial earnings gaps during periods of economic growth. Additionally, antidiscrimination enforcement of loan denial rates benefited nonprotected groups more than racial minority group members (Myers and Ha 2018).

Because there has historically not been an equal opportunity for racially and ethnically oppressed groups, current equal-opportunity approaches to reform for disadvantaged groups ensure that those groups will continue to be left behind. Furthermore, superimposing race-neutral reforms onto inherently racist mental health and criminal legal systems reforms will fail to address the root causes of inequities. Focusing on the dichotomy between race-neutral and race-conscious approaches may distract policymakers from developing effective interventions. Instead, research suggests that arguing for racially conscious programs that go beyond race significantly increases public support (Sniderman et al. 1996). Previous attempts at race-neutral criminal legal systems and mental health reforms have backfired, worsening racial inequities in these systems.

Race-Neutral Drug Treatment Courts: A Cautionary Tale

Drug treatment courts gained widespread appeal by offering to divert people from conviction, incarceration, and deeper penetration into the criminal legal system toward treatment. Individuals with drug offenses who could demonstrate their ability to complete a rigorous treatment program became natural targets of these reform initiatives, and some hailed this system-level change as a step in the right direction. Decades later, however, growing evidence suggests that White individuals with drug offenses are more likely to benefit from these programs than Black individuals with the same offenses. In fact, in one study, White individuals were more likely to complete the program and, in doing so, were more likely to get out of the criminal legal system. The opposite was also true, whereby Black individuals were less likely to complete the program and were doubly punished for it (increased sentences were given to individuals who failed to complete the program). Thus, these race-neutral interventions have worsened racial disparities not only by lowering the proportion of White individuals with criminal legal system involvement but also by increasing sentences for Black participants (O'Hear 2009).

Health and criminal legal systems can glean important lessons in how these ostensibly neutral interventions worsened racial inequities. First, drug treatment courts only addressed individuals after being arrested. As long as policing practices remain the same and Black Americans are dramatically overrepresented at the front end, racial inequities will likely remain at the back end (O'Hear 2009; Shim et al. 2021; Vinson and Dennis 2021). Any contemporary criminal legal reform for people with SMI would maximize its effects by incentivizing antiracist interventions at intercept 0 (i.e., nonpolice behavioral health crisis responders) (Myers and Ha 2018; Vinson and Dennis 2021) (see Chapter 9).

Second, Black participants' higher failure rates than White drug treatment court participants largely could be attributed to a higher bur-

den of socioeconomic disadvantage (O'Hear 2009). This disparity alone
may have exacerbated race-related disparities. But this point is further
compounded by the fact that failure or even near-failure in drug treatment courts often resulted in greater lengths of incarceration than non-
participants would have received. For example, in a study of New York
City drug courts, sentences for failing participants were two to five
times longer than for conventionally adjudicated defendants (Zhou and
Ford 2021). This inequity leads to individuals being punished twice:
first, for the initial criminal charge, and second, for subsequently failing
to comply with court-mandated treatment (O'Hear 2009).

The importance of drug treatment courts to the pursuit of equity
cannot be understated. Drug treatment courts can be effective in reducing carceral involvement and further penetration into the criminal legal
system for many individuals. But they do not do so equally. As the research demonstrates, drug treatment courts worsen disparities for
Black participants and can lengthen sentences for individuals who do
not successfully complete the program. Drug treatment court reform
should focus on ways that program interventions benefit participants
regardless of their race. General strategies for achieving equitable reform are discussed in the remaining sections of this chapter.

Thus, it is not safe to assume that all participants have equal access
to interventions or success in completing interventions when developing reforms. Whether reforming drug courts and 911 police response or
developing alternative non-police-based mental health crisis responses,
policymakers and reformers must pursue antiracist approaches that
consider the potential downstream effect of interventions on marginalized populations and seek ways to mitigate these potential disparities.
Prioritizing access to minoritized and overrepresented groups, incentivizing race-related data collection, and an earnest commitment to
address racially disparate outcomes may prevent the unintended consequences seen in drug treatment courts.

Making Equity a Focus

Many interventions that aim to divert people from the criminal legal
system toward mental health services currently lack race-related data,
and results are mixed when data do exist (Goldman and Vinson 2022).
One area of reform at the intersection of mental health access and policing that receives significant attention is mental health crisis services.
Crisis service reform initiatives have goals of diverting people away
from jails and overcrowded emergency departments toward mental
health treatment (Goldman and Vinson 2022). Thus far, equity-specific

diversion outcomes have been understudied. In a 2021 evaluation of an Indianapolis-based co-responder team composed of a mental health clinician and a police officer, Black individuals were significantly less likely to have an immediate arrest compared with Black individuals to whom the police responded as usual (Bailey et al. 2022). This reduction in arrest was not found among White participants. However, the published data do not show how the absolute arrest rates compare among White and Black participants before or after the intervention, so whether immediate arrest rates are equitable in this community remains an open question.

The lack of sociodemographic data and outcomes related to health equity likely has many causes. Collecting race and other demographic data is difficult during a crisis, especially since people in a crisis may be more reticent to give personal information. Additionally, many existing quality measures do not contain—and many public and private payors do not routinely require—these types of data (Goldman and Vinson 2022). Furthermore, national guidelines, such as the 2020 Substance Abuse and Mental Health Services Administration (SAMHSA) guidelines for behavioral health crisis care, to which crisis program funding is often linked, do not have any specific recommendations for collecting race-related data or achieving equitable outcomes (Substance Abuse and Mental Health Services Administration 2020). Although much work has been done advocating for equity to be a focus before 2020 (Nelson and Brooks 2015; Stewart and Shim 2020), the lack of national recommendations or requirements to include equity in quality metrics by funding entities likely contributes to the crisis system's current limitations.

Following the tragic deaths of unarmed Black men and women and the social unrest that ensued in 2020—including the death of Daniel Prude, an African American man who died after being placed in police custody during a mental health crisis—many institutions throughout society have made the pursuit of equity an explicit focus (Balfour et al. 2022; Goldman and Vinson 2022; Stewart and Shim 2020). Leading experts in behavioral health crises have called for incorporating an explicit commitment to racial equity in crisis response services (Balfour et al. 2022; Goldman and Vinson 2022). These recommendations include conducting racial equity impact assessments before implementing interventions to determine the potential to worsen disparities or cause unintentional trauma or harm (Balfour et al. 2022). As seen in the example of drug courts, simply creating diversion programs does not necessarily improve outcomes. Neither does improvement across groups mean that those groups improved equally. Without knowing who benefits from reform programs, who are disadvantaged by them, and to what extent, well-intentioned initiatives or studies that are not capturing racial data may exacerbate racial disparities. Moreover, without racial equity assessments, early data collection, analyses, and quality improvement, worsening racial disparities may only be discovered decades later. The Government Alliance on Racial Equity has multiple tools to help formalize the process of centering racial equity, including the Racial Equity Toolkit. The Toolkit is designed to integrate consideration of racial equity into organizational decision-making, including policies, practices, programs, and budgets with the goal of reducing racial inequities and improving outcomes for all (Nelson and Brooks 2015).

In addition to considering existing inequities and completing a racial equity impact assessment, institutions, agencies, and policymakers should make a commitment to racial equity that includes ongoing data collection, analysis, and accountability. Quality improvement assessments that include race and ethnicity allow for analyses of any disparities in outcomes stratified by race. To aid in this equity-driven pursuit, the National Council for Mental Well-Being developed behavioral health crisis service metrics that incorporate equity as a shared value and measurable standard and allow for stratification of crisis outcomes (e.g., involuntary treatment, police involvement, referrals to a higher level of care) by race/ethnicity and other variables (Goldman et al. 2023).

A grant from SAMHSA, along with the U.S. Department of Health and Human Services (DHHS) and Center for Mental Health Services (CMHS), funded a large, equity-focused study evaluating a variety of mental health measures to help inform 988 messaging and use. A three-digit mental health crisis line, 988 is another effort to divert people in crisis away from law enforcement and toward mental health treatment. The study completed qualitative and quantitative surveys of populations representing diverse demographic backgrounds about their mental health, suicidal ideation, perceptions of 988, what messaging frames would compel these groups to use 988, and what trusted messengers and resources the participants turn toward when struggling with their mental health (Feldman et al. 2023). The diverse needs assessment and explicit commitment to equity by SAMHSA in the implementation of 988 demonstrates a changing focus in the field and progress toward this ideal.

Additional recommendations include using the American Association for Community Psychiatry (AACP) Self-Assessment for Modification of Anti-Racism Tool (SMART). Developed specifically for behavioral health organizations, SMART helps address structural racism through five domains: 1) hiring, recruitment, retention, and promotion; 2) clinical care; 3) workplace culture; 4) community advocacy; and 5) population health outcomes/evaluation (Talley et al. 2021). To improve the quality of data, it is recommended that clinical staff be trained on how to collect sociodemographic data in crisis settings. It is also recommended that organizations hire clinical staff and researchers of diverse backgrounds and advocate for increased crisis service research funding to advance an equity focus in every research and quality improvement project (Goldman and Vinson 2022). These tools and recommendations are important for increasing awareness of structural racism and accountability in organizations but cannot lead to different outcomes without an explicit commitment from organization leadership to make equity a focus.

In 2020, Columbia University's public health school launched Fighting Oppression, Racism, and White Supremacy through Action, Research and Discourse (FORWARD) to address existing concerns of racism in the program and permanently commit to making the school an "antiracist, multicultural, and fully inclusive institution." Reporting directly to the dean, an accountability cabinet comprising students, faculty, alumni, staff, and academics as well as administrative leaders provides oversight to seven action corps, each with similarly diverse representation and their own focus of improvement (e.g., curriculum, student recruitment, faculty recruitment, community, goals, and measuring progress). Each action corps provides recommendations that are reviewed by the accountability cabinet and elevated to the dean for approval, implementation, and funding. Although FORWARD's programmatic functioning is completed by volunteers, the school has invested one full-time equivalent (FTE) for administrative support; one-quarter FTE for leadership salary support; five annual student stipends; six FORWARD fellows; funding for research, antiracism training, and speaker fees; as well as money to expand mentoring programs (Garbers et al. 2023). This model provides another example of a structure and process for initiating antiracist reforms on an organizational level.

Multisystem Reform

Racially equitable reform for people with SMI in the criminal legal system ideally includes concurrent mental health and criminal legal system changes. Without approaching these issues across the systems that influence them, applying a reform, even when equitable, onto fundamentally racist and siloed systems will not address the underlying causes and drivers of systemic racism (Shadravan et al. 2021). As described in the 2021 report *The Roadmap to the Ideal Crisis System* (Group for the Advancement of Psychiatry 2021), ideal systems must be more than a single program or collection of services. Rather, ideal systems are coordinated systems with a governance and accountability structure with shared values—such as racial equity—to ensure individual and population needs are met effectively and efficiently. Once defined, the shared values are incorporated into every part of the system through measurable standards. Outcome data from these standards are reported back to an accountable entity, ideally representative of the various stakeholders, including consumers of the system, for ongoing quality improvement (Group for the Advancement of Psychiatry 2021). Although these system design concepts describe the development of ideal behavioral health crisis systems in this report, they apply in practice to any system or multisystem reform.

Antiracist, multisystem reform must be bold (Group for the Advancement of Psychiatry 2021). Given that every criminal legal and mental health system is different and has its own values, and because helping people with SMI entangled in misdemeanors involves multiple systems and stakeholders, an essential first step is to convene an all-user stakeholder group. This group would include providers, payers, service users and their families, law enforcement, judges, emergency medical services, call centers, hospital systems, behavioral health crisis leaders, school superintendents, permanent supportive housing leaders, and homeless shelter directors, among others. Collectively, this group would define and codify a shared set of values, goals, and intended results, which could then serve as a framework for the reform's definition of quality benchmarks. The group would then assess their systems' inequities, determine reform components, decide how to operationalize the changes, and ultimately define success with an agreement on how it will be measured (Goldman et al. 2023; Group for the Advancement of Psychiatry 2021).

Multisystem reform that includes racial equity as its focus is a challenging task, and examples of it being successfully implemented are limited. However, promising collaborations are underway. The state of Ohio is in the process of overhauling its behavioral health crisis system. In its redesign process, it convened more than 200 stakeholder groups from many different systems and followed the collaborative steps described in the previous paragraph to create a collective vision of a crisis system that includes equity as a part of that vision and as a measurable standard (Ohio Department of Mental Health and Addiction Services 2023). Still in its nascent stages of implementation, the state's ongoing commitment to equitable reform remains to be seen. Nevertheless, the scope and design of its collaboration may serve as a model.

The Judges and Psychiatrists Leadership Initiative (JPLI), a collaboration between national leaders from the American Psychiatric Association Foundation, the National Center for State Courts, and the Council of State Governments Justice Center, is another example of an important, growing partnership focused on multisystem reform. Their core priorities focus on building enhanced connections between system leaders and increasing training and educational resources for judges and psychiatrists that include a focus on social determinants of health, implicit bias, racism, and equitable outcomes (American Psychiatric Association Foundation 2024). The goals of the JPLI are ambitious, but their inclusion of equity as a focus in mental health and criminal legal system reform exemplifies an ideal approach.

Equity Torchbearers

Racial inequity is a problem that affects everyone. Its emotional, physical, and financial repercussions reverberate from the individual to their families and communities across the country (Vinson et al. 2020). Given the pervasiveness of racial inequities, addressing them requires a high level of commitment (Stewart and Shim 2020). As previously discussed, ideal systems include racial equity as a value built into their framework. Currently, leaders of underrepresented groups are often more responsible for addressing inequities. In a practice referred to as the "minority tax," academic and other institutions, for example, disproportionately task faculty and employees of color with service to enhance diversity and inclusion (Trejo 2020). This undue and often uncompensated burden requires these individuals to balance efforts between their research and equity initiatives, frequently at the detriment of their academic success. Achieving excellence in diversity and inclusion and reaching racial equity in criminal legal and mental health reform requires *all* leaders (Shim 2021), including those from underrepresented and well-represented groups, to carry the torch.

Conclusion

Racialized people with SMI who encounter the criminal legal system are "multiply burdened" (Crenshaw 1989) by the mental health system, criminal legal system, and the other social systems that shape their lived experiences. Achieving racial equity in these systems requires an understanding of how racist processes lead to racial inequities in nearly every downstream social category—in policing neighborhood stability, in limited access to education and employment, in adverse childhood experiences that lead to poorer health and social outcomes, and in the quality of mental health care racialized people receive as adults.

Racial disparities exist even in ostensibly progressive programs, such as drug courts, and demonstrate why it is not enough to simply aspire to equity without explicitly considering the impact of race and racism in outcomes for racialized people with mental illnesses entangled in the criminal legal system. From drug courts to community policing to mobile crisis unit programs, we see the importance of knowing who benefits from programs and reforms and who is disadvantaged by them. We must closely examine racial data to ensure that these programs and policies do not further worsen racial inequities. Lastly, these efforts must be consistent across the other systems discussed in this chapter because each system has upstream and downstream consequences for racialized people entangled in the criminal legal system.

KEY POINTS

- Race, mental illness, and criminal legal system involvement play significant and intersecting roles in shaping the lived experiences and structuring the disparate outcomes of marginalized people in the United States.
- Racial inequities shape individuals' health, income, education, and employment, each of which may limit racially and ethnically oppressed people's abilities to control their own lives.
- Any system that does not include racial equity as a focus will likely not have racial equity as an outcome.
- Collecting race-related data is vital to ensuring equitable reform.
- In an ideal system, all system leaders must champion equity through coordinated, collaborative multisystem reform.

References

Al-Rousan T, Rubenstein L, Sieleni B, et al: Inside the nation's largest mental health institution: a prevalence study in a state prison system. BMC Public Health 17(1):342, 2017 28427371

Alegría M, Chatterji P, Wells K, et al: Disparity in depression treatment among racial and ethnic minority populations in the United States. Psychiatr Serv 59(11):1264–1272, 2008 18971402

American Psychiatric Association Foundation: Judges and Physicians Initiative. Washington, DC, American Psychiatric Association Foundation, n.d. Available at: https://www.apaf.org/our-programs/justice/judges-psychiatrists-leadership-initiative/. Accessed September 12, 2024.

Arias E, Tejada-Vera B, Kenneth D, et al: Provisional life expectancy estimates for 2021. Vital Statistics Rapid Release (Report No 23), August 2022. Available at: https://www.cdc.gov/nchs/data/vsrr/vsrr023.pdf. Accessed November 4, 2023.

Asad AL, Clair M: Racialized legal status as a social determinant of health. Soc Sci Med 199:19–28, 2018 28359580

Bailey K, Lowder EM, Grommon E, et al: Evaluation of a police-mental health co-response team relative to traditional police response in Indianapolis. Psychiatr Serv 73(4):366–373, 2022 34433289

Bailey ZD, Krieger N, Agénor M, et al: Structural racism and health inequities in the USA: evidence and interventions. Lancet 389(10077):1453–1463, 2017 28402827

Balfour ME, Hahn Stephenson A, Delany-Brumsey A, et al: Cops, clinicians, or both? Collaborative approaches to responding to behavioral health emergencies. Psychiatr Serv 73(6):658–669, 2022 34666512

Barnes JC, Motz RT: Reducing racial inequalities in adulthood arrest by reducing inequalities in school discipline: evidence from the school-to-prison pipeline. Dev Psychol 54(12):2328–2340, 2018 30265031

Baumgartner FR, Epp DA, Shoub K, Love B: Targeting young men of color for search and arrest during traffic stops: evidence from North Carolina, 2002–2013. Polit Groups Identities 5(1):107–131, 2017

Bennett N, Hays D, Sullivan B: 2019 Data show Baby Boomers nearly 9 times wealthier than Millennials. Wealth Inequality in the U.S. by Household Type, August 1, 2022. Available at: https://www.census.gov/library/stories/2022/08/wealth-inequality-by-household-type.html. Accessed November 4, 2023.

Bishop DM, Leiber M, Johnson J: Contexts of decision making in the juvenile justice system: an organizational approach to understanding minority overrepresentation. Youth Violence Juv Justice 8(3):213–233, 2010

Blankenship KM, Del Rio Gonzalez AM, Keene DE, et al: Mass incarceration, race inequality, and health: expanding concepts and assessing impacts on well-being. Soc Sci Med 215:45–52, 2018 30205278

Branch B, Conway D: Health Insurance Coverage by Race and Hispanic Origin: 2021 (ACSBR-012). Washington, DC, U.S. Census Bureau, November 2022. Available at: https://www.census.gov/content/dam/Census/library/publications/2022/acs/acsbr-012.pdf. Accessed November 4, 2023.

Bureau of Justice Statistics: Jail Inmates in 2021—Statistical Tables. Washington, DC, Bureau of Justice Statistics, 2021a. Available at: https://bjs.ojp.gov/library/publications/jail-inmates-2021-statistical-tables. Accessed April 4, 2023.

Bureau of Justice Statistics: Prisoners in 2021—Statistical Tables. Washington, DC, Bureau of Justice Statistics, 2021b. Available at: https://bjs.ojp.gov/library/publications/prisoners-2021-statistical-tables. Accessed April 6, 2023.

Bureau of Labor Statistics: Labor force characteristics by race and ethnicity, 2021. BLS Reports (No 1100), January 2023. Available at: https://www.bls.gov/opub/reports/race-and-ethnicity/2021/home.htm#:~:text=The%20unemployment%20rate%20averaged%208.6, was%206.8%20percent%20for%20Hispanics. Accessed November 4, 2023.

Clair M: Privilege and Punishment: How Race and Class Matter in Criminal Court. Princeton, NJ, Princeton University Press, 2020

Clark E: Conduct disorders in African American adolescent males: the perceptions that lead to overdiagnosis and placement in special programs. Alabama Counseling Association Journal 33(2):1–7, 2007

Coker TR, Elliott MN, Toomey SL, et al: Racial and ethnic disparities in ADHD diagnosis and treatment. Pediatrics 138(3):e20160407, 2016 27553219

Compton MT, Graves J, Zern A, et al: Characterizing arrests and charges among individuals with SMI in public-sector treatment settings. Psychiatr Serv 73(10):1102–1108, 2022 35378991

Cook BL, Zuvekas SH, Carson N, et al: Assessing racial/ethnic disparities in treatment across episodes of mental health care. Health Serv Res 49(1):206–229, 2014 23855750

Creamer J, Shrider EA, Burns K, et al: Poverty in the United States: 2021. Washington, DC, U.S. Census Bureau, September 2022. Available at: https://www.census.gov/content/dam/Census/library/publications/2022/demo/p60-277.pdf. Accessed November 4, 2023.

Crenshaw K: Demarginalizing the Intersection of Race and Sex: A Black Feminist Critique of Antidiscrimination Doctrine, Feminist Theory and Antiracist Politics. Chicago, IL, University of Chicago Legal Forum, 1989

Daniels TE, Victor C, Smith EM, et al: Associations of restraint and seclusion with race and ethnicity on an adolescent inpatient psychiatry service. J Am Acad Child Adolesc Psychiatry 62(5):503–506, 2023 36736689

Del Pozo B, Rich JD: Addressing racism in medicine requires tackling the broader problem of epistemic injustice. Am J Bioeth 21(2):90–93, 2021 33534692

Development Services Group, Inc: Racial and Ethnic Disparity in Juvenile Justice Processing. Washington, DC, U.S. Department of Justice, 2022. Available at: https://ojjdp.ojp.gov/model-programs-guide/literature-reviews/racial-and-ethnic-disparity#03796e. Accessed November 4, 2023.

Dotson S, Ogbu-Nwobodo L, Shtasel D: Demilitarizing hospital restraints: recognizing the stones in our glass houses. Psychiatr Serv 73(1):100–102, 2022 34074142

Dunlap E, Johnson BD: The setting for the crack era: macro forces, micro consequences (1960–1992). J Psychoactive Drugs 24(4):307–321, 1992 1491281

Edwards ML, Saenz SR, Collins R, et al: Social injustice and structural racism, in Social (In)Justice and Mental Health. Edited by Shim R, Vinson S. Washington, DC, American Psychiatric Association Publishing, 2021, pp 47–62

Ely DM, Driscoll AK: Infant mortality in the United States, 2019: data from the period linked birth/infant death file. Natl Vital Stat Rep 70(14):1–18, 2021 34878382

Fadus MC, Ginsburg KR, Sobowale K, et al: Unconscious bias and the diagnosis of disruptive behavior disorders and ADHD in African American and Hispanic youth. Acad Psychiatry 44(1):95–102, 2020 31713075

Feisthamel K, Schwartz R: Differences in mental health counselors' diagnoses based on client race: an investigation of adjustment, childhood, and substance-related disorders. J Ment Health Couns 31(1):47–59, 2009

Feldman D, Chao C, Thompson-Kuhn C, et al: 988 Suicide and Crisis Lifeline: Messaging and Communications to People at Higher Risk for or Disproportionately Impacted by Suicide. New York, Ad Council Research Institute, 2023. Available at: https://suicidepreventionmessaging.org/sites/default/files/2023–11/AdCouncil_988_Report_9_2023_FINAL.pdf. Accessed December 22, 2023.

Garbers S, Joseph MA, Jankunis B, et al: FORWARD: building a model to hold schools of public health accountable for antiracism work. Am J Public Health 113(10):1086–1088, 2023 37499199

Gatewood BJ, Muhammad BM, Turner S: Breaking generational curses: success and opportunity among black children of incarcerated parents. Soc Probl, spad026, 2023

Goff PA, Jackson MC, Di Leone BAL, et al: The essence of innocence: consequences of dehumanizing Black children. J Pers Soc Psychol 106(4):526–545, 2014 24564373

Goldhaber D, Kane T, McEachin A, et al: The Consequences of Remote and Hybrid Instruction During the Pandemic. Research Report. Cambridge, MA, Center for Education Policy Research, Harvard University, 2022

Goldman M, Shoyinka S, Allender B, et al: Quality Measurement in Crisis Services. Washington, DC, The National Council for Mental Wellbeing, 2023. Available at: https://www.thenationalcouncil.org/wp-content/uploads/2023/01/23.01.13_Quality-Measurement-in-Crisis-Services.pdf. Accessed November 4, 2023.

Goldman ML, Vinson SY: Centering equity in mental health crisis services. World Psychiatry 21(2):243–244, 2022 35524591

Group for the Advancement of Psychiatry: Roadmap to the Ideal Crisis System. Washington, DC, National Council for Mental Wellbeing, 2021. Available at: https://www.thenationalcouncil.org/wp-content/uploads/2022/02/042721_GAP_CrisisReport.pdf. Accessed November 4, 2023.

Harris AP, Ash E, Fagan J: Fiscal pressures and discriminatory policing: evidence from traffic stops in Missouri. J Race Ethn Polit 5(3):450–480, 2020

Haslam N, Rothschild L, Ernst D: Essentialist beliefs about social categories. Br J Soc Psychol 39(Pt 1):113–127, 2000 10774531

Hetey RC, Monin B, Maitreyi A, et al: Data for change: a statistical analysis of police stops, searches, handcuffings, and arrests in Oakland, Calif., 2013–2014. Stanford SPARQ, June 23, 2016. Available at: https://searchworks.stanford.edu/view/by412gh2838. Accessed November 4, 2023.

Hetey RC, Eberhardt JL: The numbers don't speak for themselves: racial disparities and the persistence of inequality in the criminal justice system. Curr Dir Psychol Sci 27(3):183–187, 2018

Hoffman KM, Trawalter S, Axt JR, et al: Racial bias in pain assessment and treatment recommendations, and false beliefs about biological differences between blacks and whites. Proc Natl Acad Sci USA 113(16):4296–4301, 2016 27044069

Jones CP, Bright CM, Laurencin CT: Segregation in Housing and Education. Washington, DC, National Academies Press, 2020

KFF: Adults who report fair or poor health status by race/ethnicity, in State Health Facts. Washington, DC, KFF, 2021a. Available at: https://www.kff.org/other/state-indicator/percent-of-adults-reporting-fair-or-poor-health-status-by-raceethnicity/. Accessed November 4, 2023.

KFF: Total diabetes deaths, in State Health Facts. Washington, DC, KFF, 2021b. Available at: https://www.kff.org/other/state-indicator/diabetes-death-rate-by-raceethnicity/. Accessed November 4, 2023.

KFF: Total heart disease deaths by race/ethnicity, in State Health Facts. Washington, DC, KFF, 2021c. Available at: https://www.kff.org/other/state-indicator/number-of-heart-disease-deaths-per-100000-population-by-raceethnicity-2/. Accessed November 4, 2023.

Kugelmass H: "Sorry, I'm not accepting new patients": an audit study of access to mental health care. J Health Soc Behav 57(2):168–183, 2016 27251890

Massey DS, Denton NA: American Apartheid: Segregation and the Making of the Underclass. Cambridge, MA, Harvard University Press, 1998

Massoglia M, Pridemore WA: Incarceration and health. Annu Rev Sociol 41(1):291–310, 2015 30197467

Morgan PL, Staff J, Hillemeier MM, et al: Racial and ethnic disparities in ADHD diagnosis from kindergarten to eighth grade. Pediatrics 132(1):85–93, 2013 23796743

Murji K, Solomos J (eds): Racialization: Studies in Theory and Practice. New York, Oxford University Press, 2005

Myers SL, Ha I: Race Neutrality: Rationalizing Remedies to Racial Inequality. Lanham, MD, Lexington Books, 2018

National Center for Education Statistics: Status dropout rates, in Condition of Education: Preprimary, Elementary, and Secondary Education. Washington, DC, U.S. Department of Education, Institute of Education Sciences, 2023. Available at: https://nces.ed.gov/programs/coe/indicator/coj/status-dropout-rates#:~:text=The%20overall%20status%20dropout%20rate,to%205.2%20percent%20in%202021. Accessed November 4, 2023.

Nelson J, Brooks L: Racial Equity Toolkit: An Opportunity to Operationalize Equity. Washington, DC, Government Alliance on Race and Equity, 2015. Available at: https://www.racialequityalliance.org/wp-content/uploads/2015/10/GARE-Racial_Equity_Toolkit.pdf. Accessed November 4, 2023.

O'Hear M: Rethinking drug courts: restorative justice as a response to racial injustice. Stanford Law Policy Rev 20(2):463–500, 2009

Ohio Department of Mental Health and Addiction Services: Landscape analysis, in Learn and Find Help: Crisis Systems. Columbus, OH, Ohio Department of Mental Health and Addiction Services, 2023. Available at: https://mha.ohio.gov/get-help/crisis-systems/landscape-analysis/landscape-analysis#background. Accessed November 4, 2023.

Omi M, Winant H: Racial Formation in the United States. London, Routledge, 2014

Pager D: Marked: Race, Crime, and Finding Work in an Era of Mass Incarceration. Chicago, IL, University of Chicago Press, 2007

Pedersen ML, Gildberg F, Baker J, et al: Ethnic disparities in the use of restrictive practices in adult mental health inpatient settings: a scoping review. Soc Psychiatry Psychiatr Epidemiol 58(4):505–522, 2023 36454269

Pérez-Stable EJ: NIMHD director statement in support of NIH efforts to address structural racism. National Institute on Minority Health and Health Disparities blog, March 2, 2021. Available at: https://blog.nimhd.nih.gov/archives-2021/news_feed/nimhd-director-statement-in-support-of-nih-efforts-to-address-structural-racism. Accessed November 4, 2023.

Pettit B, Gutierrez C: Mass incarceration and racial inequality. Am J Econ Sociol 77(3–4):1153–1182, 2018 36213171

Prins SJ: Does transinstitutionalization explain the overrepresentation of people with SMI in the criminal justice system? Community Ment Health J 47(6):716–722, 2011 21655941

Pryar W, Barkow R, Breyer C, et al: Demographic Differences in Sentencing: An Update to the 2012 Booker Report. Washington, DC, United States Sentencing Commission, 2017

Ramos NJ: Pathologizing the crisis: psychiatry, policing, and racial liberalism in the Long Community Mental Health Movement. J Hist Med Allied Sci 74(1):57–84, 2019 30576559

Raphael S, Stoll MA: Assessing the contribution of the deinstitutionalization of the mentally ill to growth in the U.S. incarceration rate. J Legal Stud 42(1):187–222, 2013

Raz M: The deprivation riots: psychiatry as politics in the 1960s. Harv Rev Psychiatry 21(6):345–350, 2013 24201824

Raz M: Psychiatrists and the transformation of juvenile justice in Philadelphia, 1965–1972. J Hist Med Allied Sci 73(4):437–463, 2018 29893867

Raz M, Dettlaff A, Edwards F: The perils of child "protection" for children of color: lessons from history. Pediatrics 148(1):e2021050237, 2021 34112658

Roehrkasse AF, Wildeman C: Lifetime risk of imprisonment in the United States remains high and starkly unequal. Sci Adv 8(48):eabo3395, 2022 36459563

Shadravan SM, Barceló NE: Social injustice and mental health inequities, in Social (In)Justice and Mental Health. Edited by Shim RA, Vinson SY. Washington, DC, American Psychiatric Association Publishing, 2021, pp 35–44

Shadravan SM, Edwards ML, Vinson SY: Dying at the intersections: police-involved killings of black people with mental illness. Psychiatr Serv 72(6):623–625, 2021 34110254

Shea T, Dotson S, Tyree G, et al: Racial and ethnic inequities in inpatient psychiatric civil commitment. Psychiatr Serv 73(12):1322–1329, 2022 35959533

Shim RS: Dismantling structural racism in psychiatry: a path to mental health equity. Am J Psychiatry 178(7):592–598, 2021 34270343

Shim RS, Vinson SY (eds): Social (In)Justice and Mental Health. Washington, DC, American Psychiatric Association Publishing, 2021

Shim RS, Compton MT, Rust G, et al: Race-ethnicity as a predictor of attitudes toward mental health treatment seeking. Psychiatr Serv 60(10):1336–1341, 2009 19797373

Shim RS, Compton MT, Manseau M, et al: Overview of the social determinants of mental health and mental illness, in The Social Determinants of Mental Health. Edited by Compton MT, Shim RS. Washington, DC, American Psychiatric Publishing, 2015, pp 1–21

Shim RS, Tierney M, Rosenzweig MH, et al: Improving behavioral health services in the time of COVID-19 and racial inequities. NAM Perspect, 2021 34901776

Skiba RJ, Arredondo MI, Williams NT: More than a metaphor: the contribution of exclusionary discipline to a school-to-prison pipeline. Equity Excell Educ 47(4):546–564, 2014

Sniderman PM, Carmines EG, Layman GC, et al: Beyond race: social justice as a race neutral ideal. Am J Pol Sci 40(1):33, 1996

Stacy C, Cohen M: Ban the Box and Racial Discrimination: A Review of the Evidence and Policy Recommendations. Washington, DC, Urban Institute, 2017

Stewart AJ, Shim RS: Achieving mental health equity. Psychiatr Clin North Am 43(3):xiii–xiv, 2020 32773083

Substance Abuse and Mental Health Services Administration: National Guidelines for Behavioral Health Crisis Care—A Best Practice Toolkit. Knowledge Informing Transformation. Rockville, MD, Substance Abuse and Mental Health Services Administration, 2020. Available at: https://www.samhsa.gov/sites/default/files/national-guidelines-for-behavioral-health-crisis-care-02242020.pdf. Accessed November 4, 2023.

Substance Abuse and Mental Health Services Administration: Highlights by Race/Ethnicity for the 2021 National Survey on Drug Use and Health. Rockville, MD, Substance Abuse and Mental Health Services Administration. 2023. Available at: https://www.samhsa.gov/data/sites/default/files/2022-12/2021NSDUHFFRHighlightsRE123022.pdf. Accessed November 4, 2023.

Swanson J, Swartz M, Van Dorn RA, et al: Racial disparities in involuntary outpatient commitment: are they real? Health Aff (Millwood) 28(3):816–826, 2009 19414892

Talley RM, Shoyinka S, Minkoff K: The Self-assessment for Modification of Anti-Racism Tool (SMART): addressing structural racism in community behavioral health. Community Ment Health J 57(6):1208–1213, 2021 34023974

Trejo J: The burden of service for faculty of color to achieve diversity and inclusion: the minority tax. Mol Biol Cell 31(25):2752–2754, 2020 33253072

U.S. Census Bureau: QuickFacts: United States. Washington, DC, U.S. Department of Commerce, 2023. Available at: https://www.census.gov/quickfacts/fact/table/US/PST045221. Accessed April 4, 2023.

Vinson SY, Dennis AL: Systemic, racial justice-informed solutions to shift "care" from the criminal legal system to the mental health care system. Psychiatr Serv 72(12):1428–1433, 2021 33979203

Vinson SY, Coffey TT, Jackson N, et al: Two systems, one population: achieving equity in mental healthcare for criminal justice and marginalized populations. Psychiatr Clin North Am 43(3):525–538, 2020 32773079

Voigt R, Camp NP, Prabhakaran V, et al: Language from police body camera footage shows racial disparities in officer respect. Proc Natl Acad Sci USA 114(25):6521–6526, 2017 28584085

Vyas CM, Donneyong M, Mischoulon D, et al: Association of race and ethnicity with late-life depression severity, symptom burden, and care. JAMA Netw Open 3(3):e201606, 2020 32215634

Wakefield S, Wildeman C: Children of the Prison Boom: Mass Incarceration and the Future of American Inequality. New York, Oxford University Press, 2013

Western B, Wildeman C: The Black family and mass incarceration. Ann Am Acad Pol Soc Sci 621:221–242, 2009

Wielen LMV, Gilchrist EC, Nowels MA, et al: Not near enough: racial and ethnic disparities in access to nearby behavioral health care and primary care. J Health Care Poor Underserved 26(3):1032–1047, 2015 26320931

Wildeman C, Muller C: Mass imprisonment and inequality in health and family life. Annu Rev Law Soc Sci 8(1):11–30, 2012

Wildeman C, Wang EA: Mass incarceration, public health, and widening inequality in the USA. Lancet 389(10077):1464–1474, 2017 28402828

Williams DR, Collins C: Racial residential segregation: a fundamental cause of racial disparities in health. Public Health Rep 116(5):404–416, 2001 12042604

Wright JD: International Encyclopedia of the Social and Behavioral Sciences, 2nd Edition. Amsterdam, Netherlands, Elsevier, 2015

Yeh M, McCabe K, Hurlburt M, et al: Referral sources, diagnoses, and service types of youth in public outpatient mental health care: a focus on ethnic minorities. J Behav Health Serv Res 29(1):45–60, 2002 11840904

Zhou H, Ford EB: Analyzing the relationship between mental health courts and the prison industrial complex. J Am Acad Psychiatry Law 49(4):590–596, 2021 34452945

Index

*Page numbers printed in **boldface** type refer to tables or figures.*

Use of force, 170, 222

Vagrancy, 99, 105
Value pluralism, 72, 75, 90, 92
Vertical sweeps, 106, 113
Veterans Crisis Line, 234
Victim preferences, and assault
  charges, 187–188
Violence. *See also* Domestic violence;
  Family violence
  biological explanations, 275
  escalating, 188
  risk factors, 177–178, 194–195

Violent crime, 175–197. *See also*
  Assault
  charges related to, 179–182, **181**
  predictors of, 177–178
  scope of problem, 176–179
  terminology, 175–176, 179–180

War on Drugs, 276
Warrants, arrests without, 26
Warren, Earl, 105
West, Louis J., 275

Zero tolerance, 269, 275